U0218518

（中英双语版）

责任与担当

MNCs'ACTIONS
IN FIGHTING COVID-19 TOGETHER
WITH CHINA

抗击
新冠肺炎疫情中的
跨国公司

中国国际跨国公司促进会

主编

李新玉

执行主编

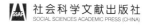

社会科学文献出版社
SOCIAL SCIENCES ACADEMIC PRESS (CHINA)

高级顾问委员会

李礼辉	中国银行原行长
	中国国际跨国公司促进会特邀副会长
孔 丹	中信集团原董事长
	中国国际跨国公司促进会特邀副会长
张建国	中国建设银行原行长
	中国国际跨国公司促进会特邀副会长
张笑宇	联合国和平大学校董
	中国国际跨国公司促进会常务副会长

Senior Adversary Board

Qinglin Du   Member of the Secretariat of the 18th CPC Central Committee

Vice Chairman, the 11th & 12th National Committee of CPPCC

Honorary President of CICPMC

Wantong Zheng   Vice Chairman, the 11th National Committee of CPPCC

President of CICPMC

Fulin Shang   Head of the Economic Committee, 19th CPPCC

Former Secretary of the Party Committee and Chairman of CBRC

Former Chairman of the China Securities Regulatory Commission

Specially Invited Vice President of CICPMC

Yizhong Li   Former Minister, Ministry of Industry and Information Techonology

Specially Invited Vice President of CICPMC

Jinzhang Li   Former Vice Minister, Ministry of Foreign Affairs

Specially Invited Vice President of CICPMC

Weizhi Qu   Former Director, the National Information Advisroy Committee & Former Vice Minister, Ministry of Information Industry

Specially Invited Vice President of CICPMC

Yunchun Hou	Former Vice Minister, the State Council Information Office
	Specially Invited Vice President of CICPMC
Yongwen Han	Former Vice Governor, Hunan Province & Former Deputy Director & Secretary of the Party Leadership Group of Standing Committee of Hunan Provincial People's Congress
	Specially Invited Vice President of CICPMC
Xiaonan Ji	Former President, the Supervisory Board of Major SOEs
	Specially Invited Vice President of CICPMC
Lihui Li	Former President, Bank of China
	Specially Invited Entrepreneur Vice President of CICPMC
Dan Kong	Former Chairman, CITIC Group Co., Ltd
	Specially Invited Entrepreneur Vice President of CICPMC
Jianguo Zhang	Former President, China Construction Bank
	Specially Invited Entrepreneur Vice President of CICPMC
Xiaoyu Zhang	Member of the University for Peace Council
	Executive Vice President of CICPMC

高级咨询委员会

尹　正　　　施耐德电气全球执行副总裁兼中国区总裁
李　强　　　思爱普全球高级副总裁兼中国区总裁
苗天祥　　　辉瑞普强大中华区主席兼总裁
周学军　　　路易达孚集团全球副总裁，北亚区董事长兼首席执行官
孟　樸　　　高通无线通信技术（中国）有限公司董事长
张志强　　　ABB（中国）有限公司总裁
倪西蔓　　　力拓集团执行委员会成员兼全球企业关系总裁
康　斌　　　安博（中国）总裁
蒋惟明　　　帝斯曼（中国）有限公司全球高级执行副总裁兼中国总裁
甄超凡　　　环球影业（中国区）执行副总裁兼董事总经理
潘　庆　　　捷豹路虎全球董事兼捷豹路虎（中国）投资有限公司总裁

Senior Consultative Board

Zheng Yin	Excutive Vice President of Schneider Electric & President of Schneider Electric China
Sam Li	Global Senior Vice President, SAP SE & President SAP China
Tianxiang Miao	Chairman & President, Greater China Region, Pfizer Upjohn
James Zhou	Global Vice President of LDC, Chairman & CEO of LDC North Asia
Frank Meng	Chairman, Qualcomm Wireless Communication Technologies (China) Ltd.
ZZ Zhang	President, ABB (China) Ltd.
Simone Niven	Group Executive for Corporate Relations of Rio Tinto
Ben Cornish	President, Prologis (China)
Weiming Jiang	Corporate Senior Excutive Vice President & China President, DSM (China) Ltd.
Jo Yan	Excutive Vice President & Managing Director, Universal China
Qing Pan	Global Board Member of Jaguar Land Rover & President, Jaguar Land Rover (China) Ltd.

编委会

刁志辉	太古（中国）有限公司董事
马　征	嘉吉投资（中国）有限公司副总裁
王　洁	施耐德电气（中国）有限公司副总裁
王海燕	帝斯曼（中国）有限公司高级经理
朱海鸾	赛诺菲（中国）投资有限公司副总裁
李　洁	捷豹路虎（中国）投资有限公司执行副总裁
苏巴鸿	大众汽车集团（中国）高级总监
张建弢	可口可乐（大中华、韩国及蒙古区）副总裁
郭　涛	高通无线通信技术（中国）有限公司副总裁
袁　凌	力拓（中国）企业关系总经理
席　庆	辉瑞投资有限公司副总裁
徐　旸	陶氏化学（中国）投资有限公司政府事务总经理
徐　俊	安博（中国）高级副总裁
谢燕琦	思爱普（大中华区）副总裁
黄志湘	环球影业（中国区）副总裁
焦　燕	路易达孚北亚区副总裁
董慧娟	ABB（中国）有限公司副总裁

Editorial Board

中国国际跨国公司促进会简介

经中华人民共和国国务院批准的专门从事跨国公司工作的非政府组织，被联合国经社理事会授予特别咨商单位，成立于 1993 年。十八届中央书记处书记，第十一届、十二届全国政协副主席杜青林兼任名誉会长。第十一届全国政协副主席郑万通担任会长。

China International Council for the Promotion of Multinational Corporations (CICPMC)

Approved by the State Council of PRC as a non-governmental organization with a focus on the promotion of multinational corporations, China International Council for the Promotion of Multinational Corporations (CICPMC) was established in 1993, and granted Special Consultative Status with the Economic and Social Council of the United Nations. Mr. Du Qinlin, member of the Secretariat of the 18th CPC Central Committee, and Vice Chairman of the 11th & 12th National Committee of CPPCC, is the Honorary President of CICPMC. Mr. Zheng Wantong, Vice Chairman of the 11th National Committee of CPPCC, is the President of CICPMC.

执行主编简介

李新玉，国际关系学博士，中国国际跨国公司促进会副会长兼秘书长，北京国际交往中心建设专家委员会委员。曾任中国人民对外友好协会民间外交战略研究中心主任等职。主要编著出版《陈翰笙文集：1919-1949》（英文）、《30 人谈 30 年——纪念改革开放 30 周年名人访谈录》、《城市外交：理论与实践》、《中国城市竞争力专题报告（1973-2015）——开放的城市，共赢的未来》、《如何讲好中国故事》等。

Xinyu Li , Ph. D in international relations, is vice president of China International Council for the Promotion of Multinational Corporations (CICPMC), also the expert for the Beijing International Communication Center. Before CICPMC, she was the Director General of Research Center for People-to-People Diplomacy of the Chinese People's Association for Friendship with Foreign Countries (CPAFFC).

Her research works includes *Chen Hanseng's Writings, 1919-1949, 30 Interviewers about 30-Year China Economic Reform, City Diplomacy:Theory And Practice, A Special Report on China Urban Competitiveness (1973-2015) -- An Open City* and *A Win-Win Future* and *How to Tell the World about China* etc.

序

  2020 年春节，一场突如其来的新冠肺炎疫情，使我们中华民族文化中一年一度最重要的节日——春节，比往年多了许多沉重和紧张的意味。疫情无情，但人间有爱。在这一艰难的时刻，全国人民在习近平主席的指挥下，举国上下携起手来，共同战"疫"，彰显了我们中华民族强大的凝聚力。在这场抗击新冠肺炎疫情阻击战中，许多长期在华发展的外资跨国公司也纷纷积极行动起来，担负起企业社会责任，主动捐款捐物，全力参与支援抗击疫情行动，展现出了企业的责任与担当。

  我还听说许多跨国公司都从各自不同专业领域，积极参与了武汉火神山医院和雷神山医院的紧急建设工作，从产品捐赠、调货、运输、组装、接线、调式、运行，都做了大量的工作，对保证医院电力系统、通信系统、数据中心系统及时安全运营发挥了重要作用，特别是许多"90 后"和"00 后"年轻人夜以继日工作奉献，有效配合了中国政府抗击新冠肺炎疫情。

  这本汇编文集《责任与担当——抗击新冠肺炎疫情中的跨国公司》，正是跨国公司爱心、责任与担当的一个缩影和记录，反映出跨国公司与中国同呼吸、共命运。另外，在积极捐款捐物的同时，许多跨国公司还积极建言献策，提出一些具有建设意义的观察与思考。在中国改革开放 40 多年的历史进程中，作为参与者、见证者、贡献者、受益者，跨国公司发挥了重要作用；在经济全球化进程中，跨国公司始终是主要的推动力量；在中国的疫情防控取得阶段性胜利、全球疫情防控形势依然严峻的情况下，相信跨国公司将继续为构建人类命运共同体，促进世界经济共商共建共享共赢发挥应有的积极作用。

我祝贺这本汇编文集的出版，希望中国国际跨国公司促进会为推动中外企业互助共赢的合作，推动世界经济持续的繁荣发展做出更多有意义的工作。

第十一届全国政协副主席

中国国际跨国公司促进会会长

2020 年 6 月 10 日

Forward

During the Spring Festival of 2020, the sudden outbreak of COVID-19 made the most important festival for the Chinese much heavier and tenser than before. The epidemic is ruthless, but people are caring. At this difficult time, under the leadership of President Xi Jinping, the people of the whole country joined hands to fight the epidemic, demonstrating the strong cohesion and solidarity of the nation. During this battle, many foreign multinationals that have been operating in China for a long time have demonstrated social responsibility, donating money and materials and taking an active part in supporting the fight against the virus.

I heard that many multinational companies have actively participated in the emergency construction of Wuhan Huoshenshan Hospital and Leishenshan Hospital, from product donation, logistics, transportation, assembly, wiring, commissioning and operation. They have been very important in ensuring the timely and safe operation of the hospital's power system, communications system and data center system. In particular, many young people born in the 1990s and the 2000s have worked with dedication around the clock to fight COVID-19.

This compilation, *MNCs'Actions in Fighting COVID-19 Together with China*, is a record and an epitome of the care, responsibility and dedication of multinationals, showing that multinationals are sharing weal and woe with China. In addition to kind donations, many multinationals have proposed constructive observations and suggestions. In the past 40 years of reform and opening-up, as participants, witnesses, contributors and beneficiaries, multinationals have played a very important role. During economic globalization, multinationals are the main driving force; in the era after the epidemic, multinationals will continue to play its part in building a community of share future for all mankind and promoting participation, consultation, sharing and win-win in the global economy.

My congratulations on the publication of this compilation. I hope that the China Council for the Promotion of Multinational Corporations will do more in the future in encouraging mutual support and win-win among Chinese and foreign multinationals for continued cooperation and common prosperity to the world economy.

Wantong Zheng

Vice Chairman, the 11th Chinese

People's Political Consultative Conference

President, China International Council for

the Promotion of Multinational Corporations

10 June 2020

目录 CONTETS

前言 / 001

Preface / 005

第一部分 | **集思广益聚智慧** / 001

Part 1 Brainstorm for Wisdom-gathering

【按照议题分类排序】

新时代危机防范体制建设的建议 / 003

The Development of China's Crisis Prevention System in the New Era / 014

新型冠状病毒肺炎疫情主要应对模式比较与思考 / 028

The Comparison of Different COVID-19 Epidemic Control Measures / 039

疫情常态化下中国数字化发展的机遇和挑战 / 052

Opportunities & Challenges of China's Digital Development under the Regular Epidemic Prevention and Control Measures / 060

政府、社会组织和企业"黄金三角"合作机制提升应急救援能力 / *072*

Golden Triangle Partnership among Government, Business & Civil Society to Enhance Emergency Response and Disaster Relief Capabilities / *079*

发挥制度优势,完善全民健康体系 / *089*

Utilize System Advantages to Improve the National Health System / *095*

新冠肺炎疫情对制定企业传染性疾病应急预案的启示 / *103*

What COVID-19 Tells about Corporate Pandemic Preparedness / *114*

应急响应机制与经验及对中国企业的借鉴意义 / *128*

Rio Tinto's Emergency Responding Mechanism / *138*

从新冠肺炎疫情看制造业供应链的应对与启示 / *149*

Response of Supply Chain in Manufacturing Sector to COVID-19 and Revelations / *159*

5G 应用赋能疫情常态化下经济转型 / *173*

Key 5G Applications: Enablers of Economic Transformation & Industry Upgrading under the Regular Epidemic Prevention and Control Measures / *186*

完善供应链建设,保障粮油物资供应
——新冠肺炎疫情的启示 / *205*

How to Improve the Supply Chain in the Grain and Oilseeds Industry to Secure Supplies for Livelihoods / *214*

互联网医疗在疫情防控与日常医疗中的作用 / *226*

The Role of Internet Healthcare in Pandemic Control & Daily Care / *230*

把握汽车行业规律,力保全球产业链 / *236*

Grasping Automotive Industry Principle & Safeguarding the Global Industry Chain / *246*

疫情对物流行业的挑战与机遇 / *258*

Challenges & Opportunities of the Epidemic to the Logistics Industry / *270*

国际突发公共卫生事件对航空业的影响及对策建议 / *286*

Impacts of International Public Health Emergency and Recommendation of Countermeasures on Aviation Industry from the Epidemic / *295*

2020 年大变局之文化影视行业新思考 / *308*

Film and Television Industry in the Disruptive Changes of 2020 / *316*

第二部分 ∣ **抗击疫情在行动** / *329*

Part II   Actions for Fighting COVID-19

【按照新闻发布时间先后排序】

齐心必胜！赛诺菲通过中国红十字基金会捐赠 100 万元人民币 / *331*

Sanofi Announced the Donation of RMB 1 Million to Chinese Red Cross Foundation / *332*

共抗疫情，嘉吉捐赠 350 万元现金及防护物资 / *333*

Cargill Donates RMB 3.5 Million to Help Fight the New Coronavirus Pneumonia / *334*

雅诗兰黛集团累计捐赠现金及物资 1500 万元人民币驰援新冠肺炎疫情 / *335*

Estée Lauder Companies has Donated Cash and Supplies in the Cumulative Amount of RMB15 Million to Support the Fight against the Novel Coronavirus-infected Pneumonia / *336*

太古集团宣布捐赠人民币 1000 万元用于支援抗击新型冠状病毒感染的肺炎疫情 / *338*

Swire Group Announcement of Donation of RMB 10 Million for Providing Aid in Combating the Novel Coronavirus Pneumonia Epidemic / *339*

抗击疫情，路易达孚在行动 / 340

LDC in Action: Fighting COVID-19 / 341

高通捐款 700 万元人民币，支持抗击新冠肺炎疫情 / 342

Qualcomm Donates RMB 7 Million in Support of Efforts to Combat the Coronavirus / 343

IBM 捐款 200 万元支持中国抗击新型冠状病毒肺炎疫情 / 344

IBM Donated RMB 2 Million to Support China's Fight against Novel Coronavirus / 345

霍尼韦尔捐赠价值 100 万美元物资助力武汉抗击新型冠状病毒肺炎疫情 / 346

Honeywell Donates US $1 Million in Equipment to Support Fight against Coronavirus in Wuhan / 348

凯雷及员工捐助 300 万元善款物资 驰援湖北疫区一线 / 350

Carlyle and Its Employees Donate RMB 3 Million in Cash and Medical Supplies to Support Frontline Medical and Support Staff in China's Most Affected Areas / 351

安博与武汉同在，与湖北同在，与中国同在 / 352

PROLOGIS with Wuhan, with Hubei & with China / 354

大众汽车集团（中国）携旗下大众、奥迪、保时捷、宾利和斯柯达等品牌，与合资企业一道，共同捐资 1.2 亿元人民币抗击疫情 / 356

Volkswagen Group China and Its Joint Ventures to Collectively Donate RMB 120 Million to Combat Coronavirus Outbreak / 358

亚马逊筹措全球逾百万件医疗物资驰援疫情严重省份，中国加油！/ 360

Amazon Donates Millions of Items to Healthcare Professionals of Affected Cities in China / 362

耐克捐资 1000 万元支持抗击疫情 / *363*

Nike Donates RMB 10 Million to Help Wuhan against COVID-19 / *364*

BP 中国捐赠逾 300 万元人民币的物资和现金，为抗击疫情贡献一臂之力 / *365*

BP Donated RMB 3 Million worth of Medical Protective Materials and Funds to the Epic Center to Fight against the COVID-19 Pandemic / *370*

与时间竞速，施耐德电气紧急援建火神山、雷神山医院 / *375*

Schneider Electric Provides Emergency Support for Huoshenshan Hospital and Leishenshan Hospital in Wuhan / *377*

高盛集团捐赠 100 万美元支持中国应对新型冠状病毒 / *379*

Goldman Sachs Committing A Total of US$1 Million to Support China's Efforts to Tackle the Coronavirus Outbreak / *380*

并肩战"疫"！力拓助力中国抗击新型冠状病毒疫情 / *381*

Rio Tinto Supports China's Fight against COVID-19 Outbreak / *382*

"蒂"结同心　共"克"时艰
　　——蒂森克虏伯积极支持抗击新冠肺炎疫情 / *383*

Be of One Mind and Overcome Difficulties Together - thyssenkrupp Actively Supports the Fight against the Coronavirus / *385*

ABB 支持抗击疫情，积极复工复产 / *387*

ABB Supports Fight against COVID-19 and Actively Resumes Work and Production / *389*

群策群力，为武汉加油！为中国加油！ / *391*

Pool the Wisdom and Efforts of All to Fight against COVID-19 / *393*

标普全球捐赠 100 万元人民币支持抗击新型冠状病毒 / 396

S&P Global Awards A Grant of RMB 1 Million to Support Frontline Health Workers and Hospitals / 398

必和必拓支援中国战"疫"，与中国共克时艰 / 399

BHP Makes a Donation to Fight Coronavirus / 400

共同抗疫，杜邦始终在前线 / 401

DuPont in the Frontline of Epidemic Control / 403

卡特彼勒陈其华：中国终将打赢这场艰难的战"疫"/ 405

Qihua Chen of Caterpillar: China will Persevere during this Difficult Time / 407

聚焦落实　放眼长远
　　——梅赛德斯－奔驰星愿基金公布首笔捐款落实细则宣布再捐 2000 万
　　　元用于持续战疫 / 409

Mercedes-Benz Star Fund Donates an Additional RMB 20 Million against COVID-19 and Shares Initial Donation Execution / 413

帝斯曼中国捐款 100 万元人民币并分批捐赠超过一亿片维生素 C 产品驰援疫情防控 / 418

DSM China Donates to Support Efforts Amidst COVID-19 Outbreak / 420

同心协力，抗击疫情 / 422

In the Fight Together / 423

众志成城，共克时艰！捷豹路虎多措并举，驰援中国抗"疫"/ 424

Jaguar Land Rover Takes Consecutive Actions to Support the Fight against COVID-19 in China / 426

辉瑞中国心系抗疫一线 / 428

Pfizer China Supported Anti-Coronavirus Battle in China / 430

马士基集团捐赠价值超 200 万元医用物资并助力救援物资运输，共抗疫情 / 432

A.P. Moller – Maersk Donates Medical Materials with Value over RMB 2 Million and Assists in the Transportation of Relief Supplies to Fight against the Epidemic / 434

阿斯利康捐赠雾化祛痰药物增援疫情防控 / 436

AstraZeneca's Added Donation of Atomization Expectorant Medicines to Fight COVID-19 / 438

思爱普追加千万抗"疫"捐赠，数字化助力湖北中小企业复产复工，再现活力 / 440

SAP Donates Millions More in Pandemic Support – Using Digital Means to Empower Hubei SMEs Regain Vitality / 442

诺基亚与中国携手共克时艰 / 444

Nokia Joining Forces with China to Go Through the Difficult Times / 446

一切都会好起来！ / 449

I Will Be There for You! / 450

UPS 向中国运送超过 400 万只口罩及防护装备，助力中国抗击疫情 / 451

UPS Airlifted More than 4 Million Masks and Protective Gear to China to Help Combat the Spread of the Coronavirus / 453

渣打捐款 260 万元支持中国抗击新冠肺炎疫情 / 455

Standard Chartered Donated RMB 2.6 Million Supporting the Fight against COVID-19 in China / 457

阿尔斯通战"疫"任务之口罩供给：一个也不能少 / 459

Alstom's Coronavirus Mask Mission – Ensuring No One is Left Behind / 461

雅培中国捐赠总额超 4100 万元现金和医疗物资助力抗击疫情 / *463*

Abbott Donates RMB 41 Million Worth of Medical Supplies and Funding to
Support Relief Efforts for the Coronavirus Outbreak in China / *465*

部分跨国公司捐赠中国"抗疫"一览 / *467*

前　言

2020 年伊始，一场突如其来的新冠肺炎疫情肆虐中华大地。疫情就是命令，防控就是责任。疫情发生以来，在以习近平同志为核心的党中央坚强领导下，举国上下众志成城，全力以赴抗击疫情。

在疫情面前，许多跨国公司紧急动员，积极捐款捐物，支持中国抗击新冠肺炎疫情，用各种方式为"武汉加油"，为"中国加油"！

跨国公司是 20 世纪 70 年代初由联合国经济及社会理事会决定统一采用的名称，主要指发达国家的大型企业，在国内通常也称"外资企业"，以本国为总部基地，在世界各地通过对外直接投资，设立分支机构或子公司，进行国际化生产和经营活动。1978 年中国开启改革开放的大门，跨国公司开始进入中国市场。在这 40 年里，跨国公司参与和见证了中国令世界瞩目的经济发展奇迹，也为中国经济腾飞做出了重要贡献。

2019 年 10 月 19 日，商务部研究院发布《跨国公司投资中国 40 年报告》（以下简称《报告》），系统梳理了 40 年来跨国公司在中国的发展历程、总结了跨国公司在中国取得的成就以及为促进中国经济发展所贡献的力量，同时展示了中国对外开放实现互利共赢的决心和信心。

《报告》显示，截至 2018 年底，中国累计设立外商投资企业 96.1 万家，实际吸收外商投资 2.1 万亿美元，已经成为全球最大的外商投资东道国之一。《报告》认为，外商投资推动了中国的改革开放，推动了思想观念更新、政府职能转变和宏观经济管理制度的改革，为建立开放型经济新体制发挥了重要作用。《报告》还指出，快速成长的中国市场，给跨国公司提供了难得的发展机遇和新的投资热土；中国的改革开放，为跨国公司全球布局、寻求增长提供了"中国机会"。

作为推动经济全球化的重要力量，跨国公司以其强大的经济实力主导着全球经济的发展走向，引导着世界经济新秩序的形成。在经济全球化过程中，一方面，各国、各地区的经济相互交织、相互影响、相互融合，形成全球统一市场；另一方面，在世界范围内建立起规范经济行为的全球规则，并以此为基础建立了经济运行的全球机制。因此，经济全球化成为一个生产要素跨越国界，并在全球范围内自由流动且相互融合、相互补充的全球统一运营的市场机制。跨国公司既是经济全球化的重要推动力量，又为经济全球化进程奠定了坚实的基础。

伴随经济全球化的脚步，跨国公司进入中国市场 40 年，经历了从水土不服到逐步适应，到主动融合，再到争取"国民待遇"的发展进程，投资规模从小到大、投资水平由低到高、投资区域从沿海到内地，已经在中国大地上形成了中国改革开放进程中一道独特而靓丽的风景线。跨国公司不仅是中国改革开放的参与者、见证者、贡献者、受益者，更是与中国一起携手前行、共创辉煌的同行者、互助者、合作者、共享者。

2020 年伊始，跨国公司携手中国追求高质量发展目标。新冠肺炎疫情没有使跨国公司却步，许多跨国公司纷纷表现出坚定信心，认为中国经济基本面和长期向好趋势不会因疫情改变，为外资创造良好条件的综合竞争优势也不会由于疫情发生变化。

2020 年 2 月 15 日，中国美国商会主席葛国瑞（Greg Gilligan）接受中国新闻网专访时表示，我们非常赞赏中国政府面对疫情的迅速反应和果断措施。截至 15 日，商会会员企业捐助的物资和现金总价值近 4.6 亿元。我们想用行动证明，我们也是中国社会一分子。葛国瑞还谈到，从商会会员企业高管们的反馈看，在华美企对中国经济信心未改。他们更关心怎么解决当前存在的问题，如何调整生产经营计划。

德国大众汽车集团董事会主席迪斯博士（Dr.Herbert Diess）分别通

过新浪微博、中央国际电视台和中国驻德国大使馆网站表示，"我看到亿万中国人民团结一心，全力以赴对抗新冠肺炎疫情。虽然形势严峻，但我深信坚强的中国人民一定会赢得这场疫情的胜利。大众汽车集团将一如既往地和中国人民在一起"。

2020 年 2 月 26 日，英国太古集团主席施铭伦（Merlin Swire）在接受中国国际电视台采访时表示，"我坚信在中央政府的强有力领导下，在数以万计勇敢而辛劳的医护人员及志愿者的努力下，中国终将克服困难，赢得挑战。太古在中国的经营历史已经超过 150 年，早已深深扎根中国。在这场抗击疫情的战斗中，太古将与中国并肩作战"。

2020 年 3 月 1 日，美国高通公司首席执行官史蒂夫·莫伦科夫通过新华网表示，"我们深知中国人民坚忍不拔，对他们有能力克服目前的挑战充满信心。作为植根中国的坚定合作伙伴，高通对中国经济发展保持长期向好的趋势充满信心"。

在疫情面前，许多跨国公司在积极捐款捐物、支持抗击疫情的同时，还从不同视角的观察、不同层面的思考、不同行业的经验，提出了他们的建议。作为 40 年来跨国公司第一本汇编报告，旨在梳理、总结、建言、启示，表达跨国公司的企业社会责任与担当、对中国的真情关切和与中国携手同行的坚定信心。

该汇编分为两部分，第一部分，"集思广益聚智慧"，精选部分跨国公司面对新冠肺炎疫情的思考与建议；第二部分，"抗击疫情在行动"，收集整理了部分跨国公司在抗击新冠肺炎疫情中的爱心奉献。汇编以中文和英文两种文字呈现。

在整个构思、收集、撰写、整理、编辑过程中，我们得到了许多跨国公司的大力支持，在此一并表示感谢。

2020 年这场席卷全球的新冠肺炎疫情，造成全球经济"停摆"，其影响超过 2008 年全球金融危机，甚至超过 1929~1933 年全球经济"大萧条"，世界正在经历人类历史上百年未有之大变局，世界经济再次走到了人类发展进程的十字路口。人类共处一个"地球村",各国命运休戚相关,构建人类命运共同体是人类社会发展进步唯一正确的方向。我们希望通过这本汇编,启迪思考,凝聚共识,用人类的智慧与勇气,转危为机,开创人类持续发展、合作共赢的新时代!

执行主编:李新玉　博士

中国国际跨国公司促进会副会长兼秘书长

2020 年 5 月 19 日

于北京

Preface

At the beginning of 2020, the sudden outbreak of the COVID-19 wreaked havoc on China. Since the outbreak, under the strong leadership of President Xi Jinping, the whole country has worked together to fight the epidemic.

In the face of COVID-19, many multinational corporations swiftly mobilized and donated goods and money to support China in fighting the epidemic, showing solidarity with Wuhan and China in various ways.

Multinational corporation is a term adopted by the UN Economic and Social Council (ECOSOC) in the early 1970s, referring primarily to large enterprises in developed countries. In China they are often referred to as "foreign-invested enterprises". Headquartered in their home country, they produce and operate globally through foreign direct investment and establishing subsidiaries or branches. As China opened the door through reform and opening up in 1978, multinational corporations gradually began to enter the Chinese market. Over the past 40 years, multinational corporations have participated in and witnessed China's astounding economic achievement, and have also contributed significantly to China's economic take-off.

On October 19, 2019, the research institute of the Ministry of Commerce CAITEC released the *Multinationals In China: 40 Years of Investment* (hereinafter referred to as the "Report"), which systematically reviewed the history of multinational corporations in China over the past 40 years and summarized the achievements of multinational corporations in China and their contribution to China's economic growth. The report also shows China's determination and confidence in opening to the world for mutual benefit and win-win results.

According to the Report, by the end of 2018, a total of 961,000 foreign-invested enterprises had been established in China, utilizing US$2.1 trillion in foreign investment. It has become one of the world's largest host country for foreign investment. The Report believes that foreign investment has promoted China's reform and opening up, i.e., the renewal of ideas and concepts, the transformation of government functions and the reform of the macroeconomic management system, and played an important role in establishing a new open economic system. The Report also pointed out that the fast-growing Chinese market has provided opportunities for the global strategy and growth of multinational companies.

As an important force in economic globalization, multinational companies with their economic prowess dominate the development trend of the global economy and guide the formation of a new world economic order. In the process of economic globalization, on the one hand, the economies of countries and regions are intertwined, influencing each other on the way towards a unified global market; on the other hand, global rules that regulate economic behaviors are set up worldwide and based on this, a global mechanism for economic operation. Therefore, economic globalization has become a globally unified market mechanism in which production factors cross national borders, flow freely around the world and complement each other. Multinational corporations are not only an important driving force for economic globalization, but also a solid foundation of the whole globalization process.

Along with economic globalization, after 40 years, multinational companies have gone through different stages: from being maladapted to gradually adapting, and then to active integration and national treatment. Investment has increased in size and the destinations spread from coastal areas to further inland. It is a unique feature in China's reform and opening-up process. Multinational corporations are not only participants, witnesses, contributors, and beneficiaries in China's reform and opening up, but also partners who walk along with China, help each other and share with each other for a better future.

While the beginning of 2020 when multinational corporations joined China in pursuing high-quality economic development goals was defined by the COVID-19 pandemic, they were nevertheless not only undeterred, but have displayed even greater confidence that China's economic fundamentals and long-term upward trend will not change due to the epidemic, nor will the comprehensive competitive advantages that created good conditions for foreign investment.

On February 15, 2020, Greg Gilligan, Chairman of American Chamber of Commerce in China, expressed in an exclusive interview with China News Network his appreciation of the Chinese government's rapid response and decisive measures in the face of the epidemic. As of 15th February, the total value of materials and cash donated by member companies of AmCham reached close to 460 million yuan, as they wanted to prove with action that they are also part of Chinese society. Mr. Gilligan also mentioned that from the feedback of the executives of member companies of AmCham, US enterprises in China remain confident in the Chinese economy. They are more interested in solving existing problems and how to adjust production and operation plans.

Dr. Herbert Diess, Chairman of Volkswagen Group, said through Sina Weibo, China Central Television and the website of the Chinese Embassy in Germany, "Currently looking at China, I see that millions of Chinese joining forces to win the battle against the coronavirus. Though the situation is very serious, I am deeply convinced that the Chinese people will overcome it with solidarity and dignity. The Volkswagen will always family stand close alongside the people of China."

In an interview with China International Television, Merlin Swire, Chairman of Swire Pacific Ltd, said on February 26, 2020, "I have full confidence that under the able leadership of the central government, and with the support of tens of thousands of brave and hardworking medical professionals and volunteers, China will overcome this challenge", "Swire has been operating in China for more than 150 years and has long been deeply rooted in China. In this battle against the epidemic, Swire will fight alongside China."

On March 1, 2020, Steve Molenkov, CEO of Qualcomm, said through Xinhuanet.com, "We know that the Chinese people are persevering and we are confident in their ability to overcome current challenges. Being a staunch partner deeply rooted in China, Qualcomm is fully confident that China's economy will maintain a long-term upward trend."

In the face of the epidemic, many multinational companies actively donated money and materials and supported the fight against the epidemic. They also gather their suggestions from different perspectives of observation, different levels of thinking and experience in different industries. As the first compilation of report of a multinational company in 40 years, it aims to sort out, suggest, enlighten, inspire, and also demonstrate corporate social responsibility of multinational companies as well as their genuine concern for China and firm confidence in working with China.

The compilation is divided into two parts. The first part, "Brainstorm for wisdom-gathing", presents multinational companies' thoughts, ideas and suggestions in fighting against COVID-19; the second part, "Actions for Fighting Epidemic", demonstrates their care and dedication during the times of the epidemic. The compilation is presented both in Chinese and English.

Throughout the process of collecting, writing, arranging and editing the reports, we have received strong support from many multinational companies, and here we would like to express to them our gratitude.

The COVID-19 that swept through the world in 2020 caused the global economy to grind to a halt. Its impact exceeded the global financial crisis in 2008 and even the global "Great Depression" of 1929-1933. The world is experiencing changes unseen in a century, and with the great changes, the world economy has once again reached a crossroads in the history of human development. Human beings live together in a "global village", the destiny of all countries being closely related, and therefore building a community with a shared future for mankind is the only right direction in the development and progress of human society. We hope that through this compilation, we can inspire thinking, build consensus, crystallize human wisdom and courage so as to turn crises into opportunities and create a new era of sustainable development and win-win cooperation for all.

Xinyu Li, Ph.D

Executive Editor-in-Chief

Vice President & Secretary General of CICPMC

19 May 2020

Beijing

第一部分
集思广益聚智慧
Part I
Brainstorm for Wisdom-gathering

新时代危机防范体制建设的建议

ABB*（中国）有限公司

中国已成为全球第二大经济体，2018 年经济总量约占全球的 16%，对世界经济增长贡献接近 30%。2020 年伊始，中国政府为阻止突发新冠肺炎疫情蔓延、救治感染患者所采取的果断、坚决措施获得世界高度赞赏。中国为世界各国抗击新冠肺炎疫情赢得了时间，取得了宝贵的经验。

本文将基于对中国应对新冠肺炎疫情的观察，分析应对过程中公共卫生基础设施、应急管理机制、防护物资的储备、复工复产的组织等情况，结合具体案例和 ABB 的自身经验，为新时代危机防范体制建设的进一步提升提出建议。

一　危机防范机制现状

中国作为全球第二大经济体，对于各种危机防范已经有了相对完善的体制，在应对地质灾害、洪涝、干旱、极端天气事件、海洋灾害、森林草原火灾等一系列重大自然灾害的风险挑战中，都显示出高效的应对能力。在应对突发的公共卫生安全事件时，对于已知的如鼠疫、霍乱等传染病，同样显示出非常强的控制能力。

从中华人民共和国应急管理部网站可以查到的重大事故案例看出，重

---

　　*　ABB 是全球技术领导企业，致力于推动行业数字化转型升级。基于超过 130 年的创新历史，ABB 以客户为中心，拥有全球领先的四大业务——电气、工业自动化、运动控制、机器人与离散自动化，以及 ABB Ability™ 数字化平台。ABB 由两家拥有 100 多年历史的国际性企业——瑞典的阿西亚公司和瑞士的布朗勃法瑞公司在 1988 年合并而成，总部位于瑞士苏黎世。

大事故的发生在近年来虽有反复，但是整体下降趋势明显，表明中国对安全生产及交通类重大事故的管控已经有相对完善的体系，并积累了丰富的经验。图 1 是根据近年来中华人民共和国应急管理部发布的特别重大事故调查报告汇总的特别重大事故数量。

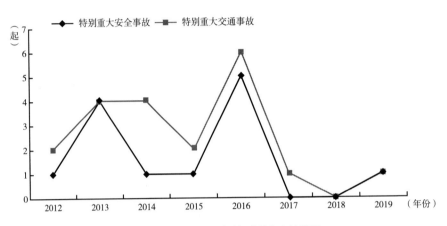

图 1　2012~2019 年特别重大事故数量

资料来源：https://www.mem.gov.cn/gk/sgcc/tbzdsgdcbg/。

新冠肺炎疫情的出现，使中国危机防范机制，特别是从疫情的初期预警、医疗设施配置到应急物资调配和生产组织等方面都经历了重大考验。在启动联防联控机制后，中国快速建设火神山医院、雷神山医院以及方舱医院，紧急增援医护人员，指导防疫物资生产企业快速复工复产，缓解防护物资供应紧缺状况，使疫情得到初步有效遏制。但是对疫情的整体应对也反映出中国危机防疫体系的建设，包括公共卫生基础设施建设、应急管理机制的运行、防护物资的储备、复工复产的组织等还有很大的提升空间。

二　公共卫生基础设施建设

新冠肺炎疫情的暴发，凸显了公共卫生基础设施的欠缺。当武汉突发新冠肺炎疫情时，武汉金银潭医院和武汉肺科医院总计仅有 600 张床位，很多患者得不到及时救治，很多疑似病例不能被有效隔离，加上公众对病毒传染性认识不足，导致疫情暴发。

面对突发的疫情，武汉市及湖北省的医疗机构顿时面临巨大压力，医疗检测设施紧缺、医护人员紧缺、医疗和防护物资紧缺。为了控制疫情，武汉将很多医院改为定点医院，并且火速建设火神山医院和雷神山医院，将很多会展中心和体育场馆改建为方舱医院，将宾馆等用于隔离人员。全国各地紧急为武汉增援医护人员，为武汉可以收治所有重症患者增加力量。轻症患者被收治到方舱医院，疑似病例及亲密接触者也有了集中管理的去处，实现应收尽收。截至 2020 年 2 月 24 日，武汉市 48 家定点医院共开放床位 23532 张，已用床位 19275 张，有了空床位 4311 张[①]。至此，疫情得到遏制。到 3 月 10 日，武汉 14 家方舱医院全部休舱，让大家真真切切看到了胜利的曙光。[②]

在世界各地人员流动如此频繁的时代，中东呼吸综合征、埃博拉病毒、登革热等各种疫情都随时可能在中国出现，那么，加大投入，设立常规防疫设施非常必要。建议对于所有医院、机场、车站都常设正规的隔离设施，包括随时可以使用的隔离室，并配有专业医护人员值守，保证所有防护设施有效运行。一旦出现传染病患者，立即将其进行隔离、转送、收治。

经过改革开放 40 多年的发展，中国已经进入高质量发展的新时代，需要满足日益增长的人民对于美好生活的追求。然而在公共消费包含教育、卫生和文化等方面的投资比重，相比在环保、交通等基础设施领域的投资比重还比较低。2018 年中国医疗卫生领域政府财政支出 1.6 万亿元，占 GDP 比重仅为 1.7%，与世界各国医疗卫生投入相比也比较低[③]，与世界第二大经济体的地位不相适应。

[①]《最新数据：武汉 48 家定点医院病床使用情况一览，金银潭医院空床位 115》，北晚新视觉网，2020 年 2 月 26 日。

[②]《方舱医院，开舱休舱同样传递希望》，新华网，2020 年 2 月 11 日。

[③] https://stats.oecd.org/Index.aspx?DatasetCode=HEALTH_STAT#http://data.stats.gov.cn/easyquery.htm?cn=C01.

我们注意到全国各地方政府的工作报告中都对医疗卫生投入有明确的任务，比如，北京市人民政府在 2020 年政府工作报告中已经提出了"研究制定公共卫生体系能力建设三年行动计划，提高传染病和突发公共卫生事件处置能力"。①

从新冠肺炎疫情发展至今，新技术的应用包括人工智能（AI）为抗击疫情发挥了重要作用。据不完全统计，人工智能防疫已经应用在防疫追踪统计、人员健康检测、物资平台调度、医生诊断辅助和各类功能型机器人等方面。武汉的部分医院使用各种机器人进行消毒、测温、巡逻、送餐、送药等，在疫情中替代了部分人力，帮助提高工作效率，同时也降低了人员交叉感染的可能性。火神山医院成为武汉使用最多 AI 产品的医院，包括肺部影像辅助诊断、合理用药系统、机器人和无人超市。②

ABB 的协作机器人未来可以应用于医院的实验室科研和物流环节，从而帮助医务人员减少重复、费时、精细的工作流程，包括加药、混药和移液任务，以及无菌仪器装配和离心机装料与卸料，提高安全性和一致性。同时可以帮助提高医疗工作效率，让医疗专家和科研人员专注于更有价值的工作，最终帮助更多患者接受治疗，回归健康生活。此外，医疗行业正面临着人口老龄化、高水平医疗人员紧缺的挑战，为了给患者提供更高效的诊疗和健康服务，很多医院也在致力于利用最新的自动化、数字化和智能化技术，进行转型升级。

建议中国政府在公共卫生领域增加投入，一方面要增加医护人员的数量，特别要提高医护人员的待遇；另一方面要增加全国各地公共卫生设施建设的投入，鼓励更多地使用包括机器人应用在内的自动化、数字化和智能化技术的应用，建设智慧医院，进一步提升公共卫生设施为公众服务的水平，提升国家整体应对突发公共卫生事件的能力。

---

① 《2020 年北京市政府工作报告全文公布！》，北晚新视觉网，2020 年 1 月 19 日。
② 《AI 防疫：机器人最受武汉医院青睐 火神山使用不同 AI 产品最多》，腾讯网，2020年 2 月 28 日，https://new.qq.com/omn/20200228/20200228A0TUQG00.html。

三　应急管理机制的运行

应急管理机制的有效运行，对于疫情的控制至关重要。当疫情出现时，各省市很快启动应急响应机制，武汉市启动"封城"措施。但是武汉封城之后的很长一段时间，医护人员的交通、住宿、饮食等很多后勤保障工作是由社会各界的志愿者在承担，防护物资的调配也非常混乱。

抗击突发的疫情如同一场战争，一线医护人员就是奔赴前线的战士，应急管理机制必须提供强有力的后勤保障。与上述混乱状况截然不同的是火神山医院建设的高效、有序管理。

2020 年 1 月 23 日武汉市政府决定建设火神山医院，参照北京小汤山医院模式用 10 天建成，集中收治新型冠状病毒肺炎重症患者。医院总建筑面积 3.39 万平方米，采用模块化、鱼骨状设计布局，进行功能分区，将医护人员治疗区和生活区分离，现场洁净区、半污染区和污染区分离；雨水、污水、氯气等多层次净化后排放，采用负压病房，空气消毒排放，医疗垃圾统一就地焚烧，进行无害化处理。[1]

为了建设火神山医院，武汉成立了武汉城建局、中建三局、参建分包单位三级指挥系统，中建三局作为牵头单位[2]，统筹制定路线图，统一策划、组织、协调，做好工序和工艺的穿插流程，为所有参建单位提供服务和施工安排，保证每家单位都能最大限度发挥专业优势，保持各单位的施工节奏步调一致[3]。建设中需要协调十几家企业数以万计的工作人员的参与。

---

[1] 《施工档案助火神山医院火速建成》，中华人民共和国国家档案局，2020 年 2 月 27 日，http://www.naa.gov.cn/daj/c100251/202002/eaebd1c977b84ddb9046167c2e4ac282.shtml。

[2] 《火神山、雷神山医院建设的"中国速度"！》，搜狐网，2020 年 2 月 6 日，https://www.sohu.com/a/370939296_120094713。

[3] 《揭秘火神山雷神山医院建设背后的"中国力量"》，人民网，2020 年 2 月 24 日，http://finance.people.com.cn/n1/2020/0224/c1004-31600744.html。

值得一提的是，现场组建起安全防疫管理团队，分两个安全小组与现场施工同步进行，24 小时不间断安全监管。在办公区、工人生活区设置 5 处固定的红外线测温仪，在施工现场设置 3 处流动测温点，安排 8 位管理人员随身携带测温仪现场巡查测温，确保作业人员每天监测体温不少于 4 次。火神山医院施工现场未发生任何安全事故，参建人员未发生一起疫情感染状况。[①]

火神山医院建设时间短，参与单位多，物资需求量大，现场人员多，感染防控难度大。唯有专业化的周到、细致而高效的管理，才能在建设过程中协调所有参与方密切配合，使物资供应、现场施工流程、时间节点都能无缝衔接，同时保证安全防护，才能在 2 月 2 日将医院建成交付使用。在整个项目建设中，无论哪一个环节出现问题，出现滞后，十天建成一座医院，都是一个无法完成的任务。如果应急管理体制可以借鉴这样项目管理的方式运行，一定可以提高未来的危机防范能力。

四 防护物资储备

防护物资的储备与调配对于应对无论是自然灾害还是公共卫生事件都至关重要。2003 年的 SARS 之后，国家完善了突发公共卫生事件应急管理体系，包括应急物资储备体系。医护人员的个人防护用品包括防护服、防护眼镜、口罩等都在储备清单内。疫情出现时，防护用品是保证医护人员抗击疫情的重要物资。

然而，在新冠肺炎疫情暴发之初，由于疫情传播速度快，感染人数暴发式增长，各方面物资很快无法支撑一线医务人员的防护需求，医务人员直接向社会求助。社会各界迅速响应，利用全球资源紧急支援。ABB 也立即决定捐款 100 万元，用来购买一线医疗救护人员所需的防护

---

① 《直击：火神山医院交付，建设过程到底有多难？》，红星欣慰，2020 年 2 月 2 日，https://baijiahao.baidu.com/s?id=1657440519510800159&wfr=spider&for=pc。

物资，同时启动海外供应资源，购买并向武汉、厦门、重庆、上海等地定点医院捐赠 1.6 万多只 N95 口罩，为一线医护人员提供安全防护保障。

在国家启动联防联控机制之后，防护物资的产能很快得到恢复，各地还出现很多新增加的产能，口罩、防护服等防护物资的紧缺状况逐渐得到缓解。但是需要反思的是，作为制造大国，也是世界上最大的口罩生产国和出口国，年产量占到全球的 50%，在疫情暴发时，却不能为一线医护人员提供足够的口罩。应急物资储备的缺口如此之大，成为国家应急管理体系的短板。

2020 年 3 月 1 日出版的《求是》杂志发表的习近平主席的文章《全面提高依法防控依法治理能力 健全国家公共卫生应急管理体系》指出，要把应急物资保障作为国家应急管理体系建设的重要内容。国家应该以此为契机，完善对涉及公共卫生突发事件所需防护物资的储备体制和机制，优化重要应急物资的储备和产能保障，从而提高危机防范能力。

五 安全有序复工

复工复产可以为疫情防控提供可靠的物资保障，维护社会经济的稳定运行。安全有序的复工需要各企业在保证生产的同时，落实疫情防控措施。在复工之初，国家各专业机构都在为交通、居家、工作场所等提供防护指南，企业要对员工安全防护进行专业性管理，保证安全复工，防止疫情复发。

1. ABB 的复工经验

在 2020 年 2 月 10 日复工的第一天，中央电视台新闻联播节目报道了 ABB 安全有序复工情况。ABB 始终将确保员工安全与健康作为企业运行的首要准则。新冠肺炎疫情暴发之初，ABB（中国）第一时间启动防疫准备工作，成立疫情防控工作小组，密切关注疫区及全国各地员工健康安全问题。

春节假期期间，ABB（中国）管理层团队及相关部门持续跟踪各地公共卫生部门政策更新，制定员工健康安全指导细则，并通过短信、邮件及微信群等方式与员工不间断内部沟通，普及新冠病毒防范措施。

根据国家各级政府的要求，公司取消或延期举行大型内部会议和活动，采用视频或电话会议的备用方案。提醒各位同事关注并且遵守所在社区及当地政府的各项防疫要求，减少外出并取消不必要的聚会。提醒员工要勤洗手洗脸、保持健康饮食与作息、适量运动、加强免疫力；保持居家环境清洁与通风；保持心情放松愉悦，避免过度恐慌和焦虑。

ABB 响应中国各级政府的号召，在严峻的防疫形势下，为应对防护物资供给挑战，在制定流程提升个人保护装备（PPE）使用效率的同时，获得集团全球供应链的支持，确保员工生产防护物资的供给。同时，做好复工培训："春节复工指南——疫情下赴工途中的卫生防护"、"疫情下办公室的安全防护"以及"春节复工指南——疫情下抗疫心理调节"。

ABB 各企业严格遵照当地政府对复工防护的要求，为员工提供防护用品，同时控制复工人数，规范现场管理。员工按照公司的管理要求，每天按时提交健康信息，按照标准佩戴口罩，保持适当的安全距离，共同保证安全复工。

复工初期，由于全国各地疫情防控的需要，人员流动受到限制，原材料供应、物流等都无法正常进行。有些重要供应商的复工审批也遇到很大问题。幸运的是，我们企业所在的很多地方政府如北京、上海、厦门等地方政府在推动企业复工的过程中，不仅帮助协调供应商企业所在地政府，推动当地对复工的审批，而且帮助协调包括长三角、京津冀、厦门周边地区的跨省、市的物流问题，使我们的供应商能够保证原材料及元器件的稳定供应，支持我们企业持续生产，并保证产品能够及时送达客户，为复工提供了巨大的支持。同时，为了鼓励安全复工复产，国家各级政府出台了很多支持政策，减少新冠肺炎疫情的暴发对企业生产造成的影响。

复工之后，仍然有很多地区，包括疫情稳定地区的很多人员都无法返回工作地，即使回到工作地，有的地区要求员工自己找地方隔离 14 天后才能回到租住的住房，对员工的生活造成极大不便，也影响企业的复工复产。建议在未来的危机防范机制中，将企业的复工复产作为重要的议题，在全国各地一盘棋的情况下，考虑人员、交通、物流对生产的影响，在做好防护的情况下，更好地保证有序、安全复工复产，降低对经济发展的影响。

2. 携手客户与合作伙伴共同抗疫

疫情出现之初，ABB 很快恢复服务热线，保证随时为客户提供线上线下服务支持，与客户及合作伙伴共同努力，积极利用自身技术、产品、供应链和服务优势，参与多项疫情防控项目，确保电力供应并提供必要的物资和服务，支持中国在抗击疫情的同时，保持经济持续稳定发展。

为及时有效防治新冠肺炎，贵阳市自 2020 年 1 月底加紧实施大水沟病区改造，改扩建贵阳版"小汤山医院"。根据贵阳市政府的部署，贵阳在大水沟院区原老病房楼址拟修建 404 个床位的隔离应急病区。ABB 团队争分夺秒，火速支援医院改扩建，为项目提供重症加强护理病房（ICU）专用隔离变压器，以及塑壳断路器、微型断路器、漏电断路器、隔离开关、接触器、双电源开关等产品。在物流快递受阻的情况下，ABB 工程师自驾车辆将必需物资由重庆运往贵阳，支持贵阳"小汤山医院"建设。

为确保抗击疫情相关应用场所的安全可靠运行，ABB 迅速启动紧急机制，为各地医院系统扩容提供解决方案，履行 7×24 小时的全方位服务承诺，保障抗击疫情一线及后方的生产需要，比如，为上海金山医院扩容积极协调各地经销商资源，第一时间调配 VD4 型真空断路器。

与此同时，我们注意到，ABB 为客户企业打造的全自动生产线在安全复工时体现了很大的优势。机器人的使用不仅减少了用工成本，降低车间内人员密集度，还能更高效地恢复生产。例如，2018 年 ABB 为海拉电子打造的先进的遥控汽车钥匙生产线，使用了 11 台 ABB 机器人。在许多企业受到疫情暴发带来的各种影响时，工人返乡以及返乡后无法回到工作岗位成为一大难题。而海拉电子的这条生产线，自动化程度高，不需要直接操作工，因而春节期间也未完全停产，很快就完全恢复正常生产。

机器人与自动化技术的应用，包括远程服务，在疫情出现时，保证了企业的持续运行。

六 建议

新冠肺炎疫情暴发之后，举国行动，展示了中国抗疫的力度、速度和透明度，得到国际社会各界的赞赏。应对过程中出现的问题和取得的经验，对于未来危机防范机制的建设都非常有借鉴意义。基于对中国应对新冠肺炎疫情的观察，提出如下参考建议。

第一，2020 年，国家各级政府将启动"十四五"规划的制定，建议制定规划时增加公共卫生基础设施建设的投入，以提高应对重大公共卫生突发事件的能力。

第二，进一步完善应急保障机制，包括所有涉及的后勤保障，制定更加详细的执行细则，使机制有更强的可操作性、可执行性。执行层面可借鉴项目管理的模式，提高应急保障机制的运行效率。

第三，完善应急物资储备体系，把应急物资保障作为国家应急管理体系建设的重要内容，优化重要应急物资的储备和产能保障。

第四，借鉴地震、火灾等自然灾害的培训、演练经验，对疫情的防范加大宣传力度，并增加公众的参与度，为公众提供培训，安排公众演练。借助应对新冠肺炎疫情的契机，将对公众的培训常态化。

第五，加强各领域的职业安全防护。专业的职业安全健康保障体系可以保证企事业单位的安全运营和人员安全，帮助应对突发自然灾害及公共安全事件，支持灾后或疫情之后恢复安全生产。

第六，更多地鼓励包括机器人应用在内的自动化、数字化和智能化技术在工业和医疗卫生领域的应用，提升社会的整体危机防范能力。

七 结束语

ABB 衷心感谢中国为遏制疫情所付出的巨大努力，同时，向奋战在疫情救治和防控一线的人员致以崇高的敬意！

中国是 ABB 全球第二大市场，伴随中国改革开放，ABB 不断成长壮大，持续扩大在华投资，支持中国经济发展，如近年投入运营的创新研发与制造基地 ABB 厦门工业中心，以及上海在建的 ABB 全球最先进的机器人新工厂等。未来，我们将继续投资中国市场，推动业务长足发展。

ABB 对新时代中国经济的未来充满信心。中国经济拥有坚实的基础和强大的韧性，足以战胜疫情带来的挑战。我们愿与中国的同事、客户、合作伙伴以及所有中国人民一起携手，风雨同舟，共克时艰。

The Development of China's Crisis Prevention System in the New Era

By ABB (China) Co., Ltd.

China as the second largest economy in the world, China accounts for about 16 percent of the global economy, contributing roughly 30 percent of global growth in 2018. At beginning of 2020, the Chinese government took decisive and resolute measures to prevent the spread of the novel coronavirus (COVID-19) and treat infected patients, gained valuable time and experience for the world. From which, China was highly appreciated by the international community.

This paper provides an overview of current situation of China's responses to the COVID-19 epidemic. It then discusses the key factors of its responding system, such as public health infrastructure, operation of emergency management mechanism, reserve of protective supplies, and resumption of production and operation. By combining international practices, case study and ABB's practical business experience, this paper presents the suggestions for further developing the crisis prevention system of China in the new era.

1　Situation analysis

China is the world's second largest economy. While responding to a series of major natural crises, such as geological disasters, floods, droughts, extreme weathers, oceanic disasters, forest and prairie fires etc., China has demonstrated high efficiency and capability with the well-developed crises prevention system.

China has also made very good control on preventing the known infectious diseases, such as plague and cholera etc.

Over the past decades, China has set up a mature system and accumulated rich experience on managing and controlling the major work safety and traffic accidents, which helped reduce the number of major accidents significantly. This can be seen from investigation reports of extremely major accidents released by Ministry of Emergency Management of the People's Republic of China (MEM) in recent years.

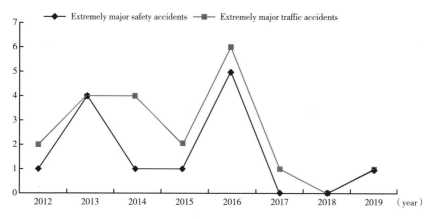

Figure 1　The number of extremely major accidents in 2012-2019
Source: https://www.mem.gov.cn/gk/sgcc/tbzdsgdcbg/.

In the course of responding to the outbreak of COVID-19, China's crisis prevention system faced many challenges, such as early warning of epidemic, allocation of medical facilities, deployment of medical supplies, and production organization. After activating the Joint Prevention and Control Mechanism of the State Council, China effectively controlled the spread of epidemic by taking various emergent and decisive measures including rapidly building Huoshenshan Hospital, Lcishenshan Hospital and shelter hospitals, sending emergency medical assistance teams to Hubei province, and guiding the manufacturers of epidemic prevention materials to accelerate production resumption to ease the pressure of shortage in protective supplies.

The experiences of tacking the epidemic challenges presented that there is much potential for China's crisis prevention system to further improve, especially in the areas of public health infrastructure, operation of emergency management mechanism, reserve of protective supplies, and organizing work and production resumption.

2　Improve public health infrastructures

When the COVID-19 epidemic broke out in Wuhan, there were a total of 600 beds available in Wuhan Jinyintan Hospital and Wuhan Pulmonary Hospital. As a result, many confirmed cases of COVID-19 were not treated in time, many suspected cases were not in effective quarantine. Coupling with insufficient public awareness of the virus's strong infectivity, the epidemic quickly erupted. It highlighted the shortage of China's public health infrastructures.

The medical institutions in Wuhan and Hubei Province faced with huge pressure due to the shortage of medical testing facilities, the medical staff, and the medical and protective materials. In order to control the virus spread, Wuhan took the decisive measures on changing many hospitals into designated ones, building the Huoshenshan Hospital and the Leishenshan Hospital at top speed, transforming many convention and exhibition centers and sports venues into shelter hospitals, and using hotels to put suspected cases in quarantine. In addition, all provinces, autonomous regions, and municipalities sent emergency medical assistance teams to help Wuhan and Hubei province. With these resolute efforts, the patients in critical condition were treated in regular hospitals, while the patients with mild symptoms were treated in the shelter hospitals, and the suspected cases and close contacts were sent in centralized quarantine facilities with no one unattended. As of February 24, 48 designated hospitals in Wuhan had a combined capacity of 23,532 beds, including 19,275 ones in use and 4311 ones [1] available – the epidemic was preliminarily contained. As of March 10, all the 14 shelter hospitals in Wuhan wrapped up their operation, giving us the truly dawn in sight. [2]

In the era of frequent mobility, various epidemics including MERS, Ebola virus and dengue may occur in China at any time, therefore it is highly necessary to increase investments to construct regular epidemic prevention facilities. It is suggested to set up standing and regular isolation facilities, including ready-to-use isolation rooms attended by medical professionals responsible for effective operation of all protective facilities in all hospitals, airports and stations. In this way, once an infectious disease patient is observed, immediate actions including isolation, transfer and treatment can be taken professionally.

Over 40+ years of development after the reform and opening up, China has stepped into a new era featuring high-quality development, and be working on meeting people's increasing demand for a better life. But China's government investments for education, health and culture are relatively lower than that for the environmental protection and transportation infrastructures. In 2018, the fiscal expenditure in China's healthcare registered CNY 1.6 trillion, accounting for only about 1.7% of the GDP, a level lower than some other countries [3] . This is not compatible with the country's position as the world's second largest economy.

We have noticed that the work report of every local government defines a specific task of investments in healthcare, for example, Beijing government has put forward that "Beijing will formulate a three-year action plan to build

---

[1]　https://baijiahao.baidu.com/s?id=1659562953722427344&wfr=spider&for=pc (Takefoto.cn. 2020-02-26. Latest data: Bed uses in 48 designated hospitals of Wuhan at a glance: Jinyintan Hospital has 115 beds available).

[2]　http://www.xinhuanet.com/comments/2020-03/11/c_1125693669.htm (www.xinhuanet.com 2020-02-11. Shelter hospitals deliver hope with its opening and wrapping up).

[3]　https://stats.oecd.org/Index.aspx?DatasetCode=HEALTH_STAT#http://data.stats.gov.cn/easyquery.htm?cn=C01.

up capacity of the public health system to improve the capability of handling infectious diseases and public health emergencies" in its Report on the Work of the Beijing Municipal People's Government 2020. [①]

Since the COVID-19 outbreak, the deployment of new technologies like artificial intelligence (AI) has been playing an important role in fighting against the epidemic. According to incomplete statistics, the AI-driven epidemic prevention approach has been applied in epidemic tracking and statistics, personnel health detection, material supply platform, diagnosis assistance and various functional robots etc. In some hospitals of Wuhan, various robots were deployed for disinfection, temperature measurement, patrol, and food and medicine delivery, which partly replaced manpower, improved work efficiency and reduced the risk of cross infection. The Huoshenshan Hospital in Wuhan deployed the most AI products during the battle against the virus, including pulmonary imaging assisted diagnosis, rational drug use systems, robots and automated supermarkets. [②]

In the days to come, ABB's collaborative robots like YuMi® can be adapted to assist medical and laboratory staff with laboratory and logistics tasks in hospitals. It has the potential to undertake a wide range of repetitive and time-consuming activities, including preparation of medicines, loading and unloading centrifuges, pipetting and handling liquids and picking up and sorting test tubes. It will allow medical experts and researchers to focus on more valuable work and ultimately treat more patients.

---

① http://www.beijing.gov.cn/gongkai/jihua/zfgzbg/t1613862.htm (The Report on Work of Beijing Municipal People's Government 2020: II Major Tasks (7) Making steady progress in ensuring people's access to childcare, education, employment, medical services, elderly care, housing, and social assistance, as well as ensuring convenience, livability, diversity, fairness and safety to allow more sense of gain, happiness and security for people).

② https://new.qq.com/omn/20200228/20200228A0TUQG00.html (QQ.com. AI-driven epidemic prevention: Robots are most popular in Wuhan hospitals and Huoshenshan Hospital deploys the most AI products).

The healthcare sector is undergoing significant transformation as the diagnosis and treatment of disease advances, while coping with an aging population, increasing costs and a growing worldwide shortage of medical staff. To provide more efficient diagnosis and health services, many hospitals are working to deploy the latest automated, digital and intelligent technologies for transformation and upgrading.

Therefore, it would be very important to increase investments in the public health field, including the increase of the number of medical staff and their compensation package, increase of public health facilities with automated, digital and intelligent technologies for intelligent hospitals. This will further improve the service level of public health institutes and boost the country's overall capability of responding to public health emergencies.

3 Operation of emergency management mechanism

The effective operation of emergency management mechanism is critical to the epidemic control. While fighting against the sudden outbreak of the epidemic, the emergency management mechanism must ensure the supply of all necessary materials for the frontline medical staffs since they are similar with the soldiers at this stage.

When the COVID-19 occurred, all provinces, autonomous regions, and municipalities rapidly triggered their emergency response mechanism, and the city of Wuhan was locked down. However, for a long time after the lockdown, many logistical support including transportation, accommodation and food for medical professionals etc. were undertaken by the volunteers, and the allocation of protective supplies was in messy situation. In the contrast, the construction of Huoshenshan Hospital went through successfully with high efficient and orderly management.

On January 23,2020, the Wuhan government decided to build the Huoshenshan Hospital for centralized treatment of critical confirmed cases by following the practice of Beijing Xiaotangshan Hospital within 10 days. With a total floor space of 33,900 square meters, the hospital adopts modular and fishbone-shaped layout. It has such strictly separated functional divisions as medical treatment section, ward section, site cleaning section, partially contaminated section and contaminated section. Moreover, the rainwater, waste water and chlorine can only be discharged after multilevel purification, and the wards under negative pressure must go through high-standard disinfection. The medical wastes must be incinerated in situ in a centralized way and disposed in a harmless manner. [1]

A three-level command system comprising Wuhan Urban and Rural Construction Bureau, China Construction Third Engineering Bureau Co., Ltd. and participating subcontractors, was established for the construction of Huoshenshan Hospital. Specifically, the China Construction Third Engineering Bureau as the general contractor [2] , was responsible for the roadmap development, overall planning, organizing and coordinating, connection and alternating of working procedures and technological processes, providing services and construction schedules for all participating organizations to ensure each party to bring their expertise into full play, and maintain aligned construction pace [3] . Tens of thousands of workers from more than ten organizations experienced a good collabration during the construction.

Thanks to the onsite safety and epidemic prevention management team, no safety accident or COVID-19 infection was reported during the project. The team comprised two subgroups for 24/7 continuous safety supervision over construction site. There were five fixed infrared thermometers in the office

---

① http://www.naa.gov.cn/daj/c100251/202002/eaebd1c977b84ddb9046167c2e4ac282.shtml (National Archives Administration of China 2020-02-27: Construction archives contributes to rapid completion of Huoshenshan Hospital).

② https://www.sohu.com/a/370939296_120094713 (2020-02-06: China speed in building Huoshenshan Hospital and Leishenshan Hospital!).

③ http://finance.people.com.cn/n1/2020/0224/c1004-31600744.html (people.cn 2020-02-24: A look at the "China Power" under rapid construction of Huoshenshan Hospital and Leishenshan Hospital).

area, the living quarters for workers, and three mobile temperature checking stations. The team has 8 supervisors assigned for site inspection and temperature measurement with the portable thermodetector to ensure four times of body temperature checking for every people on site. [①]

Due to extremely short construction time for the Huoshenshan Hospital project, there were many challenges for the participating organizations including ensuring high quantity of material supply, safety of numerous site workers and smooth connection of various processes etc. Given this, only professional, well-considered and efficient project management can coordinate for a close collaboration of all participating parties in the construction processes, so that the material supply, site construction process and time nodes can be seamlessly connected, while ensuring the safety protection. Then the hospital can be completed and delivered for operation on February 2. This could be an impossible task if any part went wrong or lagged behind. The emergency management system may draw from such an efficient project management approach, to further improve the crisis prevention capacity in the future.

4   Reserve of protective supplies

The reserve and allocation of protective supplies are very critical role for dealing with both natural disasters and public health emergencies. Since the SARS outbreak in 2003, China has improved its emergency management system for public health emergencies, including the reserve system for emergent supplies. The personal protective equipment (PPE) for medical professionals, including protective garments, safety goggles and surgical masks, are included in the list of protective supplies. When an epidemic breaks out, these PPE serve as

---

① https://baijiahao.baidu.com/s?id=1657440519510800159&wfr=spider&for= pc (Red Star News 2020-02-02. Live: How difficult is the construction and delivery of Huoshenshan Hospital?).

an important line of defense for medical professionals to combat the epidemic.

However, at the beginning of the COVID-19 outbreak, due to the rapid virus spread, early warning deviation was biased, the number of infected people increased dramatically, all kinds of protective materials quickly fell short to meet the demand of frontline medical professionals. It caused that the medical staffs had to directly seek help from the community. Immediately, all walks of life made a rapid response and mobilized global resources available to provide emergency supports. ABB immediately decided a donation of 1 million yuan to support the needs of frontline medical staff. We have since used our global supply chain to secure and deliver more than 16,000 N95 masks to hospitals in Wuhan, Xiamen, Chongqing, Shanghai and Beijing.

After the implementation the national level of Joint Prevention and Control Mechanism, the production capacity of protective supplies was quickly recovered and new production facilities were put on stream, the shortage of such protective supplies as masks and protective garments were gradually alleviated. However, what needs to be rethought is that as the world's largest mask producer and exporter with annual production accounting for 50% of the world's total, China could not sufficiently provide masks for the frontline medical professionals in quite a period since the epidemic outbreak, which highlights the gap in reserve of emergency supplies of China's emergency management system.

As stated in Comprehensively Boosting China's Prevention and Control Capability in Accordance with Laws & Regulations and Continuously Improving China's Public Health Emergency Management System, an article of President Xi published in QiuShi magazine, China should take the security of emergency supplies as one important task of developing the national emergency management system. Based on the top level attention, it is time to further improve the reserve system and mechanism of protective supplies, optimize the reserve of critical emergency supplies and guarantee production capacity for public health emergencies, thus enhancing China's crisis prevention capability.

5　Resuming work and production safely and orderly

Work and production resumption is conductive to providing reliable supplies for the epidemic prevention and control, and ensuring social and economic stability. The safe and orderly resumption of work requires enterprises to implement epidemic prevention and control measures while ensuring production. At the beginning of returning to work, many professional organizations in the country have made protection guidelines for transportation, home, workplace etc. Enterprises should carry out professional management on employee safety protection to ensure safe return to work and prevent rebound of the epidemic.

(1)　ABB's work resumption experience

The health and safety of its employees is a top priority of ABB. At the initial stage of the COVID-19 outbreak, ABB China timely started the preparation for epidemic prevention, set up a team for virus prevention and control, and closely monitored the safety and health situation of ABB employees in the affected areas and across China. On February 10, ABB started to resume work and production, which was reported by CCTV news as a good example.

During the Spring Festival holiday, the management team of ABB China and relevant functions continuously tracked the policy updates released by public health authorities, worked out detailed guidance for employees' health and safety, and communicated with employees internally via SMS, email and WeChat groups to inform COVID-19 prevention & control measures.

In line with the government requirements, ABB China decided to cancel or postpone business travel unless it's business critical; cancel or postpone the recent large-scale internal and external meetings and events, recommended employees to use Skype or teleconference options. During the holiday, the company also recommended the employees to follow the local community and government's preventative measures and safeguard the health of themselves and their family.

ABB provided all necessary personnel protection equipment (PPE) to employees by the support of global resources, and arranged trainings for protection, including the Guide for Work Resumption after the Spring Festival Holiday – Health Protection in Travel to Work Site Under COVID-19 Outbreak, the Safety Protection at Office Under COVID-19 Outbreak, and the Guide for Work Resumption after the Spring Festival Holiday – Psychological Adjustment During National Fight Against Epidemic.

After resuming normal operation, HSE precaution measures were properly implemented and shuttle buses and catering services ran smoothly across many ABB companies and factories in China. In addition, the employees returning to work also submit their health information every day, wear masks in a standard way, keep proper safety distance. ABB team have been making concerted efforts to ensure safety.

At the initial stage of work resumption, people movements were restricted to meet the epidemic prevention & control requirements across China. The raw material supply and transportation didn't work in a normal way. Moreover, some key suppliers had difficulties in production resumption. Fortunately, the local government of many cities where ABB businesses are located, for example, Beijing, Shanghai and Xiamen, provided strong support in coordinating with government approval and logistics system via the mechanism of Yangtze River Delta, the Beijing-Tianjin-Hebei region etc., to ensure timely delivery and business continuity. In addition, Chinese government has released many supportive policies to minimize the epidemic impacts on business sectors.

After the work resumption, in many cities, including the ones where no confirmed cases were reported, many people were not able to return to their work sites, or they were only allowed to return to their rented apartments after a 14 days quarantine in some other places. It caused much inconvenience and impacts the production recovery. Therefore, we would like to recommended that the resumption of production should be taken as an important topic in the future crisis prevention system. Moreover, an overall consideration in terms of safety and orderly production resumption, transportation and logistics across the whole country, will help reduce the epidemic's impact on economic development.

(2) Working with customers and partners to fight against COVID-19

In the early days of the COVID-19 outbreak, ABB timely resumed its online service and provided remote support to ensure the impact for the customers is as minimal as possible. Meanwhile, ABB team has contributed to many virus-prevention projects by working closely with the customers and partners and leveraging its advantages in technology, products, services and supply chain, to ensure sustainable economic development.

The projects included the construction of hospital in Guizhou. To timely and effectively prevent the virus spread, Guiyang decided to accelerate the upgrading of Dashuigou inpatient area and expanded it to a Guiyang-version "Xiaotangshan" Hospital. According to the plan, an emergency isolation section comprising 404 beds would be constructed in the location of the previous Dashuigou inpatient building. ABB team raced against time to provide dedicated isolation transformer for the ICU for critical cases, as well as the products like MCCBs, MCBs, RCCBs, disconnectors, contactors, and ATSs. In the face of restricted logistics and courier services, ABB engineers drove from Chongqing to Guiyang to deliver the necessary products, which strongly supported this project.

To ensure safe and reliable operation of the infrastructures, ABB rapidly activated its emergency mechanism to provide solutions for system capacity expansion of relevant hospitals, offered 7*24 all-round service, to ensure the frontline production and medical services, for example, successful supported the capacity expansion of Shanghai Jinshan Hospital, with timely delivery of VD4 vacuum circuit breakers.

The fully automated production lines deployed by our customers enjoyed great advantages in safe work resumption. The robots helped not only reduce labor costs and worker density in workshops, but also recover production more efficiently. For instance, ABB helped Hella Shanghai Electronics Co., Ltd. build an advanced production line for remote car door opener with 11 ABB robots in 2018. Thanks to its high automation level and zero requirements for direct operators, the production line didn't fully shut down even during the Spring Festival Holiday, and quickly resumed normal production after the holiday. This made a sharp contrast to the companies who suffered when their employees being not able to return to work due to the COVID-19 outbreak.

The deployment of robots and automation technologies, including remote services, helps ensure continuous operation of enterprises in the context of the epidemic outbreak.

6 Suggestions

The decisive measures China has taken to combat the epidemic have fully demonstrated the country's strength and resolve to take on responsibilities. It is highly appreciated by the international communities. During last period, the findings and learnings would be very meaningful references for the development of national crisis prevention system. Based on the observations of China's response to the epidemic, we would like to provide following recommendations:

- In 2020, China will start to work out the 14th Five-Year Plan. It would be a good opportunity for the country to plan increasing investments in public health infrastructures to further improve the capability of responding to major public health emergencies.
- The society would be benefited from further improving the emergency management mechanism including the system of ensuring the materials supply. The mechanism operation may refer to the project management model to increase its efficiency.

- As an important part of the national emergency management system, the reserve system for critical emergency supplies production capacity shall be optimized.
- The public shall have the opportunity to get regular trainings on how to react for preventing the epidemic, in accordance to the experiences of the training in responding to natural disasters like earthquake and fire, especially after the experience of fighting against COVID-19.
- The professional safety protection shall be an important part of the daily work of the enterprises and public institutions in ensuring safe operation and personal safety. This will help people to take efficient response to emergent natural disasters and public health incidents, and support safe production resumption afterwards.
- The adoption of more automated, digital and intelligent technologies including robots in industrial and medical fields shall be encouraged to boost the overall crisis prevention capability of the country.

7　Closing remarks

ABB extends sincere thanks to China for the extraordinary efforts to contain the spread of the virus. We would like to express our admiration for the people on the front line.

China is ABB's second-largest market and we have been growing together with China since the reform and opening up. To support China's growth and economic development, ABB has made significant investments over the years, most recently in an innovation and manufacturing hub in Xiamen and in the world's most advanced robotics factory, currently under construction in Shanghai. We will continue to invest in China to drive further growth.

We are absolutely confident in the future of the Chinese economy, which is strong enough to withstand the impact of the coronavirus outbreak. We will stand firm alongside our Chinese colleagues, customers, partners and all Chinese people to defeat this virus.

新型冠状病毒肺炎疫情主要应对模式比较与思考

朱海鸢　赛诺菲[*]（中国）副总裁

于静怡　辉瑞^{**}（中国）高级经理

2020 年 3 月 31 日，根据世界卫生组织（WHO）的数据，新冠肺炎确诊病例数达 85 万人，涉及全球 206 个国家和地区^①。这个疫情逐步发展的过程给了我们一个观察各种防控措施在不同社会、经济、文化和政治体系下比较其利弊的很好的机会，更是为今后公共卫生灾难的应对规划和布局提供了现实的依据。

一　几种主要疫情防控措施比较

2020 年，面对这场新冠病毒肺炎引起的全球范围危机，各国应对疫情所采取的公共卫生防控措施根据各国疫情的具体情况和防疫侧重点而各有不同，具有代表性的几个模式所取得的效果也各不相同。其中，中国和新加坡对疫情的防控都取得了不错的成效，得到了世界卫生组织总干事的高度认可[1]。美国作为一个具有全球最领先医疗技术的国家，其应对措施也一直颇受关注。

---

* 赛诺菲是一家全球领先的医药健康企业，以患者需求为本，研究、开发并推广创新的治疗方案。主要业务涵盖三个领域：制药、人用疫苗和动物保健。于 1982 年成立，总部位于法国巴黎。

** 辉瑞公司是一家以研发为基础的生物制药公司，创建于 1849 年，总部位于美国纽约市。公司产品包括降胆固醇药、口服抗真菌药、抗生素等。

① 数据来自世界卫生组织官网 https://www.who.int/。

表 美国约翰霍普金斯大学 2020 年 4 月 30 日新冠肺炎病例统计

单位: 人

国家	累计诊断	累计治愈	累计死亡
中国	82828	77578	4233
新加坡	15641	1188	14
日本	13736	1899	394
美国	1063123	147114	61603

资料来源:《4 月 30 日全球新冠肺炎（GOVID-19）疫情简报，确诊超 321 万，昨日新增死亡过万例》，梅斯，2020 年 4 月 30 日。

从新冠肺炎疫情的防控总体来看，中国模式的特点是疫情大规模暴发后的全体总动员，新加坡和日本模式侧重早期防控精准细腻，美国模式侧重考量防疫对经济和选举的影响。以下是各国模式的具体分析。

1. 中国防控：以人为本

一个人口 14 亿的国家，中国在疫情暴发后，在中共中央统一决策和部署下，以人民健康为第一要务，立即启动国家应急响应，明确要求防控新冠病毒疫情是当前各级政府的首要任务。一声令下，全国防控工作由前期在武汉等湖北重点地区迅速拓展到全国范围，成为疫情暴发后迅速成功控制的经典案例。虽然防控措施与手段开始有争议，但之后被许多国家不同程度借鉴采用。

《中国－世界卫生组织新型冠状病毒肺炎（COVID-19）联合考察报告》[2] 对中国的抗疫措施有着详细的阐述。根据疫情地特点制定防疫策略。围绕武汉等湖北省重点地区防输出、全国其他地区防输入的防控目的，以控制传染源、阻断传播、预防扩散为主要策略。1 月 20 日将新冠肺炎纳入法定报告乙类传染病和国境卫生检疫传染病，实行体温监测和健康申报制度，采取依法监测与交通场站检疫。[2] 2020 年 1 月 23 日，武汉实行严格限制交通的措施。根据疫情发展，中国果断采取延长春节假期、实施交通管制、控制运能等措施，减少人员流动，取消人群聚集性活动；统筹调配医疗物资，新建医院，启用储备床位和征用相应场所，确保应收尽收；生活物资保供稳价，维护社会平稳运行等综合性防控措施。出台"医保支付、异地结算、财政兜底"的医保政策；以全面的措施保障抗疫策略的有效执行。[2]

令人瞩目的是，面对共同威胁时，全体社会凝聚共识团结行动。每一个机构组织都能够有力地落实防控措施，提升关键措施效果。例如，不断提高病例检测、隔离及早期治疗的速度；积极利用前沿科技促进防控措施的创新，比如将常规医疗和教学工作转移到在线平台上、使用5G平台支持农村地区的防控工作。每个省、每个城市在社区层面都团结一致，帮助和支持脆弱老年人群及社区。尽管本地区也同样发生了疫情，但各省市仍不断向湖北省和武汉市派遣了数以万计的医务人员，并支援了大量宝贵的个人防护用品。在个人层面，面对此次疫情中国人民表现出极大的勇气和信念。每一个人都接受并坚持了最严厉的疫情防控措施——包括暂停公众集会、长达数月的"居家"以及禁止旅行等。

面对这种前所未知的病毒，中国采取了历史上最勇敢、最积极的防控措施。全体动员，高效推进的速度和力度都令人叹为观止。从目前进展来看，中国对疫情的防控是相当出色的，3月10日武汉所有方舱医院全部休舱。[3]湖北省除武汉市以外的地区已连续7日无新增确诊病例。[4]中国新冠肺炎疫情确诊病例数的显著下降既保护了国家安全，也为全球疾病国际传播赢得了宝贵的时间。

自2月上旬开始，中国政府已经开始逐步将"管控"转变为"服务"，出台了多项措施，协助企业尽快全面恢复业务活动。

2. 新加坡防控：侧重早期防控

根据新加坡卫生部网站(https://www.moh.gov.sg/COVID-19)的信息，2020年1月23日，新加坡确诊首例输入性新冠肺炎患者。直至3月21日，新加坡确诊新冠肺炎432例。截至3月底，新加坡没有建议全体公众戴口罩，采用不停工停课等"佛系抗疫"举措。世界卫生组织总干事谭德塞表示，新加坡在探测病例、追踪接触者和阻断传播方面的举措非常有

效。[5]随着全球疫情发展导致输入病例增加，4月14日新加坡政府也开始要求在公共场所必须戴口罩[6]

新加坡早期防疫手段有"快、准、狠"的特点。

（1）快速反应并行动，最大限度堵住外来输入病例。虽然第一例输入性确诊病人是在2020年1月23日，但在1月2日，新加坡卫生部就发布应对新冠肺炎病例的预防措施[7]，提醒所有医护人员注意来自武汉的新冠疑似病例，如有疑似患者将其隔离以防传播。并宣布从1月3日起对从武汉飞来的航班在机场入境处进行体温测量，如有疑似患者交由医院进行评估，同时对从武汉飞来的所有旅客提供详细的健康指导[8]。1月23日出现第一例确诊病例后卫计委于1月24日宣布在水路和陆路入境口均实施体温测试。随着确诊病例数的增加，1月28~30日，政府进一步启动了一系列包括限制入境和入境后隔离的相关政策。[8]

（2）"准"是指以循证作为基础的科学决策，措施针对性强，且根据疫情发展精准调整。

- 首先，高度重视检测，精准筛查患者及疑似患者。其次，精准定义"密切接触者"，全力追踪传播链。该国使用基于蓝牙技术的手机小程序，能够在保障个人隐私的情况下，找出在特定地点与确诊病例有过密切接触的人员。重视检测的另一个例子是韩国。不仅对检测十分重视，而且更重要的是通过检测来指导密切接触者追踪以及通过对早期病例来源的调查，找出病例的来源和感染高发的场所。[9]
- 分类调查，分级诊疗，既防止了在医院容易形成的交叉感染，又能保障医疗资源的有效使用。①
- 措施指导详细易懂，包括个人防护方案和责任，是否需要戴口罩，如何佩戴，如何居家隔离及强制休假等。[10]

---

① 新加坡卫生部网站，https://www.moh.gov.sg/COVID-19。

（3）"狠"指的是新加坡的法制严明。这是世界闻名的，在这次疫情防控期间更是一种有力的保障。[11]

新加坡的精细化防控措施，加上及时详细公开信息，在早期最大限度地减少了国民对疫情的未知和因未知而引起的恐慌，使防控措施得到全社会的理解和认可，并有条不紊、一丝不苟地实施。

3. 日本防控：侧重重症病例

日本的防控举措除了信息充分公开，依据科学和循证做决策外，其特点是收缩战线力保重点。

日本对新冠的检测是聚焦重点人群（持续4天发烧37.5度，老年和有基础疾病的持续发烧37.5度2天）。[12]有数据显示，从2月18日至3月29日，日本全国的检测数为54万例[13]，平均每天只有1000多例。而日本每天实际的检测能力在3月底应该过万[14]。

在疫情防控上采取轻症患者居家控制传染速度、重症入院减少死亡的原则[15]。对社会活动的管理采用限制或取消大型人群聚集性活动。即便在出现社区传染后不得已宣布紧急状态时，也没采取封城、闭户、全行业停摆的措施。

截至3月31日，日本死亡病例共56人①。有美国媒体这样评论，日本没有极端地限制人员移动，也没有进行对经济有害地大规模封锁，甚至都没有尽心广泛地核算检测，但没有出现像意大利和纽约那样的惨状。

4. 美国防控：侧重对经济和社会影响的考量

美国从2020年1月21日确诊第一例新冠病人[16]（对此目前仍有争议，甚至在2019年11月出现更早病例），到1月30日世卫组织将中国疫情定为国际公共卫生紧急事件（Public Health Emergency of International Concern–PHEIC）[17]后，美国随即宣布进入国家卫生紧急状态。[18]其采取的措施，个人防控方面仅强调洗手、避免用手乱摸脸

---

① 数据来自世界卫生组织官网 https://www.who.int/。

部、避免与病人近距离接触（6 英尺），不提倡健康公众戴口罩，也没有取消大规模活动。遗憾的是，自 3 月开始美国的新冠肺炎发病数飙升至全球之首。《纽约时报》在 3 月 28 日以"美国错失的一个月"为题，分析了美国因检测技术落后、法规不配套，白宫领导无方，政府官僚作风失去了疫情防控的黄金 30 天。[19]

美国乔治·华盛顿大学卫生政策与管理系教授杰弗里·莱维斯说："美国政府如果能更早开展广泛的病毒检测，完善检测系统，我们就不会走到今天这样的境地。"除去技术原因和法规原因，"检测标准过高"中应该也有对成本效益的考虑。如果非常低的患病率测出阳性值会给病人、医生乃至社会带来不必要的负担。所以，美国 CDC 之前给医生的指南是建议在高危人群中进行检测，其结果对诊治更有指导意义[20]。另外，在对无症状新冠病毒携带者的传染性比例和强度无法判断的情况下，美国 CDC 可能觉得对每一个无症状携带者进行追踪是对公共资源的浪费。

以上四个国家疫情防控措施的差异反映出各自防控目标的不同，而各自的防控目标是基于各国的疫情进展情况，以及由政治、经济、体制、文化来决定的。中国将以人为本、完全控制疫情作为首要目标，体现了中国对生命的尊重，对全球的责任。新加坡、日本和美国则更多根据各自国情确定各自的目标，并在平衡各种影响的过程中调整措施。面对一个全新的、不确定性的传染病疫情，对政府而言，规则举措的成本是可以确定的，但风险和收益却不确定。同时，除了传染病的传播是跨国界的，在全球化的背景下，每个国家的经济活动也会相互影响。疫情在全球暴发时，没有一个国家可以独善其身，置身其外不受影响。

疫情还没有结束，病毒也还有继续各种变异的可能，因此对于防控措施除疫情以外的整体影响还需等全球疫情接近尾声后再进行评估。不管各种措施的结果如何，都将为今后的预案提供真实的数据和参考的资料。

二 思考和建议

这次全球的公共卫生危机事件给大家留下了很多深刻的体会和感悟，以下几点尤其深刻：①疫情防不胜防，千变万化，提前预案和预案的质量十分重要；②资源不是无限的，科学分析理性决策有助于在有限的资源下以最小的代价来承受负面结果；③危急时刻，再次见到信任的力量和效能。在此，倡导加强国家完善公共卫生灾难应急规划及"备灾"方案。鼓励企业建立业务持续性规划，以降低风险、稳定就业。呼吁全社会、全人类重视信任的建设。

1. 国家公共卫生灾难应急规划

公共卫生事件具有偶然性，通常这些事件的性质和范围是事先不可知的，需要试图去识别和计划。利用专业知识库建立预测模型，包括疾病发生发展的各种场景以及相应的影响，这里需要包含对时间敏感的场景分析。同时，这些数学计算模型的建立需要保持更新。高质量地分析可以帮助以数据和证据为基础的科学决策，制定理性、聚焦兼具灵活性的防控措施。比如，在控制疫情与避免恐慌、影响经济和日常生活之间如何找一个平衡点。采用极端措施会有助于预防感染者和死亡者，但也会因经济下滑、患有其他疾病的患者得不到及时救治等带来其他损失。这需要与疾病相关的临床医学和基础医学专家外的多学科专家共同参与，包括公共卫生和卫生经济专家。同时，如何在保证人民健康的同时又不影响社会和经济的发展是一门科学，更是一门艺术，这也对今后政府部门的决策和治理水平提出了更高的要求。

2. 企业业务持续性规划

很多跨国公司都有"业务持续性规划"（Business Continuity Planning，BCP）。BCP是企业为应对自然灾害或网络攻击等潜在威胁而建立预防和恢复系统的过程。企业持续性规划设计的目的是保护人员和资产，确保人员在灾难来袭时能够快速工作。BCP 通常是预先构想的，同时规划应进行测试，以确保不存在可识别和可纠正的缺陷。

因为企业容易遭受一系列灾难，从轻微到灾难性的程度各不相同。业务的威胁和中断意味着收入的损失和更高的成本，这将导致赢利能力的下降。企业不能仅仅依靠保险，因为它不能覆盖所有的成本和那些转向竞争对手的客户。BCPs 与灾难恢复计划不同，后者侧重于在危机后恢复公司的业务。当然因疾病暴发导致大量人口受到影响，BCP 可能不会那样有效，但也能尽可能地减少负面影响。

在创建业务连续性计划时，业务影响分析、恢复、组织和培训都是企业需要遵循的步骤。

- 业务影响分析：在这里，业务将识别对时间敏感的功能和相关资源。
- 恢复：在这一部分中，业务必须识别和实现恢复关键业务功能的步骤。
- 组织：必须创建一个连续性团队。这个团队将制订一个计划来应对破坏。
- 培训：连续性团队必须经过培训和测试。团队成员还应该完成复习计划和策略的练习。
- 另外，列出一份清单是很有用的，其中包括紧急联系信息、连续性团队可能需要的资源列表、备份数据和其他必要信息的存放或存储位置，以及其他重要人员等关键细节。

除了测试连续性团队，公司还测试 BCP 本身。对它进行多次和定期测试，以确保它可以应用于许多不同的风险场景，这将有助于查明计划中的任何弱点，然后加以查明和纠正。

为了使业务连续性计划取得成功，所有的员工——甚至那些不在连续性团队中的员工——都必须了解这个计划。

业务连续性影响分析是开发 BCP 的一个重要部分。它确定业务功能和流程中断的影响。它还利用这些信息来决定恢复的优先级和策略。

3. 关注信任的建立

信任，也许会带来一些风险，但也会大大提高社会治理的效率，降低治理的成本。

危急时刻，人们往往会突然发现隐藏的信任和善良，比如疫情期间的医患关系不再是对立，更多的是信任与帮助。各国应对疫情过程中，面对未知甚至失控的局面，当人们被告知科学事实，大家更容易信任当局，也愿意追随并响应其号召，积极配合，主动合作。

同时也要看到一些个体与个体之间、个体与集体之间的信任不足，导致防控措施层层加码，社会资源负担加重的情况；国与国之间的不信任，导致关键产业、技术和资源在全球范围合作和分配的效率降低的风险。

信任虽然不能一夜之间就能建立或重建，但需要开始行动。3 月 26 日，国家主席习近平在北京出席二十国集团领导人应对新冠肺炎特别峰会上提出的四点倡导中更是对各国加强信任打破边界去合作的积极呼吁，建立"新冠肺炎疫情防控网上知识中心，向所有国家开放"，正是积极促进信任建立的具体举措。倡导"积极支持国际组织发挥作用"。[21]

俗话说，没有人愿意遭遇危机，但是，危机常常是不邀而至。而且，每次危机出现的时间、方式和形式也是不可预期的。随着全社会都来重视风险，加强各自风险防控的能力建设，我们的国家一定会发展得更加稳健。同时，各界如能建立更多的信任与合作，我们身处的社会一定会更加温暖和美好。

正如习近平主席所说，人类是一个休戚与共的命运共同体，国际社会应该守望相助、同舟共济，共创人类发展更加美好的明天！[22]

参考文献

1. 《谭德赛为何多次称赞中国抗议举措》[2020-02-24]，中国新闻网，https://

m.chinanews.com/wap/detail/zw/gj/2020/02-24/9103169.shtml。

2. 《中国 – 世界卫生组织新型冠状病毒肺炎（COVID-19）联合考察报告》[2020-2-29]，国家卫生健康委员会官方网站，http：//www.nhc.gov.cn/jkj/s3578/202002/87fd92510d094e4b9bad597608f5cc2c.shtml。

3. 《3月10日武汉所有方舱医院全部休舱》[2020-3-10]，中华人民共和国中央人民政府网，http：//www.gov.cn/xinwen/2020-03/10/content_5489713.htm#1。

4. 《"新型冠状病毒感染的肺炎疫情防控工作"新闻发布会第四十四场》[2020-3-13]，湖北省人民政府网站，http：//wjw.hubei.gov.cn/fbjd/dtyw/202003/t20200313_2181090.shtml。

5. Tedros Adhanom Ghebrey Twitter [2020-2-18]，https：//twitter.com/drtedros/status/1229711415319179266?s=12.

6. What should I wear a mask? [2020-4-14]，新加坡卫生部网站，https：//www.moh.gov.sg/article/when-should-i-wear-a-mask Gov.sg.

7. PRECAUTIONARY MEASURES IN RESPONSE TO SEVERE PNEUMONIA CASES IN WUHAN, CHINA [2020-1-2]，新加坡卫生部网站，https：//www.moh.gov.sg/news-highlights/details/precautionary-measures-in-response-to-severe-pneumonia-cases-in-wuhan-china。

8. MOH STEPS UP PRECAUTIONARY MEASURES IN RESPONSE TO INCREASE IN CASES OF NOVEL CORONAVIRUS PNEUMONIA IN WUHAN [2020-1-20]| ADDITIONAL PRECAUTIONARY MEASURES IN RESPONSE TO NOVEL CORONAVIRUS PNEUMONIA IN CHINA, [2020-1-21]| MOH ISSUES PUBLIC HEALTH TRAVEL ADVISORY IN RESPONSE TO CASES OF NOVEL CORONAVIRUS IN CHINA [2020-1-22]| Temperature Screening To Be Implemented At The Land Checkpoints From 24 January 2020 [2020-1-24] | Temperature Screening at Sea Checkpoints [2020-1-24] | Update on Additional Measures by the Ministry of Manpower to Minimise the Risk of Community Spread of the COVID-19 [2020-1-31] | EXTENSION OF PRECAUTIONARY MEASURES TO MINIMISE RISK OF COMMUNITY SPREAD IN SINGAPORE [2020-1-31] | 新加坡卫生部网站，https://www.moh.gov.sg/COVID-19/past-updates。

9. 【专题报道】《抗击新冠疫情：韩国和新加坡的成功经验》[2020-5-1]，联合国新闻，https://news.un.org/zh/story/2020/05/1056402。

10. CONTENT YOU CAN USE，新加坡卫生部网站，https://www.moh.gov.sg/COVID-19/resources。

11. COVID-19 (TEMPORARY MEASURES) (CONTROL ORDER) REGULATIONS, 新加坡卫生部网站, https://www.moh.gov.sg/policies-and-legislation/COVID-19-(temporary-measures)-(control-order)-regulations。

12. 《防控感染症和就诊基准》，日本厚生劳动省网站，https://www.mhlw.go.jp/stf/seisakunitsuite/bunya/newpage_09534.html。

13. 《有关国内·国外疫情》，日本厚生劳动省网站，https://www.mhlw.go.jp/stf/seisakunitsuite/bunya/newpage_09534.html。

14. 《厚生劳动省拟扩容核酸检测能力》[2020-4-9]，NHK World Japan，https://www3.nhk.or.jp/nhkworld/zh/news/231090/。

15. 《新型冠状病毒感染症对策基本方针：(4)医疗提供体制》，日本厚生劳动省网站，https://www.mhlw.go.jp/content/10900000/000608655.pdf。

16. First Wuhan Coronavirus Patient Identified in the United States, Rabin, Roni Caryn. [2020-01-21], The New York Times, https://www.nytimes.com/2020/01/21/health/cdc-coronavirus.html.

17. Situation report - 11 Novel Coronavirus (2019-nCoV), [2020-1-31], 世界卫生组织, https://www.who.int/emergencies/diseases/novel-coronavirus-2019/situation-reports。

18. WHO declares coronavirus outbreak a global health emergency, [2020-01-20], Statnews, https://www.statnews.com/2020/01/30/who-declares-coronavirus-outbreak-a-global-health-emergency/.

19. The Lost Month: How a Failure to Test Blinded the U.S. to COVID-19, [2020-03-28] https://www.nytimes.com/2020/03/28/us/testing-coronavirus-pandemic.html.

20. Transcript for CDC Telebriefing: Update on COVID-19 [2020-02-21] United States CDC https://www.cdc.gov/media/releases/2020/t0221-cdc-telebriefing-COVID-19.html.

21. 《习近平在二十国集团领导人特别峰会上的重要讲话（全文）》[2020-03-26]，新华网，http://www.xinhuanet.com/politics/leaders/2020/03/26/c_1125773764.htm。

22. 《习近平复信世界卫生组织总干事谭德塞》，[2020-3-26]，中国政府网，http://www.gov.cn/xinwen/2020-03/26/content_5495902.htm。

The Comparison of Different COVID-19 Epidemic Control Measures

By Hailuan Zhu, Vice President of Sanofi (China) & Jingyi Yu, Senior Manager of Pfizer (China)

According to WHO, the number of confirmed COVID-19 cases reached 850,000 in 206 countries and regions worldwide (data source: WHO website https://www.who.int/) as of March 31. It is time to analyze the advantages and disadvantages of the infectious disease prevention and epidemic control measures in different economy, cultural, and political systems, and it can serve as supportive evidence for the future public health emergency preparation.

1 Comparison of major pandemic control measures

During the breakout of COVID-19 in 2020, different epidemic control measures have been adopted across the countries and regions in response to the virus. Some worked well, and some are less efficient. Both China and Singapore have achieved positive results, which was recognized by the Director General of the WHO.[1] The United States has attracted considerable attention in its response to COVID-19, as it has the world's most advanced technology.

Table   COVID-19 Cases on April 30[th 2020] by John Hopkins

Country	Total Diagnosed	Total Recovered	Total Death
China	82,828	77,578	4,233
Singapore	15,641	1,188	14
Japan	13,736	1,899	394
United States	1,063,123	147,114	61,603

Source:http://www.medsci.cn/article/show_article.do?id=467619323301.

In general, China strictly controlled mobilization by implementing large scale lock down right after the outbreak; Singapore and Japan focus on precisely tracking and containing epidemic at the early stage; whereas, the United States tried to balance the epidemic control and economic impact.

(1) China's approach: people's lives first

In a country with more than 1.3 billion population, central and provincial government took immediate response to COVID-19 under the unified decision-making and deployment of the Central Committee of the Communist Party of China. All levels government were clearly requested to make containing COVID-19 as their primary task. With order from central government, the epidemic control tasks were quickly expanded from Wuhan and surrounding arears in Hubei to all over China. China approach is a successful epidemic control case, which has quickly contained the spread of COVID-19 right after the outbreak in Wuhan. Given the controversy of the massive lock down, this approach has been adopted by multiple countries during the global outbreak.

The "China -- World Health Organization New Coronavirus Pneumonia (COVID-19) Joint Investigation Report" elaborated described China's anti-epidemic measures: set anti-epidemic strategies according to the spot of the COVID-19 cases, focusing on preventing export cases from key areas in Hubei Province, such as Wuhan, and tracking import cases in other areas of the country.[2] The purposed of the strategy is to control the source of infectious disease, block transmission, and prevent proliferation. On January 20, COVID-19 was classified as Class B infectious diseases in China, which requires mandatory report, and as national border quarantine infectious disease. [2]According to the regulation, traffic quarantine stations were set up to monitor passengers' temperature and health declaration. On January 23, strict traffic restriction was imposed in Wuhan. To reduce the mobility of population, government decisively extended Chinese New Year holiday and cancel crowd gathering activities. Central government coordinated the supply and deployment of medical supplies, built new field hospitals, used reserve hospital beds, and expropriated lands and buildings to ensure all patients are hospitalized. In addition, the stability of grocery supplies and operation in the community are maintained well. China government considered thoroughly when making policies to contain virus. An example is the government promulgate the medical insurance policy -- "medical insurance payment, off-site settlement and financial aids" -- to expand coverage of COVID-19.[2]

What remarkable in China is that when the country is under crisis, the entire society quickly reach consensus and take unified actions. Each organization can effectively implement and even enhance epidemic control measures, such as continuously improving the speed of diagnosis, quarantine, and early treatment. The local government proactively adopted cutting-edge technology to promote innovation in COVID-19 containment, such as launching the online medical platform to provide consultation and using the 5G platform to support epidemic control in rural areas. Provincial and city government worked together to support vulnerable group in the communities during the crisis. Although the epidemic occurred in the places outside Hubei, other provinces and cities continuously dispatched tens of thousands of medical personnel to Hubei and Wuhan to treat COVID-19 patients. Tons of medical supplies were sent to Hubei when there were severe shortage of masks and preventive clothing. The Chinese people have demonstrated great courage and conviction in the face of the epidemic by complying with strictest containment measures -- whether it was public gathering suspension, "stay at home" for more than a month, or a travel ban.

In the face of this previously unknown virus, China has taken the bravest and most proactive epidemic control measures in history. It surprised the world with the speed and scale of efficient pandemic containment. By far China's epidemic control is quite outstanding. On March 10, all square cabin hospitals in Wuhan were closed.[3] That day in Hubei, the areas outside Wuhan reported zero new cases for 7 days.[4] This sharp decline of new cases contributed to health of the entire nation and earned time for the foreign government to prepare for the outbreak in their countries. During this period, COVID-19 has costed many lives and huge amount of resource in China, including the economy impact from the nation's shutdown for almost one month and the supply shortages of medical supplies and protective materials.

Since mid-February, China government has begun to gradually transform "control" into "service". It has introduced a number of measures to assist companies to resume business activities as soon as possible.

(2) Singapore approach: quick intervention in the early stage

On January 23, 2020, Singapore confirmed the first case of imported COVID-19 case. Until March 21, Singapore had 432 cases diagnosed, with the first two deaths. Singapore has successfully controlled the epidemic without implementing large scale lock down. Until the end of March, the government didn't recommend wearing masks in public, or closing the schools and offices. WHO Director General Tanker said Singapore is a good example of all government approach, which effectively identifies sick individuals, strictly tracks close contacts, and prevents disease transmission.[5] With the increasing imported COVID-19 cases, Singapore government required everyone to wear mask in public from April 15th.[6]

Singapore's epidemic control approach is the characteristics of "fast, precise, and strict":

1) Fast response and quick actions. Singapore implemented strict travel control

to prevent imported cases. Although the first imported patient was diagnosed on January 23, 2020, on January 2, the Singapore Ministry of Health issued "Precautionary measures in response to severe pneumonia cases in Wuhan, China" to alert all medical practices to pay attention to Suspected cases of new crowns in Wuhan.[7] Once patient with suspected COVID-19 is identified, the patient is quarantined immediately. From January 3, all passengers from Wuhan must take temperature at airport and are provided with detailed health guidance when entering Singapore, and the passengers with fever are sent to hospital for further evaluation. The first COVID-19 case was confirmed on January 23, the next day the Ministry of Health announced that it will take temperature of passengers at both waterway and land entry points.[8] With the increasing the number of cases, from January 28 to January 30, the government further implemented a series of policies including travel restrictions and quarantine when entering Singapore from overseas.[8]

2) "Precise" refers to evidence-based scientific decision-making measures, precisely adjusted the strategy during epidemic in accordance with the development of the situation

- First, emphasize on diagnosis and screening. Precisely screen patients and patients suspected with COVID-19. The government uses a Bluetooth app to locate patients and people who contact with the patients without infringing privacy. South Korea also used similar approach to track patients, paying attention to diagnose and track patients as early as possible to identify the spot where is highly contagious.[9]
- Hierarchical diagnosis and treatment guidance prevented infection transmission cross hospital and ensured the efficient medical resources utilization. (Source: Singapore MOH https://www.moh.gov.sg/COVID-19)

- Detailed and easy-to-understand guidance includes personal protection schemes and responsibilities including whether it's necessary to wear a mask and the correct way to wear it, how to make judgement whether to stay at home or take compulsory leave, etc.[10]

3) "Strict" refers to Singapore's world-famous strict legal system, which benefits the government in response to COVID-19.[11]

Singapore's streamlined epidemic control approach is coupled with timely and detailed public information, which has improved the transparency and, as a result, reduced the public panic. The epidemic control measures are widely accepted and strictly implemented, successfully controlled the epidemic at the first stage and avoiding community transmission. At the same time, it left limited the impact to daily life and economy.

(3) Japan's approach: focusing on critical cases treatment.

In Japan pandemic information is fully disclosed, decisions are made based on scientific evidence, and precisely screen and track patients to prioritize resource allocation.

The diagnosis was only recommended to high risk populations (fever over 37.5 centigrade for 4 days, 37.5 centigrade for 2 days in the elderly and with underlying diseases).[12] Statistics show that from February 18 to March 29, there were 540,000 tested for COVID-19 nationwide, with an average of just over 1,000 tests per day.[13] The actual daily testing capacity increased to over 10,000 cases in March in the early days of the outbreak.[14]

In Japan, only critical cases are hospitalized, and the mild case are quarantined at home.[15] The government limited or canceled public gatherings. Business wasn't shut down even when community infection happened, and emergency status was announced.

There were 56 deaths in Japan as of March 31 (Data Source: WHO Website https://www.who.int/) The New York Times mentioned that Japan hasn't extremely restricted the mobilization of people, nor has it conducted a massive lock down which is harmful to the economy, and it has not even done extensive testing, but Japan hasn't been as tragic as it is in Italy and New York.

(4) The United States approach: attempting to balance epidemic control and economy impact

In the United States, the first COVID-19 patient was diagnosed on January 21 (There aremany arguements regarding this point, even the first COVID-19 patiet in the US starts in Nov. 2019).[16] After WHO declared COVID-19 as an International Public Health Emergency (PHEIC) on January 20,[17] US States declared a national health emergency.[18] At the beginning, Americans were suggested to wash hands more often and carefully, avoid touching the face with hands, and keep social distance of 6 feet. The government didn't suggest healthy individuals to wear masks, nor did it ban the large-scale gatherings. The New York Times, entitled "A Missed Month in the United States" on March 28, analyzed the United States' lack of leadership in the White House due to low efficiency diagnostic technology and inadequate regulations.[19] The government's bureaucracy has caused the United States to lose 30 days for epidemic control.

Jeffrey Levi, a professor at the Department of Health Policy and Management at George Washington University in the United States, said, "If the US government could carry out extensive virus detection earlier and improve the detection system, we wouldn't have gone to such a situation today." Besides diagnostic technology and regulations, federal government also has cost-effective considerations. Testing for low prevalence rate disease will bring unnecessary burdens to patients, doctors and even communities. Therefore, the previous guidelines provided to doctors by the CDC suggested them to provide COVID-19 diagnostic testing to high-risk patients suspected with COVID-19 only.[20] In addition, there wasn't enough evidence to prove the portion asymptomatic carriers among the population and their ability to carry and spread disease. The US CDC considered tracking each COVID-19 asymptomatic carriers as a waste of public resource.

The differences in the epidemic control measures in the above countries reflect the different status in virus containment, which are determined based on the epidemics, politics, economy, infrastructures, and culture of each country. As one of the centers of COVID-19 breakout, China has taken the fully epidemic control as its primary goal, reflecting the country's willingness to take global responsibility and respect lives. When facing a new pandemic situation of infectious diseases, it is not clear for the government to determine the outcome and risk of epidemic control measures, but the costs are clear. In the context of globalization, not only the virus can spread across countries, but also one country's economy can affect that of one another's.

COVID-19 isn't over yet, and the virus is likely to continue to mutate. Regardless of the results of various epidemic control measures, it will provide data and reference for future plans.

2 Thoughts and suggestions

This global public public health incidence has brought profound experience and insights for everyone. 1. The epidemic is hard to defend from and is ever-changing, and plan in advance and the quality of the prevention is the key. 2. Resources are not unlimited; we must carefully analyze the evidence to make rational decisions, minimizing the impact with limited resources. 3. During the crisis, the power of trust has shown significant impact. It is important that each country has a public health emergency plan as part of the disaster preparedness plan. Enterprise need to establish business continuity plan to keep business continue operations and avoid unemployment. Humanity need to trust each other when facing the disasters.

I. Establish a national emergency plan for public health disasters. Public health disaster occurs accidentally with unknown nature and scope, which requires attempts to identify the epidemic and plan for the containment. Scientists can build and maintain the predictive models with various scenarios of disease occurrence and development and the corresponding impacts, especially time-sensitive scenario analysis. Based on data and evidence, high-quality analysis can help policy makers to make rational, focused, and flexible prevention and control measures. For example, an approach that can balance between controlling the epidemic and avoiding panics. The extreme measures will help prevent infected and deceased people, but it will also induce other losses due to the economy downturn and the lack of timely treatment for patients with other diseases. This requires the participation of multidisciplinary professional experts in addition to clinical and medical experts, such as public health and health economics experts. Finally, how to ensure people 's health without affecting economy is a science as well as an art, which has put forward higher requirements for the future decision-making and governance level of government.

II. Enterprise business continuity planning. For enterprises, many multinational companies have "Business Continuity Planning" (Business Continuity Planning, BCP). BCP is the process of the prevention and recovery system established by enterprises in response to potential threats such as natural disasters or cyber-attacks. The purpose of enterprise continuous planning and design is to protect people and assets and ensure that they can work quickly when disaster strikes. BCP is usually pre-conceived, and the planning should be tested to ensure that there are no identifiable and correctable defects.

Enterprises are vulnerable disasters; the degree of impact varies from mild to catastrophic. The disruptions of business mean loss of revenue and higher costs, which will lead to a decline in profitability. BCPs are considered as important parts of companies' business. Enterprise cannot only rely on insurance alone, since it covers part of the costs and customers will turn to competitors. BCPs are different from disaster recovery plans, which focus on restoring company business after a crisis. Of course, when a large number of people are affected by the outbreak of the disease, BCP may not be as effective, but it can reduce the impact as much as possible.

When creating a business continuity plan, enterprises need to follow the steps including business impact analysis, recovery, organization, and training.

- Business impact analysis: the business identifies time-sensitive functions and related resources.
- Recovery: the business identifies and implements steps to recover critical business functions.
- Organization: a continuity working team should be created continuously working on it. This team will develop a plan to deal with the damage.
- Training: the continuity team must be trained and tested. Team members should also complete the practice of reviewing plans and strategies.
- In addition, it is useful to make a list, including emergency contact information, a list of resources that the continuity team may need, storage or storage locations for backup data and other necessary information, and other key details such as important personnel.

In addition to testing the continuity team, the enterprise should test the BCP itself. It should be tested multiple times and regularly to ensure it can be applied to different risk scenarios by identifying the flaws in the plans and correcting them.

In order for the business continuity plan to succeed, all employees—even those who are not on the continuity team—must understand the plan.

Business continuity impact analysis is an important part of developing

BCPs. It determines the impact of business function and process interruption. It also uses this information to determine the priority and strategy of recovery.

III. It is necessary to the establish of trust among the countries. Trust may expose a country to risks, but it will also greatly improve the efficiency of governance and reduce the cost of governance.

At this moment of crisis, people often suddenly find trust and kindness. The doctor-patient relationship during the epidemic is no longer a confrontation, but more trust and support. Facing an unknown situation, people are more likely to trust the authorities and proactively follow guidance when informed with scientific facts.

Lack of trust between individuals or between individuals and collectives can lead to overwhelming repetitive investments and increasing burden. The mistrust between countries will cause the nationalization of key industries and technologies reducing productivity and the efficiency of resource allocation.

Trust isn't built or rebuilt overnight. However, the actions must be taken right away. During G20 on March 26, President Xi Jinping proposed to establish a COVID-19 knowledge center and open to all countries as part of the partnership among all countries in epidemic control. He also suggested all countries should support the role of international organizations. This is an attempt to establish trust and encourage partnership with other countries. [21]

Disaster usually arrives when we are not expecting one. We wouldn't know when and how it comes, therefore, improving the capability to prevent disasters and partnership across countries have become fundamental to the stability of the global politics and economy.

Just as President Xi said, humanity is in a community of shared destiny, and we should watch for each other and work together to create a better tomorrow for everyone. [22]

References

1. Why Tedros Adhanom Praised China COVID-19 Containment Several Times [2020-02-24], China News https://m.chinanews.com/wap/detail/zw/gj/2020/02-24/9103169.shtml.

2. China -- World Health Organization New Coronavirus Pneumonia (COVID-19) Joint Investigation Report [2020-2-29], China MOH http://www.nhc.gov.cn/jkj/s3578/202002/87fd92510d094e4b9bad597608f5cc2c.shtml.

3. All Wuhan Mobile Cabin Hospitals Are Clear On March 10th [2020-3-10], China Government Net http://www.gov.cn/xinwen/2020-03/10/content_5489713.htm#1.

4. 44th COVID-19 Epidemic Control Press Release [2020-3-13], Hubei Government Site, http://wjw.hubei.gov.cn/fbjd/dtyw/202003/t20200313_2181090.shtml.

5. Tedros Adhanom Ghebrey Twitter [2020-2-18], https://twitter.com/drtedros/status/122971 11415319179266?s=12.

6. What should I wear a mask? [2020-4-14], Singapore MOH, https://www.moh.gov.sg/article/when-should-i-wear-a-mask Gov.sg.

7. PRECAUTIONARY MEASURES IN RESPONSE TO SEVERE PNEUMONIA CASES IN WUHAN, CHINA [2020-1-2] Singapore MOH https://www.moh.gov.sg/news-highlights/details/precautionary-measures-in-response-to-severe-pneumonia-cases-in-wuhan-china.

8. MOH STEPS UP PRECAUTIONARY MEASURES IN RESPONSE TO INCREASE IN CASES OF NOVEL CORONAVIRUS PNEUMONIA IN WUHAN [2020-1-20]| ADDITIONAL PRECAUTIONARY MEASURES IN RESPONSE TO NOVEL CORONAVIRUS PNEUMONIA IN CHINA [2020-1-21]| MOH ISSUES PUBLIC HEALTH TRAVEL ADVISORY IN RESPONSE TO CASES OF NOVEL CORONAVIRUS IN CHINA [2020-1-22]| Temperature Screening To Be Implemented At The Land Checkpoints From 24 January 2020 [2020-1-24] | Temperature Screening at Sea Checkpoints [2020-1-24] | Update on Additional Measures by the Ministry of Manpower to Minimise the Risk of Community Spread of the COVID-19 [2020-1-31] | EXTENSION OF PRECAUTIONARY MEASURES TO MINIMISE RISK OF COMMUNITY SPREAD IN SINGAPORE [2020-1-31] Singapore MOH https://www.moh.gov.sg/COVID-19/past-updates.

9. [special report] fighting a new epidemic: success stories from South Korea and Singapore. [2020-5-1], United Unions News, https://news.un.org/zh/

story/2020/05/1056402.

10. CONTENT YOU CAN USE, Singapore MOH, https://www.moh.gov.sg/COVID-19/resources.

11. COVID-19 (TEMPORARY MEASURES) (CONTROL ORDER) REGULATIONS, Singapore MOH, https://www.moh.gov.sg/policies-and-legislation/COVID-19-(temporary-measures)-(control-order)-regulations.

12. Benchmark of Disease Prevention and Control, Japan Ministry of Health, Labor and Welfare, https://www.mhlw.go.jp/stf/seisakunitsuite/bunya/newpage_09534.html.

13. About National and International Pandemics, Japan Ministry of Health, Labor and Welfare, https://www.mhlw.go.jp/stf/seisakunitsuite/bunya/newpage_09534.html.

14. Ministry of Health, Labour and Welfare plans to expand the nucleic acid detection capacity, [2020-4-9], NHK World Japan, https://www3.nhk.or.jp/nhkworld/zh/news/231090/.

15. COVID-19 Basic Policy: (4) Health Provider, Japan Ministry of Health, Labor and Welfare, https://www.mhlw.go.jp/content/10900000/000608655.pdf.

16. First Wuhan Coronavirus Patient Identified in the United States, Rabin, Roni Caryn. [2020-01-21], The New York Times, https://www.nytimes.com/2020/01/21/health/cdc-coronavirus.html.

17. Situation report - 11 Novel Coronavirus (2019-nCoV), [2020-1-31], WHO, https://www.who.int/emergencies/diseases/novel-coronavirus-2019/situation-reports.

18. WHO declares coronavirus outbreak a global health emergency, [2020-01-20], Statnews, https://www.statnews.com/2020/01/30/who-declares-coronavirus-outbreak-a-global-health-emergency/.

19. The Lost Month: How a Failure to Test Blinded the U.S. to COVID-19, [2020-03-28], https://www.nytimes.com/2020/03/28/us/testing-coronavirus-pandemic.html.

20. Transcript for CDC Telebriefing: Update on COVID-19, [2020-02-21], United States CDC, https://www.cdc.gov/media/releases/2020/t0221-cdc-telebriefing-COVID-19.html.

21. Xi Jinping Gives Important Speech On G20, [2020-03-26], Xinhua Net, http://www.xinhuanet.com/politics/leaders/2020-03/26/c_1125773764.htm.

22. A Letter Replied by Xi Jinping To WHO Director-General Tedros Adhanom, [2020-03-26], China Government Net, http://www.gov.cn/xinwen/2020-03/26/content_5495902.htm.

疫情常态化下中国数字化发展的机遇和挑战

谢燕琦　思爱普*（中国）有限公司大中华区副总裁

彭俊松博士　思爱普（中国）有限公司大中华区副总裁、首席数字官

2020 年伊始，新型冠状病毒肺炎疫情在中国暴发以来，神州大地为抗击疫情所做的不懈努力获得举世关注。世界卫生组织（WHO）等国际机构和多国政要高度评价中国政府为抗击疫情所展示的坚定性决心和实施的强有力措施，对中国人民早日战胜疫情充满信心。在华外资企业踊跃为疫情重点地区捐款捐物，组织调动资源保障防疫用品的生产。针对此次突发的社会重大事件，思爱普（SAP）深度践行"在中国，为中国"的美好愿景，积极履行企业社会责任。我们坚信，"沉舟侧畔千帆过，病树前头万木春"，疫情困难终将过去，历史车轮一定会继续向前。2020 年 2 月 14 日，习近平主席再次针对疫情防控、加强社会治理做出"建立 15 种体系、9 种机制和 4 项制度"的重要部署，为此后系统性应对指明了方向。思爱普将就疫情相关情况进行系统梳理，分享一点思考与建议。

一　助力抗疫注重实效，防控疫情技术先行

思爱普成立于 1972 年，总部设在德国的沃尔多夫市，是全球最大的

---

　*　思爱普公司成立于 1972 年，是德国市值最高的企业、欧洲最大的科技公司，目前为全球最大的企业应用软件提供商。总部位于德国沃尔多夫。

　特别感谢纪秉盟（Mark Gibbs）和李强对本文的贡献。

企业管理、商务解决方案和云供应商之一。作为欧洲品牌价值最高的企业，全球 77% 的贸易交易都跟思爱普产品和服务有关。思爱普不仅是德国工业 4.0 战略规划的发起者和核心领导企业，更是中德合作的主要推动者。思爱普 1992 年进入中国，总部位于上海市静安区，公司在华业务的迅速发展受益于中国的改革开放，此次参与抗疫义不容辞、全力以赴。

1. 积极参加现金捐助，送抵一线

就在 2020 年 1 月 24 日，中国传统佳节的除夕守岁时，针对在湖北武汉发生的新冠肺炎疫情，思爱普全球管理层紧急召集大中华区的高管研讨对策，发出动员令并启动应急措施。通过湖北慈善总会，第一批捐赠的 300 万元善款到位，分别送达华中科技大学同济医学院附属同济医院、华中科技大学同济医学院附属协和医院、武汉市中心医院、武汉市第一医院、武汉市金银潭医院等五家主力抗疫医院。同时，思爱普落实第二期 100 万欧元捐款，并捐赠为此次抗疫量身定制的价值 100 万欧元的管理软件（含人才培训和后期维护服务）。

2. 增强城市综合免疫，识时达变

随后，思爱普迅速协调资源，发挥自身的高科技优势，利用参与疫病监测的经验，全力支持抗击疫情以及城市生产和生活功能的有效恢复等工作。公司再次紧急调动在数字化、云计算、智能应用方面的能动基因，基于思爱普软件管理系统提供城市应急防控解决方案和卫健人才培养长效机制计划，贡献专业智慧，主要效用如下。

（1）建立健全全能型医疗人才档案库和应急防控人才培养体系，借助大数据与智能匹配构建高效应急队伍。

（2）实施动态跟踪与考核，保障应急防控知识与技能随时在线，智能分析应急防控人才储备、人员配备和相关资源调配。

（3）完善公共卫生风险隐患信息预警与监控机制，智能辅助调查隐患，实时报告疫情防控动态走势。

同时，针对疫情初步得以控制后生产恢复面临的困难，如人员流动阻隔、复工条件受限、上下游产业链断裂等负面因素，思爱普出台"区域劳动力优化配置解决方案"，主要以园区为管理边界搭建劳动力资源共享及配置平台，通过"政府端""企业端""用户端"信息联动解决复工过程中的诸多现实困难。这些努力实践均已落地到中长期的实施规划中，并为今后的疫情防控乃至其他社会突发紧急事件的"数字治理"积累了有益经验。

3.增强企业守法意识，强化合规

遵照全国人大法工委的相关要求，贯彻中央网信办、工信部的统一部署，思爱普在员工春节返回京沪的相关隔离观察要求、办公场所的疫情防控、业务恢复和监督管理等方面，认真组织相关部门和人员系统学习了《传染病防治法》《突发事件应对法》《网络安全法》《突发公共卫生事件应急条例》《中央网络安全和信息化委员会办公室关于做好个人信息保护利用大数据支撑联防联控工作的通知》等规定，切实提高企业自身的守法和合规意识。同时结合公司自身的业务优势，根据国务院联防联控机制的要求，依法依规开始尝试在公司内部采集分析用于疫情防控的相关数据，并研发相关程序和软件，服务、支撑国务院卫生防疫主管部门和地方政府的需求。此外，在分析使用数据的过程中，思爱普依据国家个人信息保护的有关法律法规，严格落实数据安全和个人信息保护的相关措施。

二 痛定思痛寻痛源，防患未然研举措

当前，中国经济增长处于增速放缓、转型升级、结构改革的关键时期，此次疫情将导致消费承压、投资不振、财政收入减少等问题雪上加霜。受人口红利和加入世界贸易组织双重利好的影响，2003 年年初出现的"非典"疫情并没有阻滞当时中国经济的总体上升趋势。但此次新型冠状病毒肺炎疫情较为严重，确诊感染人数，患病离世人数，波及的地理范

围，因隔离观察等造成延迟工人复工、学生开学、职员上班等带来的连锁型经济社会负面影响已经远超"非典"，几乎涵盖了我国所有经济活跃且服务业发达省市，特别是对民众心理预期冲击很大。从持续时间、影响范围、受损程度等多维度多场景分析，COVID-19疫情的叠加影响将数倍于非典（SARS）疫情。

自2003年非典疫情之后，至本次新冠肺炎疫情之前，国际范围内还发生了五次世界卫生组织宣布的国际关注的突发公共卫生事件（PHEIC），依次为：2009年甲型H1N1流感、2014年脊髓灰质炎疫情、2014年西非埃博拉疫情、2015~2016年寨卡疫情、2018年刚果（金）埃博拉疫情（2019年7月宣布）；此外再加上2015年韩国暴发的中东呼吸综合征（MERS），这些均表明突发性高传染的病毒疫情在地球村中从未停止，这一直是现代国际社会面临的共同性难题，发生地国家很难做到靠一己之力而力挽狂澜，客观上需要各国通力合作，携手应对此类尖锐性、严重性、复杂性挑战，"人类命运共同体"价值观的务实践行愈发显得弥足珍贵。目前的重中之重是牢牢稳定疫情，集数国乃至全球之力加大疫苗和专项性药物的研制力度，其次是密切与相关国家和国际机构的经济协作，加强相互理解和支持，坚决杜绝"甩包袱"和以"疫"为壑的狭隘做法。正如世界卫生组织总干事谭德塞所言，中国实施武汉封城，一天后湖北、北京、上海、安徽、天津、重庆等多个省份连续启动重大突发公共卫生事件一级响应，付出如此大的代价严厉管控疫情，为其他国家和地区防止疫情蔓延提供了宝贵的机会窗口期和缓冲时间。

综上，从国家层面考量，我们确实应前瞻此次疫情得以防控后的三方面事情。

（1）强化底线思维和红线意识，提高国家综合防范疫情并发或多发情况的能力。针对最严峻的情况准备最艰苦的应对预案，比如人类疫情和动植物疫情同时暴发的应对，再如突发疫情、自然灾害、经济危机甚至地缘政治冲突等不可预判因素两个或多个同时暴发的有效有序应对；

坚持科学防控，坚决避免在抗疫过程中出现的过分乐观和持续悲观的两个极端想法。

（2）一方面持续加大"由外输入"的疫情防控力度，另一方面精心筹划防控"内在自生"的疫情风险，继续以大国担当的宝贵勇气和提高现代国家综合治理水平的手段，提高各级政府的治理水平，提高国民科学素养，增强国民自觉防范疫情意识，提前谋划布局，扎实筹备，以更高效周密的系统处置规划、更专业精准的科学防范措施、更扎实稳健的应急预案保障应对未来可能出现传染性更强的病毒疫情。

（3）及时谋划好未来十年乃至更长时间的"国家重大安全风险评估、预防和应对机制"建设，做好相关研究预判和应对演练，因为这个阶段正是实现中国提出"两个一百年"宏伟奋斗目标的关键历史时期，切实提高国家的总体承载能力以及化解能力，特别是增加应对各类突发重大公共事件的救济供给和战略储备，坚决避免此类意外紧急事件给国家经济社会发展带来的严重损害和进程干扰。

三　立足完善数字治理，保障发展建言献策

思爱普结合自身从事企业应用软件的开发、销售和服务业务的经验，同时深度考虑在抗疫期间各级政府及时出台的大量帮助和扶持相关企业的有益政策，针对这次疫情应对中得到的经验和教训，主要从"数字化社会治理"的角度出发，给政府与企业提出一些参考建议。

1.这次疫情的暴发暴露出数字化基础建设上的较多薄弱环节

面对疫情，缺少口罩一类的关键物资的产能储备数据；面对经济，多少工厂需要复工，多少工厂需要产能，供应链上下游如何实现供需平衡？这些均无数据的支撑。缺少这些关键性重要数据，为国家的集中调配和快速响应带来了很大的困扰。现在各地政府包括金融机构，陆续出台了很多中小企业扶持政策。在数字化基础欠缺的情况下，缺少数据支持，很难做

到精准施行。希望政府部门能够从本次的疫情中，进一步认识到数字化基础建设的重要性和必要性，把遗漏的短板补足完善。

2. 疫情暴发前的预警和暴发后的处置过程直接暴露出国家应急管理系统上的配备不足

国际上有一项称作"危机与应急管理平台"的专门系统，缩写是C/EMP（Crisis/Emergency Management Platform），其主要功能是帮助政府管理大型公共安全危机。目前，国外的企业也越来越多地开始应用这一系统，包括电力、交通、医疗和金融等行业。C/EMP可以在企业组织面临危机的时候对任务、资源、通信、协同和数据进行管理。此外，它还可用于分析危机期间不断变化的情况，随时了解状态，确保采取的程序符合政府应急管理标准。随着危机的数量、频率、范围、影响和类型的不断增加，由国家牵头，加强不同地方、区域、组织、企业的C/EMP系统协同，进行相互沟通，对于提高应急响应和处理水平，无疑是十分必要的。思爱普认为应该深刻吸取这次的教训，一方面立即开展C/EMP的建设工作，另一方面也要设计相关的标准，确保不同企业和组织的C/EMP实现对接。

3. 从更高层面的技术角度分析，C/EMP也是危机管理技术生态系统的七大子项中的一个

目前阶段，广大企业需求最相关的是七大子项中的业务连续性管理。大量的企业因为员工、交通、场地、供应等限制条件，不能及时恢复到正常的经营和生产。很多企业虽然在数字化上进行了一些投入，但对于"业务连续性管理"这个概念却一直很陌生。"业务连续性管理"简称BCM（Business Continuity Management），在国外已经发展了20多年。早期的BCM仅仅是IT的一个灾难备份，对关键的IT设备和数据中心提供保护。但是，随着业务的发展变化以及面临新的挑战，如一些企业提供的24×7服务承诺、业务流程运营全球化、自然灾害、病毒传播等，BCM也扩展到了业务领域。针对这次疫情的防控，很多企业都希望通过远程办公来减少传播风险，同时也希望接下来业务能够迅速复原，供应商中断的

供应也能够得到恢复，这些都是 BCM 的管理目标。

4. 此次疫情将会推动"无接触"与"低接触"的工作模式和商业模式的发展

这对于众多企业而言会是一个很好的发展机遇。原来的商务人员满天飞、不见客户不成单的模式被迫做出变革，这次疫情驱动大家深度思考是否通过数字化的手段使销售业务更加透明、直接和高效，让业务人员不再沉迷于面见客户，而是更加专注于争取价值和理念的共鸣。对于消费者来说，这次疫情也相当于进行了一次消费习惯的普及，相信未来电商渠道将更接地气，注重实效，蓬勃发展。

5. 此次疫情既是"危"也是"机"，更是检测企业数字化创新能力的"试金石"

对于一些疫情急需和催生出来的新产品，从需求响应到研发、试制、测试、投产、产能爬坡等诸多环节都需要有机协同。对于每一次新的危机，如果企业能够迅速有效地通过数字化创新能力快速做出响应，将对自身和社会带来很大帮助。这一次建筑行业表现出来的协同设计、现场管理能力都有目共睹。极端事件下的产品交付一定需要配备数字化手段进行保障，否则武汉火神山医院的前期筹划阶段将无法在 78 分钟内整理完 17 年前北京小汤山医院的建筑设计方案和施工图纸，24 小时完成协同设计，60 小时敲定施工计划，6 天内完成诸多细节的协同现场施工，最后按时投入使用。

6. 以大数据、人工智能、云服务平台为代表的高新技术是此次抗疫过程中政府鼓励发展应用的重点方向，也是国家数字经济发展的重要组成部分

外商投资企业在此领域具有长期技术开发和业务经营的丰富经验，也非常渴望能够积极参与、促进中国信息通信产业的跨越式发展。我们非常理解"自主可控"政策对于保障国家经济安全的重要性和必要性，但中国改革开放 40 年所取得的伟大成就证明，跨国公司的技术投入、管理水平

和经验分享是提升中国相关产业总体发展水平的重要一环，外商投资企业希望能够获得更多的直接参与机会并做出自己的贡献。

我们坚信，通过深入贯彻习近平主席关于疫情防控工作的重要讲话和指示批示精神，积极落实党中央、国务院决策部署，中国必将打赢疫情防控的人民战争，同时必能统筹做好疫情防控和经济社会发展，也必会完成"稳就业、稳金融、稳外贸、稳外资、稳投资、稳预期"的"六稳"工作，把疫情对国家生产生活的负面影响降到最低。思爱普作为广大外资企业的一员，将与中国市场"同呼吸共命运"，秉持自己"思无界、行有方"的理念，在提供数字化抗疫应急能力和高科技手段领域，以至助力推动中国数字经济的长远发展方面，不断做出自己的贡献。

Opportunities & Challenges of China's Digital Development under the Regular Epidemic Prevention and Control Measures

By Yanqi Xie, Vice President &

Dr. Junsong Peng, Chief Digital Officer & Vice President of SAP Greater China

Since outbreak of COVID-19 in China, the efforts to fight the epidemic has gained worldwide attentions. Accordingly, many International organizations, including the World Health Organization (WHO), and political figures from many countries spoke highly of the firm determination and strong measures that Chinese government has taken to fight the epidemic. They also expressed their confidence in assuring early victory of the Chinese people. In China, Foreign-Invested Enterprises (FIEs) have been enthusiastically contributing to key epidemic areas and organizing the mobilization of resources to ensure steady production of anti-epidemic supplies.

In response to this unexpected social event, SAP has deeply practiced the good vision of "In China, For China" and actively fulfilled its corporate social responsibility. As a famous poem in Tang Dynasty described, "a thousand sails pass by the wrecked ship, ten thousand saplings shoot up beyond the withered tree." We should envisage that the epidemic-created difficulties will eventually pass away and the wheel of history will roll forward. On 14th February 2020, President Xi Jinping once again put forward "the 15 systems, 9 mechanisms and 4 policies" for the prevention and control of epidemic situation and strengthening social governance, which points out the overall direction for systemically coping with the similar emergent incidents. SAP also comprehensively combed after thinking deeply about this and then shared it with you.

1 Facilitating timely anti-epidemic actions and ensuring advanced technology go ahead

SAP is one of the world's largest providers of enterprise application software, business solution and cloud service, which was founded in 1972 and headquartered in Germany. As the most valuable brand in Europe, 77% of the worldwide transaction revenues touch SAP systems. SAP is not only the initiator and core-leader of German Industry 4.0, but also the main promoter of Sino-German cooperation. SAP entered China in 1992 and is headquartered in Jing'an District, Shanghai. The rapid development of SAP's business in China thanks to China's reform and opening up. Therefore, it is incumbent upon SAP to contribute in the fight against this epidemic.

(1) Positively participating in the fund donations to support frontline

On January 24th, Chinese New Year's Eve, SAP global management convened Greater China executives to discuss countermeasures, and initiated emergency measures to support. In the first phase, SAP has donated 3 Million RMB¥ to Hubei Charity Federation, and 78k EUR for five critical hospitals in Wuhan, which are Tongji Hospital, Tongji Medical College, Huazhong University of Science & Technology; Union Hospital affiliated to Tongji Medical College of Huazhong University of Science and Technology; The central hospital of Wuhan; Wuhan Hospital of Traditional Chinese and Western Medicine; Jin Yintan Hospital of Wuhan. In the meantime, SAP is implementing a donation of 1 million EUR, and of management software tailored for the epidemic, which is worthy of 1 million EUR that includes talent training and post-maintenance services.

(2) Enhancing the city's comprehensive immunity by adaptation to circumstances

Subsequently, SAP coordinated resources, leveraged its own high-tech advantages and experiences in participating in disease surveillance to fully support the fight against the epidemic outbreak and the restoration of urban production and living functions. Again , SAP urgently activated the genes in digitalization, cloud computing and intelligent applications to provide urban emergency prevention and control solutions and health personnel training long-term mechanism plan based on SAP's software management system. The cores are:

① Establish a sound and well-rounded medical personnel archives and emergency prevention and control personnel training system, to build an efficient emergency response team by means of big data and intelligent matching;

② Implement dynamic tracking and assessment to ensure emergency prevention and control knowledge and skills are offered anytime online, and intelligently analyze emergency prevention and control talent reserves, staffing and related resource allocation;

③ Improve the information early-warning and monitoring mechanism for potential risks for public health, and intelligently assist in investigating hidden risks and reporting real-time trends in epidemic prevention and control.

At the same time, according to difficulties that appear to during the process of production recovery upon preliminary epidemic under control: such as restrictions of employee's mobility, conditions of limited work resumption, and fracture of the upstream and downstream industrial chains, SAP developed "Optimized Configuration Solution of Regional Labor Forces", which mainly utilize the Industrial Park as the management boundary to set up a platform for sharing and allocating labor resources. This platform solves many practical problems in course of returning to work through the information linkage of "government end", "enterprise end" and "user end". All these efforts have been carried out in the medium- and long-term implementation planning, and have accumulated useful experience for "digital governance" on future epidemic prevention and control and other social emergencies.

(3) Boosting corporate law-abiding consciousness and strengthening compliance awareness

In accordance with the relevant requirements of Legislative Work Committee of the National People 's Congress, to implement the unified deployment by Office of the Central Cyberspace Affairs Commission and the Ministry of Industry and Information Technology, SAP organized relevant departments and staffs to systematically study *Infectious Disease Prevention Law, Emergency Response Law, Cybersecurity Law, Emergency Regulations on Public Health Emergencies, Central Cyber Security and Informatization Commission Office on the Protection of Personal Information and the Use of Big Data Support Notice of Joint Prevention and Control Work*. Consequently, the concerned regulations are observed in the fields of employees' quarantine and observation of returning to Beijing and Shanghai office after the Spring Festival, office epidemic prevention and control, business recovery, as well as supervision and management, all of which are for the purpose of enhancing the company's awareness of law-biding and compliance. Meanwhile, by making full use of SAP's own business advantages, and in comply with the requirements of the State Council's joint prevention and control mechanism, SAP attempted to collect and analyze relevant data for epidemic prevention and control within the company in line with laws and regulations. In addition, SAP developed related software to meet the needs of the State Council's health and epidemic prevention department and local governments. Furthermore, in the process of analyzing data, SAP strictly implements data security and personal information protection measures according to national laws and regulations in relation to protecting personal information.

2 Solving the problem by locating sources and being prepared for a rainy day

Before the breakout of the COVID-19 that is currently raiding the entire world, the economy of China was just going through a critical time — the general indicators of economic growth were going down, the transformation and upgrade were ongoing, along with the well-planned revolutionary change on the economic structure. Hence, this epidemic situation will undoubtedly lead consumer market, investment market, state's financial incomes into an even darker place. This is not the SARS in early 2003 , while China was still on the honeymoon with WTO and enjoying a rapidly growing population and all those benefits that come in with it. SARS was too little of an impact on China's upraising economy. COVID-19 is spreading in a speed the world has never witnessed with the performance of affecting China in the worst possible way. It has rapidly spread over the entire country, with no province left behind. People get sick, quarantined and even killed, while factories, schools and office buildings were left empty. Needless to say, the chain effects triggered by COVID-19 is crushing all major economic activities in developed cities. More importantly, judging more its duration, scope, and destructiveness, the COVID-19 will have a much more significant influence on China than the SARS.

Between the SARS (2003) and the COVID-19 (2020), the world has been through five other epidemics that were proclaimed as "Public Health Emergencies of International Concern" (PHEIC) by WHO. Chronologically, they are Pandemic H1N1 (2009), Polio (2014), Ebola in West Africa (2014), Zika (2015-16), and Ebola in Congo (2018-19). Plus the MERS outbreak in Korea (2015), it is fair to say that the world was never safe from highly contagious epidemics and has never stopped facing the challenges. It is clear that despite our best effort, the world simply can afford to sit aside and let one or two particular countries facing such disease all by themselves. International cooperation works better than wishful thinking. When facing challenges that are of such urgency, severity and complicacy, the world has no choice but to join hands with each other. For all of us, "Community of Shared Future for Mankind" is a vision that is far too precious to be missed. For now, the most crucial task is to control the outbreak and join all the powers we can to speed up the development and production of the vaccine. Secondly, it is more important than ever for all involved countries, regions and institutes to understand, support and help each other. And keep in mind, hatred and bullying are not only distractive but also counter-productive. As Doctor-General of WHO, Dr. Tedros Adhanom Ghebreyesus, has said, China put Wuhan on lockdown, and serval mega-provinces including Hubei, Beijing, Shanghai, Anhui, Guangdong, Tianjin, and Chongqing on the highest level of public health concern alert. The price is painfully huge, as it often is when you are making the right decision. China quarantined itself with no hesitation, not to protect the nation that was already plundered by the epidemic. But to close the door from the inside, in a room that caught on fire.

In conclusion, from the state government point of view, now it is time to look beyond this particular epidemic, reflect the past and take precautions for the future.

① Improve bottom line thinking and red line thinking. Build stronger resilience on the national level, particularly against epidemic and complex emergent situations caused by the epidemic outbreak. To accomplish that, we need positive thinking and preparations for the worst possible scenarios. In other words, we need emergency response plans for either epidemic outbreaks or natural disasters, economic crises, geopolitical conflicts, and even possible cases that they might overlap or interact with each other. Trust scientific prevention and rehabilitation as the primary guide to our action, avoid both over-positiveness and excessive pessimism.

② Take precautions and develop emergency response plans against both imported cases and domestic epidemic outbreaks. Keep taking the leading role as a major power in the international community. Reinforce China's image as the living example of a modern state with advanced instruments of governing. Build stronger and more effective governance capabilities in all levels of local government, raise awareness of public health concerns among the general population. Put resilience theory into practice by establishing and implementing emergency response plans, to tackle worse possible epidemic outbreaks.

③ Establish long term plans for the next ten years or even longer by building a major national security risk assessment system and the response plan accordingly. Considering the significance of the next decade period for achieving the "Two Centenary Goals", it is essential to push forward the related scientific researches, then develop and enforce prevention drills. We are looking into a critical time for China, and it is of paramount importance that China makes the best effort to improve its overall resilience capacity, especially in dealing with major public emergencies. Emergency acts such as disaster relief and strategic reserve should be refined and reinforced with great determination so that the society can quickly recognize, respond, stay resilient, and thrive from possible disasters in the future.

3　Based on improving digital governance and offering advice to ensure development

Combining with its own experience in enterprise application software R&D, sales and service, and considering deeply the beneficial policies issued by governments to support related enterprises during the epidemic, SAP makes suggestions to government and enterprises from the perspective of "digital social governance".

(1) This outbreak has exposed many weak links in digital infrastructure

In the face of the epidemic, there is a lack of capacity reserve data for key materials such as masks. In the face of the economy, how many factories need to resume work, how many factories need capacity, and how can balance of supply and demand be achieved upstream and downstream in the supply chain? No data supports. The lack of these key and important data has brought great trouble to the country's centralized deployment and rapid response. Governments around the world, including financial institutions, have successively issued policies for supporting small and medium-sized enterprises. In the absence of both digital foundation and data support, it is difficult to achieve precise implementation. SAP hopes that government could further recognize the importance and necessity of digital infrastructure from this epidemic situation, and make up for the missing shortcomings.

(2) The early warning before the outbreak and the disposal process after the outbreak directly shows the insufficient equipment on the national emergency management system

There is a special system called "Crisis and Emergency Management Platform"(abbr. C/EMP). Its main function is to support government to manage large public safety crisis. At present, more and more foreign companies have begun to apply this system, including fields of power, transportation, medical and financial industries. C/EMP is capable to manage tasks, resources, communications, collaboration, and data when an organization is facing a crisis. In addition, C/EMP could be used to analyze changing conditions during a crisis, to keep abreast of the status, and to ensure that the procedures adopted meet government emergency management standards. As the number, frequency, scope, impact, and types of crises continue to increase, government will take the lead to strengthen the coordination and communication of C/EMP systems in different places, regions, organizations, and enterprises. It is undoubtedly necessary to improve emergency response and handling. SAP believes that we should learn deeply from lessons of this epidemic. On the one hand, the construction of C/EMP should be carried out immediately. On the other hand, relevant standards should be designed to ensure that the C/EMP of different enterprises and organizations are connected.

(3) From a higher-level technical perspective, C/EMP is also one of the seven sub-items of the crisis management technology ecosystem

At present, the most relevant requirement for the majority of enterprises is business continuity management in the seven sub-items. A large number of enterprises are unable to resume normal operations and production in a timely manner due to constraints such as employees, transportation, site, and supply. Although many companies have made some investments in digitalization, they have always been new to the concept of "Business Continuity Management" (abbr. BCM), which has been developed abroad for more than 20 years. The early BCM was just IT disaster recovery, providing protection for critical IT equipment and data centers. However, with the development of business and new challenges, such as the 24 7 service commitments provided by some companies, the globalization of business process operations, natural disasters, and virus transmission, BCM has also expanded into business areas. In response to the prevention and control of this epidemic, many companies hope to reduce the risk of transmission through remote office work. At the same time, they also hope that the business can be quickly restored and the supply interrupted by suppliers can be restored. These are BCM's management goals of.

(4) This epidemic will promote the development of "non-contact" and "low-contact" working models and business models, which will be a good opportunity for many enterprises

The traditional business model "Only Seeing Customers Can Sign Contracts" would be forced to make changes. This epidemic has driven everyone to think deeply about whether digital sales can be used to make sales operations more transparent, direct and efficient. By this way can businessmen no longer focus on meeting customers, but more focus on the resonance of value and philosophy. And for consumers, this epidemic is also equivalent to the popularization of consumption habits. SAP believes that in the future, e-commerce channels will be more grounded, target on practical results and flourish.

(5) The epidemic brings us not only "a danger" but also "an opportunity", which also constitutes a touchstone to test the digital innovation ability of enterprises

Regarding some new products urgently needed and expedited by the epidemic, many links require organic coordination, which typically comprise demand response, R&D, trial production, testing, full operation and ramping-up of capacity. Regarding every new crisis, if enterprises can respond quickly and effectively through digital innovation capability, it will bring great help to themselves and society. During the specific time-span of anti-epidemic, the collaborative designs and site management capabilities of China Construction Industry are predominant to all. The delivery of products under extreme events must be guaranteed by digital means, otherwise the preliminary planning stage of Wuhan Huoshenshan Hospital will not be able to finish within 78 minutes the architectural design scheme and construction drawings of Beijing Xiaotangshan Hospital that happened 17 years ago, to complete the collaborative design within 24 hours, to finalize the construction plan within 60 hours. All aforesaid factors guarantee accomplishing the collaborative field construction containing many details within 6 days and eventually putting into use on time.

(6) The high-tech, which is represented by big data, artificial intelligence and cloud service platform, is the key direction for the government to encourage the development and application in the anti-epidemic process

Meanwhile, it also constitutes an important part of the development of national digital economy. In this professional field, FIEs have accumulated rich experiences in long-term technology development and business operation. Accordingly, they are eager to actively participate in with the aim of promoting the leapfrog development of China's Information and Communication Industry (ICT). We fully understand the importance and necessity of "Autonomous and Controllable" policy for safeguarding national economic security. However, the technology investment, management level and experience sharing of multinational companies make up an essential part of improving the overall development level of relevant industries in this great country, which is proven by the outstanding achievements of China's reform and opening-up over the past 40 years. FIEs hope to get more opportunities for direct participation and make their own contributions.

We firmly believe that China will win the people's war against epidemic prevention and control through in-depth implementation on President Xi Jinping's important speeches and instructions in this realm and carrying out the decision-making of the Central Committee of CPC and deployment of China State Council. At the same time, we are confident that China can coordinate anti-epidemic and economic and social development by means of "Maintaining Six Stabilities", i.e., stabilizing employment, finance, foreign trade, foreign investment, domestic investment and expectation. All these endeavors are focused on minimizing negative impact of epidemic on national production and life. As a member of the vast number of FIEs, SAP will "Share the Same Breath and Destiny" with the Chinese market, adhere to his concept of "Boundless Thinking, Well Behaved", make unremitting contributions to enhancing digital emergency response capabilities of anti-epidemic and providing high-tech means, as well as helping to promote the long-term development of China's digital economy.

政府、社会组织和企业"黄金三角"合作机制提升应急救援能力

张建弢　可口可乐[*]大中华、韩国及蒙古区　副总裁

　　新冠肺炎疫情是对国家应急救援能力的严峻考验，中国政府采取了果断措施，取得了很好的效果。正如中国－世界卫生组织（World Health Organization）新冠肺炎联合专家考察组所说，这些努力避免或至少推迟了数十万新冠肺炎病例，为世界各国采取积极的防控措施争取了宝贵的时间，提供了值得借鉴的经验。[①]

　　在这场举国战"疫"中，各界有一个共同的感受：调动全国力量在武汉这样一个上千万人口的城市和湖北各市县提供大规模医疗救助和生活保障，企业和公益组织等社会力量在配合以政府为主导的各项工作中，发挥了各自的优势，打出了漂亮的组合拳。

　　为了保障前方医务人员的饮用水，正月初一当天，可口可乐在武汉启动了"净水24小时"应急饮用水救援机制：由合作伙伴壹基金和云豹救援队评估了几个医院的需求量，然后派专业志愿者驾车前往可口可乐湖北厂武汉仓库，仓库的值班员提前把饮用水和其他饮料运到厂区外，再由志愿者将物资运到医院指定安全区，全程无人员接触。既充实了一线的饮水供应，又没有占用政府在救援指挥中的组织和物质资源。

　　＊　可口可乐是世界最大的全品类饮料公司，成立于1886年，总部位于美国佐治亚州亚特兰大市。

　　①　《中国－世界卫生组织新型冠状病毒肺炎（COVID–19）联合考察报告》，2020年2月29日。

一 "黄金三角伙伴关系"理念

可口可乐公司前任董事长兼首席执行官穆泰康（Muhtar Kent）先生总结了公司多年来与政府和社会组织合作解决可持续发展问题的经验，提出了"黄金三角伙伴关系"（Golden Triangle Partnership）的理念，并于 2013 年在可口可乐基金会推出了"黄金伙伴基金"。穆泰康指出，当今世界面临的很多问题非常复杂艰巨，单单依靠一家企业甚至一个行业的力量，很难产生巨大的影响，必须依靠能有效结合政府、企业和社会组织三方力量的"黄金三角伙伴关系"推动三方合作联动。

在"黄金三角"这个创新体系中，企业提供科技、资金、产品和业务模式的支持，社会组织负责招募和培训志愿者，确保广泛参与和直接服务，政府则扮演引导、监督、物资采购以及建设和逐步完善相应政策环境的角色。三方精诚合作，可以充分发挥市场机制的专业高效和社会组织的灵活性的优势，推动各界相互取长补短，有效解决问题，也有助于促进社会和谐。

在全球，践行"黄金三角伙伴关系"著名案例之一就是非营利机构 ColaLife 配合赞比亚公共卫生当局开展的偏远地区痢疾防治工作。赞比亚基础设施落后，将痢疾防治药品分发到乡村的问题一直没有解决。英国非营利机构 ColaLife 的创始人 Simon Berry 早年从事非洲援助工作的时候注意到，在非洲大陆的偏远地区，可口可乐依然随处可见。Berry 想道，为何不把相关药品放在可口可乐箱里，随可口可乐下乡呢？2008 年他在社交媒体上发布了这个想法，很快得到了 BBC 等英国媒体的关注和可口可乐公司的支持。2010 年，在可口可乐同意进行试点后，Berry 和他的妻子创立了 ColaLife，专注于解决非洲等贫困地区的儿童痢疾药品短缺问题。他设计了一个小药匣子，嵌在可口可乐货箱的瓶子中间，解决了药品供应的"最后一公里"问题。该项目落地赞比亚的第一年就惠及该国 45%

的偏远地区儿童，这是世界卫生组织、联合国儿童基金会等大型组织在此努力多年都未达到的比例。

"黄金三角"框架下的战略合作可以有效推动社会公共事业的创新，促进可持续发展——这已经成为公共管理学界和政界的一种主流声音。联合国在《2030 年可持续发展议程》中明确提出为实现 2030 年可持续发展目标，需要"借鉴伙伴关系的经验和资源配置战略，鼓励和推动建立有效的公共、公私和民间社会伙伴关系"①。

二 "黄金三角"案例："净水 24 小时"应急救援饮用水机制

众所周知，饮用水是救灾中最急需的物资之一。在传统的救灾模式下，灾难发生后再开始组织采购、运输，很难在第一时间满足救援需求。为切实解决这一问题，2013 年，可口可乐与壹基金、壹基金救灾联盟以及各地政府部门合作推出了一个结合中国实际的"黄金三角伙伴关系"项目"净水 24 小时"应急饮用水救援机制。承诺在灾害发生的 24 小时内，将救灾最需要的瓶装饮用水送达救灾一线。

黄金三角组合的合作模式将原本相互独立的商业运营网络、民间救灾网络、地方民政部门进行了结合，实现各方联动，发挥所长，确保机制安全高效地运行。

可口可乐中国、装瓶商及遍布全国的装瓶厂达成共识，设置了高效的财务、人员联动和灾害评估机制，确保灾害发生时，可口可乐的商业生态系统能迅速转化为社会灾害响应网络的一部分。

当灾害发生时，"净水 24 小时"机制的各个合作方都可以启动该机制。由可口可乐中国可持续发展团队、壹基金和其他专业救灾伙伴的成员组成的执行团队首先评估灾区应急饮用水的需求情况和灾区的交通情况，制定

---

① 《变革我们的世界：2030 年可持续发展议程》，联合国大会 2015 年 9 月 25 日第 70/1 号决议通过。

救援规划并启动应急机制，酌情报备当地政府的救灾指挥部门。执行团队与灾害发生地的装瓶集团和装瓶厂对接后，由装瓶厂根据执行团队提供的需求和情况分析，从距离灾区最近的货舱、物流中心或零售点调拨产品，安排最合适灾区运输条件的车辆和人员，向灾区运送瓶装水。

在"净水24小时"机制下，壹基金、壹基金救灾合作伙伴充分利用专业救灾能力，将可口可乐系统供应的安全饮用水安全送达救灾一线。各装瓶厂可选择本区域内具有专业能力和响应力的官方或民间机构作为有机补充。

在一场场"与时间赛跑"的救援行动中，"净水24小时"累计响应各类灾害超过224次，为222万灾民提供了1875万瓶饮用水，多年来共有超过200家地方政府和社会组织及4000多名社区志愿者参与。

"净水24小时"机制获得了可口可乐董事会的年度大奖，同时也经可口可乐基金会推广到其他国家，展示了"中国创造"的魅力。

三　探索救灾新机制，"黄金三角"大有可为

综观全球，企业和社会组织在应急救援行动中的贡献也越来越受到各国政府的重视和社会的认可。中国"十三五"发展规划纲要提出，要"建成与公共安全风险相匹配、覆盖应急管理全过程和全社会共同参与的突发事件应急体系"，积极探索政府主导、企业联动、社会力量精准参与的救灾新机制。

作为公共管理问题专家，清华大学苏世民学院院长薛澜也出现在全国新冠肺炎专家组的名单上。他在2020年3月接受采访时指出，"对中国来说，这次疫情是一堂风险社会的启蒙课"。[①] 他主张，为了消除风险，应该发挥政府、社会和市场的积极性，其中社会力量的参与至关重要。

---

① 《薛澜：这是一堂风险社会启蒙课》，《财经》杂志，2020年3月11日。

"今天中国的基层社会已经有很强的自主意识了，引导这种力量在突发事件应对方面更好地发挥作用，需要尽快提到日程上。党的十九届四中全会决定提出要'建设人人有责，人人尽责，人人享有的社会治理共同体'。这段话非常好，也非常重要，应当成为社会组织参与应急管理的指导。"薛澜认为，如果说市场经济就是通过市场，把每个人内在的激励机制和全社会利益最大化有机连接起来，那么，社会公益的"市场"同样可以发挥类似作用，把社会力量动员起来。人人都有自利的一面，也有利他的一面。自利的一面可以通过市场机制这个"看不见的手"来解决，利他的一面可以通过社会公益市场来释放。把个体向善的力量通过社会公益组织和公益服务"市场"整合起来，会形成良好的社会秩序，为风险治理提供重要的补充。一些国家已经着手开展这一领域的制度建设。2005 年卡特里娜飓风之后，美国联邦应急管理署（Federal Emergency Management Agency）成立了私营部门分部，专门负责应急管理中的公私合作；日本则在国家防灾组织中设有中小企业厅，专司协调企业参与灾害应对和救援。

可以预见，未来企业和社会组织在积极配合政府工作，参与应急援助、慈善事业和推动社会进步方面会发挥越来越大的影响力。在这样的时代背景下，"黄金三角"等经过多年实践，极大释放企业和社会能量的公益模式可以为全球建设因地制宜的救灾机制提供灵感和借鉴。

四 发挥"黄金三角"优势，提高应急救援能力

在中国，结合多年来同各方伙伴通力协作的经验和战"疫"后的思考，我们希望就通过推动"黄金三角伙伴"合作，进一步提升中国社会的应急救援能力，提出一点建议。

1. 设立虚拟货舱

地方政府可以和灾备物资的生产企业签订合作协议，设立虚拟货舱，

平时企业将虚拟货舱的货物纳入正常销售流程，在危机出现时及时激活虚拟货舱机制，按需调拨，同公益组织密切合作，投入救援。

通过这种灵活的运作方式，政府避免了设立和管理赈灾物资供应链的种种麻烦和资金占用，以及常备货舱覆盖面有限，以及由此可能产生的救灾中"远水不解近渴"的尴尬情景。同时也避免了维持常备货舱经常发生的货物过期、变质等问题造成的巨大浪费。"虚拟货舱"机制充分发挥了企业物流系统遍布全国城乡的全覆盖优势，又能充分发挥企业和公益组织的优势，确保最高效率实现物资按需及时供应和分配。

2. 分工协作，各司其职

在危机事件发生时，由政府协调，充分调动企业的积极性，激活民间潜伏的多股专业力量，发挥各自的专业特长，在政府的统一指挥下，互相配合，开展工作。在应急救援中政府应最大限度地发挥"掌舵"的作用，可以避免分散精力到"划桨"上。这样可以充分发挥各类企业和社会组织在日常运营中建立和日益优化的物资和服务生产和分配能力，利用现有的高效运营的商业网络，实现物资和服务的有效调配。

在本次中，一个紧迫的任务是保证来自各方面的救灾资金的组织管理、物资的运送和清点、按需分配和及时分发。有多家企业为此充分发挥优势，在救灾中高效运作，火线立功。例如，在全国运营了700多个货舱的京东利用在武汉地区的亚洲一号仓库，充分施展无人分拣技术，并利用智能车、机器人和无人机实现无人配送。2020年2月4日，京东物流仅用一天多时间便将钟南山团队援助汉口医院的100台制氧机顺利送达，钟南山院士写信感谢京东团队。在全国范围内，从1月20日至2月28日，京东累计向全国消费者供应了2.2亿件超过29万吨的生活用品，并在全国累计承运医疗应急物资约5000万件 [①]。

国家市场监督管理总局于1月29日启动的声势浩大的"保价格、保

---

① 《京东推多项"硬核"技术助力抗疫》，《北京青年报》2020年3月4日第5版。

质量、保供应"系列行动，则诠释了政府的高屋建瓴和精准指挥带动企业发挥出了巨大威力。这个号召甫一发出，就得到各界积极响应。截至2月27日，已经有超过7000家企业参与其中，尤其是电商平台、商场超市、连锁便利店等龙头企业旗下的门店达20多万户，遍及大中小城市和乡村。特别值得注意的是，承诺"三保"的企业中近一半都是规模以上的龙头食品企业，它们带动食品全行业推进复工复产，有力地维护了市场和国家秩序稳定，在这场行动中发挥了中流砥柱作用[①]。

3. 加强公益组织建设和志愿人员培训

支持各地和细分领域的公益组织以及企业基金会建设。鼓励成立专业志愿者人才库，利用互联网平台开展定期的培训和交流，不断提高各方面人员的各项能力和协作配合，提高人员组织和物资调动能力。

例如，壹基金在全国各地和当地社会组织一起建立了覆盖广泛的救灾联合网络。2017年壹基金救灾联合网络参与救灾90多次，只有5次需要壹基金员工到场，大部分救灾行动都是由壹基金联动企业和筹款平台支持当地社会组织开展的属地救援。"在国家减灾委、民政部和地方灾害管理部门的指导和支持下，构建这个系统后使得社会组织有序、规范、高效运作，细分化解决问题，真正做到帮忙不添乱。"壹基金秘书长李弘在采访中说[②]。

这一场新冠肺炎疫情是对我国应急救援能力一次极大的考验。作为改革开放后第一个回到中国大陆市场的国际消费品牌，可口可乐对这一场战役感同身受，竭尽力量投入其中，见证了中国政府、人民的高度团结和智慧，也为世界卫生组织高级顾问艾尔沃德先生所感慨的社会各界展现出的"纯粹的利他主义精神"深深感动。期待我们的一点建言能够抛砖引玉，对中国建设更加美好的未来有所裨益。

---

① 《价格稳定供应有序"三保"行动助力疫情防控战》，中国新闻网，2020年2月27日。
② 《灾害应对需要更多枢纽性救援平台》，《公益时报》2017年10月24日，第6版。

Golden Triangle Partnership among Government, Business & Civil Society to Enhance Emergency Response and Disaster Relief Capabilities

By Jiantao Zhang, Vice President of the Coca-Cola Company, Greater China, Korea and Mongolia

COVID-19 has been a major test to China's emergency response and disaster relief capabilities. Thanks to the effective measures adopted by the government, the achievements have been very encouraging. The WHO (World Health Organization)-China Joint Mission estimates that the truly all-of government and all-of-society approach that has been taken in China has averted or at least delayed hundreds of thousands of COVID-19 cases in the country. By extension, the reduction that has been achieved in the COVID-19 infection in China has also played a significant role in protecting the global community and creating a stronger first line of defense against international spread. [1]

Reflecting on the "all of society" battle against the virus, people applauded the effective partnership between government, business enterprises and civil society in responding to COVID-19 in Wuhan, a city with over 10 million population and providing medical relief and everyday support across the entire province, which has been centrally orchestrated by the government to enable each party to bring into full play their own expertise.

---

[1] Report of the WHO-China Joint Mission on Coronavirus Disease 2019 (COVID-19), released by WHO on Feb 24th, 2020.

To provide drinking water for medical workers at the frontline, The Coca-Cola Company (hereafter referred to as TCCC) activated "Clean Water 24", a disaster relief drinking water mechanism on the first day after the Chinese New Year in Wuhan: One Foundation and their local partner YB Rescue first appraised the demand of drinking water in a number of hospitals before they dispatched trucks with volunteers to fetch the water from the warehouse of TCCC's Wuhan Bottling Plant, where people on duty had put the water outside the factory premises, as previously agreed, to be picked up by volunteers and delivered to a safety zone outside the hospitals, with no human touch in the entire process. This operation ensures drinking water supply for medical workers without taking up any resources or bandwidth of the government.

1   The concept of golden triangle partnership

Inspired by years of partnering with both government and civil society to address challenges of sustainable development, former Chairman and CEO of TCCC, Muhtar Kent put forward the concept of Golden Triangle Partnership and launched Golden Triangle Fund in 2013 within the Coca-Cola Foundation. According to Mr. Kent, "Given the scale and complexity of today's issues, it is challenging for one business or even one industry to make a material difference on its own. Instead we must rely on partnership that connects across what I call the Golden Triangle of business, governments and civil society."

Under the innovative Golden Triangle Partnership, business brings in technology, funding, products and business models and civil society looks after volunteer recruiting and training while the government plays the role of guiding supervisor, in charge of product and service procurement and building and optimizing the policy environment. The three-party partnership brings out the full market tested efficiency of business and flexibility of civil society to enable the parties to complement each other to effectively address the challenges and promote the building of a harmonious society.

A very good example of Golden Triangle Partnership is when non-profit organization ColaLife worked with the public health authority of Zambia to prevent dysentery in remote rural area, where infrastructure is very primitive. It is a challenge to deliver medicine to the remote countryside. The founder of ColaLife Simon Berry noticed in his earlier years of volunteering in Africa that even in the most remote corners there are Coca-Cola beverages everywhere. Why not free load the distribution network of Coca-Cola to deliver medicine? Berry posted his idea in the social space in 2008 and very soon BBC and other British media picked up the idea. The Coca-Cola Company was ready to assist. After Coca-Cola agreed to pilot his idea, Berry and his wife established ColaLife, an NGO fully dedicated to bringing dysentery medicine to poor children in rural Africa. Barry designed a small packet that could be put between Coca-Cola bottles in the beverage cases, delivering medicine to the rural population, thus solving the problem of the last mile. Within a year after this program was launched, over 45% of children in the remote area were covered, more than what WHO and UNICEF achieved after years of working in the country.

It has been the consensus between the academia in public administration and the governments that strategic cooperation under Golden Triangle Partnership could effectively drive innovation in sustainability and public service. The 2030 Agenda for Sustainable Development of the United Nations stated that in order to realize the sustainable development goals of 2030, we should encourage and promote effective public, public-private and civil society partnerships, building on the experience and resourcing strategies of partnerships. [1]

---

[1] Transforming Our World: The 2030 Agenda for Sustainable Development, A/RES/70/1, UN General Assembly. Goal 17.

2　Golden triangle partnership best practice: clean water 24 disaster relief mechanism

Drinking water is one of the most needed supplies in disaster relief. In the traditional disaster relief process, procurement and transportation only starts after a disaster has stricken and it is very difficult to provide sufficient drinking water in time. To solve this problem, Coca-Cola China and One Foundation launched Clean Water 24 disaster relief mechanism, pledging to deliver bottled water to the disaster victims and relief workers within 24 hours of the disaster.

The Golden Triangle Partnership connects the originally independent business operation network, civil society network and local governments in such a way that all parties could work together, each bringing out the full potential of their competitive advantages to launch very effective disaster relief efforts.

Under this partnership, TCCC China, the bottling partners and bottling plants across the country reached an alignment to set up a very effective mechanism that involves both people and finance management. The mechanism is automatically activated once a disaster strikes to switch the business ecosystem of Coca-Cola into an emergency response and disaster relief network.

All partners of Clean Water 24 could activate the mechanism. A taskforce consisting of people from TCCC China Sustainability and Social Impact team, One Foundation and external partners will first assess the needs for drinking water and the transportation conditions before they work out a plan. If necessary, they will file a report with the local government agency in charge of orchestrating the emergency responses. The taskforce will then get in touch with the local bottler, which will allocate bottled water from the nearest fulfillment center or even retail outlets and arrange for the most suitable vehicle and people to dispatch the drinking water to the disaster area.

Under Clean Water 24, One Foundation and their local partners help deliver the clean drinking water provided by the Coca-Cola system to the frontline of disaster relief. Bottling plants also have the option to recruit local NGOs and government agencies to support. Since the launch, Clean Water 24 has been activated for 224 natural disasters, bringing 18.75 million bottles of water to 2.22 million people. More than 200 local governments, NGOs and 4,000 volunteers have helped in the efforts.

Clean water 24 won the Board of Directors Special Award and The Coca-Cola Foundation has been promoting the practice to other countries.

3　Calls for innovation in disaster relief. Golden Triangle Partnership has a lot to offer.

Contributions of business enterprises and civil society to disaster relief efforts have been highly recognized by both governments and the general public all over the world. The 13th Five-Year Plan of China also called for building a full cycle emergency response and disaster relief mechanism that is compatible with public security risks and encourages full participation of different actors of the society. The aim is to build a mechanism guided by the government with very active participation from both business enterprises and civil society.

Professor Xue Lan, President of Schwartzman College of Tsinghua University and a leading expert in public administration, sits on the National Advisory Committee against COVID-19. In an interview conducted in March [1] , Professor Xue Lan pointed out the outbreak is a moment of enlightenment in risk management. According to him, preventing and minimizing risks requires the active participation of the government, civil society and market actors. It is crucial to recruit the partnership and participation of the civil society.

"The grassroot communities of China have developed very strong self-consciousness. We should mobilize such actors to play a more active role in

---

[1]　Caijing Magazine, March 11th, 2020, Xue Lan: This is a Moment of Enlightenment in Risk Management.

emergency responses. The Communiqué of The Fourth Plenary Session of the 19th Party Congress called for the establishment of a social governance mechanism where everybody is accountable, everybody makes their contributions and enjoys the benefits. This is very important and should be the guideline to encourage social organizations to participate in emergency responses."

According to Xue Lan, market economy connects personal motivation and maximizing social benefits. There should be a market for social well-being to connect different actors of the society to motivate them to contribute to social good. Besides driving their own self-interest people also want to help and benefit others. The self-serving aspects could be looked after by the invisible hand of the market economy while the need to benefit and help others could be looked after by a market mechanism of social well-being. If we could create a "market mechanism" where people's need to do good and help others could be harnessed, we could create great complementary for the risk mitigation mechanism. Other countries have been exploring in this space. After the 2005 hurricane Katrina, FEMA (Federal Emergency Management Agency) of the US set up a department to look after private public partnership in emergency responses. Japan has a special bureau in the government looking after partnership with small and medium business in disaster relief and aid.

We anticipate that in the future business enterprises and non-profit organizations can play a more important and impactful role in emergency response and disaster relief, charity and driving social progress working with the government. Mechanisms like Golden Triangle that has proven effective in unleashing the great prowess of business and civil society would be a source of inspiration and reference.

4　Leveraging golden triangle partnership to enhance emergency response capabilities

Inspired by experience of TCCC China working with a range of partners on sustainability and social impact initiatives and based on our reflections about the experience of fighting COVID-19 in close partnership, we would like to put forward the following proposals on how to further develop and strengthen Golden Triangle Partnership and enhance China's emergency response and disaster relief capabilities.

(1) Set up virtual warehouse and preemptive stockpile.

Local governments can sign agreements with business enterprises that produce supplies for disaster relief to set up virtual warehouse, where the enterprises could keep the products covered in the agreements in their ecosystem of distribution and retail. Once an emergency strikes, the virtual stockpile can be dispatched for disaster relief purposes.

The flexibility of this partnership helps the government to avoid the trouble of setting up and managing disaster relief supplies and all the work and the capital investment needed. Besides regular stockpile has very limited coverage and when disaster strikes it could well be that the stockpile far away takes too long to help solve the problems in real time. By setting up virtual warehouse and stockpile, local governments emergency response authorities do not have to worry about tracking the shelf life to replenish the supply on a regular basis. Virtual stockpile could fully leverage the country's well-developed business ecosystem of distribution that reaches the very grassroot communities where business enterprises and NGOs could bring their initiatives into a full play to ensure efficient and timely supply of disaster relief products.

(2) Division of labor improves efficiency.

When disaster strikes, under the coordination of the governments, both business and civil society could be mobilized to work together and do their best to assist while the government could maximize their focus on piloting the boat, so to speak, and avoid wasting their energy and bandwidth paddling the oars. Such Golden Triangle Partnership could fully mobilize the capabilities of business enterprises and NGOs of producing and distributing products and services, which has been tested and optimized in their everyday operation.

In the fight against COVID-19, a daunting task is to ensure that all disaster relief products are sorted and distributed in a timely manner. Quite a few business enterprises have done a great job. For an instance, JD.com, which operates over 700 fulfillment centers across the country, has their most hi-tech equipped Warehouse Asia One in cities including Wuhan. They engineered automated sorting and delivery process leveraging smart vehicles, robots and drones. On February 4th, the fulfillment team of JD.com delivered 100 oxygen generators to hospitals in Hankou that Professor Zhong Nanshan's team donated. Professor Zhong hand wrote the team a letter of appreciation. From January 20th to February 28th JD.com delivered over 220 million parcels of over 290,000 tons of daily supplies, among which 50 million health emergency products [①].

The pledge of "stabilizing price, quality and supply" launched by the market supervision authorities on January 29th is a good example of how the government could mobilize the business community. Within a month over 7,000 enterprises have committed their support, among them e-commerce platforms, shopping malls and supermarkets, covering over 200,000 chain convenient stores in both big cities and small and medium cities and the countryside. Over half of the companies are large food and beverage companies with an annual output above 20 million RMB. Under their leadership and inspiration, the food and beverage sector gradually reopened, which ensured market and social stability. [②]

(3) Enhance civil society and volunteer capability building.

We would like to propose encouraging the development of NGOs focused

---

① Beijing Youth Daily, Page 5, March 4th, 2020, JD.com Hardcore Technologies Contributing to the Battle against COVID-19.

② www.Chinanews.com, Feb 27th, 2020, Stable Prices and Orderly Supplies under Three Stabilizing Pledge to Assist the Fight against Virus.

on regional issues, niche issues or demographic groups and business enterprises affiliated foundations. We would also like to propose that China set up a volunteer talent pool and leverage the Internet platform and technologies to rollout regular training and sharing to help enhance the capabilities of people from different organizations and their abilities to coordinate and work together.

One Foundation boasts a national network of emergency response and disaster relief alliance with local NGOs around the country. In the year 2017, One Foundation and its partners participated in the relief efforts for 90 disasters. Out of those 90 operations, One Foundation employees were present onsite for 5 of them. Most of the disaster relief efforts were conducted with One Foundation's assistance by local NGOs that One Foundation has sponsored or supported. Under the guidance of National Disaster Mitigation Commission, Ministry of Civil Affairs and their local branches, this network has enabled orderly and efficient operations where highly segmented taskforces will undertake different challenges. "Only by working in this way can we offer to help without causing any problems or disruptions," Secretary General Li Hong of One Foundation confirmed in an interview. [①]

COVID-19 has been a major test of China's capabilities of emergency response and disaster relief. As the first international consumer brand to have returned to the Chinese Mainland, TCCC China has played a very active role in the disaster relief efforts and we witnessed the solidarity and wisdom of the government and the ordinary people. We are also deeply touched by the spirits of helping others displayed by the general public, as highly applauded by the senior advisor Bruce Aylward of WHO. It is our sincere hope that our proposal would inspire more innovative ideas and we can all work together to build a better China.

---

① Social Welfare Times, Page 6, Issue of October 24th, 2017. More Hub Platforms Needed for Disaster Relief.

Summary of contributions by the Coca-Cola system in China's battle against COVID-19

Till March 1st, The Coca-Cola China System has contributed 4.5 million RMB to assist the efforts fighting the virus and provided some 1.26 million bottles of beverage via Clean Water 24, a disaster relief mechanism aiming to bring clean drinking water to disaster victims within 24 hours.

The Coca-Cola Foundation has donated half a million US dollars and another half a million US dollar worth of medical protective supplies, including 1.5 million masks and 40,000 protective gowns.

发挥制度优势，完善全民健康体系

帝斯曼[*]（中国）有限公司

2020 年中国农历鼠年之初，一场突如其来的新冠肺炎疫情给中国人民的生命健康造成重大伤害，也让经济发展面临严峻的挑战。在逆境之下，我们看到中国政府在打赢这场防疫阻击战的过程中，能够有效应对，快速反应，在动员能力、协调能力、组织能力和执行能力上凸显了制度优势，彰显了中国速度、中国规模和中国效率，得到国际社会的普遍好评和认可。

但是不能否认的是，这场疫情不仅给人们的正常生活带来严重影响，也对国民经济正常运转带来极大的困难。因此，在疫情面前我们必须要进行认真反思，以使我们能够在疫情之后长期保持经济繁荣，保障人民的幸福生活和实现全面小康。亡羊补牢，从疫情中吸取教训，总结出可以改进和完善的空间，也不失为一件好事。为此，我们就如何发挥制度优势，更好贯彻习近平主席的以人民为中心的发展理念，结合健康中国 2030 规划纲要，以提高人民健康水平为目的和宗旨，拟提出以下建议。

一 强化和提升国民卫生和健康教育

2019 年 12 月 28 日,《中华人民共和国基本医疗卫生与健康促进法》经十三届全国人大常委会第十五次会议表决通过，将于 2020 年 6 月 1 日

---

　　* 荷兰皇家帝斯曼公司是一家以使命为导向，在全球范围内活跃于营养、健康和绿色生活的全球科学公司，致力于以缤纷科技开创美好生活。成立于 1902 年，业务涵盖为人类营养、动物营养、个人护理与香原料、医疗设备、绿色产品与应用提供创新解决方案。总部位于荷兰海尔伦市。

　　特别感谢蒋惟明、诸琳瑛对本文的贡献。

正式实施。其中第六十八条指出："国家将健康教育纳入国民教育体系。学校应当利用多种形式实施健康教育，普及健康知识、科学健身知识、急救知识和技能，提高学生主动防病的意识，培养学生良好的卫生习惯和健康的行为习惯。"结合这次疫情来看，此法的颁布非常重要且恰逢其时！因此，我们建议把国民的健康教育列入大中小学教育的必修课，从娃娃做起，甚至从幼儿园开始，提倡个人卫生习惯和遵守公共场所的卫生要求，把饮食、营养和运动等健康常识性教育纳入教学大纲。培养和树立他人意识，例如，在自己身体不舒服时主动戴上口罩，这不仅仅是保护自己，也是保护他人，这是一种习惯，更是一种素质培养。

同时，除了在校园中的教育之外，面对社会大众的不间断教育也同等重要。健康教育是以预防为主方针最直接的体现，掌握了健康知识和技能就可以预防和减少疾病的发生。随着人民生活水平的提高和技术的进步，广播、电视、网络、手机这些媒介的触角已经延伸到绝大部分人群，这些大众媒介承担着公共信息传递、交流和共享的任务，充分利用这个媒介去有针对性地开展公共健康教育是最好的办法，对国民大众健康知识的提高和对疾病的预防都会产生积极的影响。目前我国微信用户数量达 11 亿，使用这个平台进行面对社会大众的健康教育和公共卫生信息宣传普及可以取得事半功倍的效果，也是充分利用制度优势实施和落实以人民为中心的理念的最佳途径。此外建议广播电视上也要增加健康知识和行为的公益广告，让良好的习惯成为人们的自觉行动。

二 加强和扶持社区健康服务系统，合理利用资源，改善服务功能

从此次新冠肺炎疫情在武汉暴发和蔓延的初期阶段来看，几乎所有二级以上医院都受到了巨大的冲击，可以说，完全不能满足瞬间扩散的疫情需要，而本应该在疫情暴发初期扮演最基础也是最重要角色的社区医院，却似乎并未起到它本应该起到的作用。从其他一些国家的经验来看，一些

流行病和传染病按照防控程序，患者可以先向家庭医生和社区医院报告，经初步诊断和筛查后，根据情况对需要送往上级医院的患者进行预约就诊，来开展进一步检查治疗。特别是在重大突发公共卫生事件中，社区医院扮演着第一道关口的角色，应该起到快速反应机制的作用，使疫情能够得到早期控制。但如果社区的医疗系统处在薄弱环节，其医疗水平和公信力方面都不能得到民众的充分信任，甚至起不到筛查、分流病人的作用，那就难以避免人们蜂拥去大医院扎堆就诊，无形中增加了交叉感染的概率，加大了医疗系统和医生的压力，失去了控制疫情迅速扩散的最佳窗口期。

实现全民健康覆盖的一个关键组成部分是确保所有人口都能获得高质量的卫生保健。中国作为世界第二大经济体，近年来在医疗保健体系方面也得到了长足的发展，权威医学杂志《柳叶刀》2018年发布的全球医疗可及性和质量指数排行榜[①]，对全球195个国家和地区在1990~2016年医疗可及性和质量的变迁情况进行了研究和比较，中国位列第48。从研究中可以了解到中国境内各地区发展不平衡问题突出：HAQ最高值与最低值相差了43.5；东部省份的HAQ指数要优于西部省份。我们认为，这可能与我们医疗资源配置不均衡、医药卫生服务和医疗保健能力有关，例如，在城乡之间，在沿海和内陆地区之间仍然存在很大的差距，北上广的医疗系统或许能够达到欧美水平，但在其他省市和一些相对贫困地区，水平就大有不同。特别是基层的卫生保健系统存在的问题就尤为突出。

我们欣喜地看到，2020年2月25日，中共中央、国务院颁发了《关于深化医疗保障制度改革的意见》，在协同推进医药服务供给侧改革方面明确指出：健全全科和专科医疗服务分工合作的现代医疗服务体系，强化基层全科医疗服务。我们认为这正是当务之急，利用制度的优势，加强和扶持社区健康服务系统，合理配置和利用资源，改善和提高服务功

---

① Measuring performance on the Healthcare Access and Quality Index for 195 countries and territories and selected subnational locations: a systematic analysis from the Global Burden of Disease Study 2016.

能，充分利用现代信息技术，建立大数据居民健康数据库，开展网上问询和远程诊断，制定有针对性和个性化的服务。建议重视并加强社区医疗机构的人才培养，包括对全科医生的培养，鼓励医科毕业生和医生到社区卫生服务中心就业工作等，切实提升社区医院的医治能力和设施建设水平，让居民享受到社区医疗的便捷和水准，努力提高人民大众的就医体验和幸福指数。

三　关注营养不良和隐性饥饿问题

从《"健康中国 2030"规划纲要》中我们看到：全民健康是建设健康中国的根本目的。立足全人群和全生命周期两个着力点，提供公平可及、系统连续的健康服务，实现更高水平的全民健康。要覆盖全生命周期，针对生命不同阶段的主要健康问题及主要影响因素，确定若干优先领域，强化干预，实现从胎儿到生命终点的全程健康服务和健康保障，全面维护人民健康。为实现此目标，我们认为预防疾病应该比治疗显得更为重要，而预防疾病最有效的途径是提升人们的免疫水平和营养水平。为此建议如下。

1. 关注生命早期以及学龄前儿童的营养健康干预

国外科学研究表明，生命最初的 1000 天，从怀孕到 2 岁的母婴营养影响人一生的健康。早期开展营养干预，是提高健康素质的机会窗口期。2012 年 6 月卫生部发布了《中国 0~6 岁儿童营养发展报告（2012）》，报告向公众介绍中国儿童营养发展状况，引起全社会对儿童营养问题的重视和关注。儿童的营养状况是衡量整个人群营养状况的最敏感指标，也是人口素质的基础。国际上通常将 5 岁以下儿童营养状况作为衡量一个国家社会经济发展的重要指标，作为关系人类生存与发展的重要问题给予关注。

2018 年国家卫健委等部门联合制定印发了《健康扶贫三年攻坚行动实施方案》，实施贫困地区儿童营养改善项目，国家免费为 6~24 个月龄儿童每天提供一个营养包，有助于婴幼儿获得最佳的生长、发育和健康状态。此外随着经济社会发展，我们也要关注一些新的儿童营养问题，如流动儿童、留守儿童等弱势群体儿童营养状况亟待改善，这些都需要多个部门的关注和支持，需要全社会的共同努力。

目前国家对于6~24个月龄贫困地区儿童有营养包干预政策，对6岁开始义务教育的贫困地区学生有营养餐项目，但在3~5岁这个年龄段的贫困儿童营养不良问题上仍然缺少成熟的帮扶政策，只有一些公益慈善组织在填补和覆盖这个空白，但受益的儿童人数有限。我们认为营养扶贫重要而迫在眉睫，营养不良问题不仅会导致国家GDP的损失，并且会在人口中产生代际传递，造成贫困导致营养不良再导致贫困的恶性循环。应该关注学龄前3~5岁这个群体，有更好的政策可以精准干预。改善贫困地区儿童营养和健康状况关系到我国未来人口素质、经济社会发展进程和国际竞争实力，也是落实健康中国2030年规划纲要、真正实现纲要中的目标需要去努力的具体行动。

2. 关注和重视"隐性饥饿"，提高全民健康质量

世界卫生组织将营养摄入不足或营养失衡称为隐性饥饿。现代医学发现，70%的慢性病包括心血管疾病、糖尿病、癌症和肥胖、亚健康状态等都与人体营养元素摄入的不均衡相关，隐性饥饿已经成为人类健康的致命杀手。2015年，国家卫计委组织专家编写了《中国居民营养与慢性病状况报告》，报告显示：中国居民脂肪摄入过多，平均膳食脂肪供能比超过30%！与此同时，相当一部分中国居民还缺乏钙、铁、维生素A、维生素D等营养素。营养专家指出："城市居民动物性食物吃得过多，一些人群害怕发胖不吃主食，杂粮吃的更少。"如果说，显性饥饿是由于缺乏能量、蛋白质、脂肪等营养物质而造成的，可以通过"充饥""吃饱"来解决，而隐性饥饿则是由营养不均衡和缺乏微量元素、维生素、矿物质而造成的，需要通过"吃对""吃好"来解决。

中国《国民营养计划（2017-2030年）》指出，近年来，我国人民生

活水平不断提高，营养供给能力显著增强，国民营养健康状况明显改善，但仍面临居民营养不足与过剩并存、营养相关疾病多发、营养健康生活方式尚未普及等问题，成为影响国民健康的重要因素。

为此，建议要加强公民的健康饮食教育、提倡合理的平衡的食品组成以及适当的膳食补充，全面普及膳食营养知识，引导国民形成科学的膳食习惯；形成合理的膳食结构。要宣传和执行中国《国民营养计划（2017–2030年）》的策略和行动，要提倡无病主动预防来取代有病被动治疗的理念。

《"健康中国2030"规划纲要》和《国民营养计划（2017–2030年）》的颁布，使国民营养健康上升为国策。荷兰皇家帝斯曼集团长期以来，是专注于营养、健康、绿色生活的全球科学企业，同时也是全球最大的营养素供应商，一直致力于与政府、国际组织和行业协会的合作，在营养改善方面做出积极贡献。帝斯曼与中国营养学会共同设立了"中国营养学会营养科研基金——帝斯曼专项科研基金"。其宗旨就是：促进我国营养科学与技术的发展，为推动营养健康食品的发展提供科学依据，改善人群营养健康状况。自2007年以来，帝斯曼与联合国世界粮食计划署结为战略合作伙伴关系，利用我们在营养和食品强化方面的专业知识，为有需要的人开发具有成本效益、可持续和营养的食品解决方案，也为实现联合国可持续发展目标做出贡献。帝斯曼在中国积极与政府部门、非政府组织、私营部门合作，为营养缺乏的人群提供可持续的营养促进模式，包括参与全国妇联、卫生部、中国儿童少年基金会共同开展"消除婴幼儿贫血行动"项目，参与中国发展研究基金会在青海省和云南省试点"社会公平——贫困地区儿童早期发展项目"，提供全面的技术支持和高质量的营养包产品。参与安利公益基金会联合中国发展研究基金会、中国儿童少年基金会等机构，共同开展"为5加油——学前儿童营养改善计划"，针对中国贫困地区3~5岁儿童免费发放儿童营养咀嚼片，帮助贫困儿童健康成长。

帝斯曼公司希望与中国在营养改善解决方案上一起合作，贡献我们的知识和经验，为中国人民的健康和福祉保驾护航！

Utilize System Advantages to Improve the National Health System

By DSM (China) Co., Ltd.

The beginning of 2020 witnessed the unexpected outbreak of COVID-19 which has caused great harm to Chinese people's health and implicated severe challenges to Chinese economy. In adversity, the Chinese government has effectively responded to the epidemic, showing its system advantages in mobilization, coordination, organization and implementation. The remarkable speed, scale and efficiency of China have been highly praised and recognized by the international community.

Undeniably, the epidemic has seriously affected not only people's normal life but also the operation of national economy. Therefore, we must reflect on the epidemic and learn from it to maintain long-term economic prosperity after COVID-19 in order to safeguard people's well-being and achieve a moderately prosperous society in all respects. The epidemic is also an opportunity for us to identify and make improvements in areas that are lacking. To this end, according to the *Healthy China 2030 Planning Outline*, we focus on how to give play to system advantages and better implement President Xi Jinping's people-centered development concept and propose to improve people's health.

1　Improve national health education

The *Law of the People's Republic of China on the Promotion of Basic Medical and Health Care* passed at the 15th session of the Standing Committee of the 13th National People's Congress of the People's Republic of China on December 28, 2019 will come into force on June 1, 2020. According to Article 68 of the law, "the state shall incorporate health education into the national education system. Schools shall use various forms to implement health education, popularize health knowledge and the awareness of proactive prevention of diseases, and develop good health habits and healthy behaviors." In view of this epidemic, the promulgation of this law is very important and timely. Therefore, we would like to propose the incorporation of national health education into the mandatory courses of primary schools, middle schools and universities; Furthermore, we advocate the education of personal hygiene habits and observation of sanitary requirements for public places starting from kindergartens, and to include basic knowledge about diet, nutrition and sports in the syllabus. We also propose to educate people to become more considerate of others, for example, wearing a mask when feeling under the weather, which can protect both ourselves and others. This is not just about forming good habits but also becoming better citizen.

In addition to school health education, continuous social health education is of equal importance. Health education is the most direct fulfillment of the principle of "prevention first", preventing and reducing diseases with health knowledge and skills. With the improvement of people's living standards and technology, media such as radio, television, Internet and mobile phones have covered the majority of people. These media undertake tasks of disseminating, exchanging and sharing public information. And it is the best way to make full use of them to carry out targeted public health education, which will have a positive impact on the improvement of people's health knowledge and the prevention of diseases. Currently, considering the 1.1 billion WeChat users in China, using this platform for public health education and disseminating public health information will get more results with less effort, and this is the best way to make full use of system advantages to implement the people-centered concept. In addition, we propose that public service advertisements on health knowledge and behaviors be increased on radio and television, so that good habits can become people's unconscious actions.

2 Support the community health service system

In the initial stage of the outbreak and spread of COVID-19 in Wuhan, almost all hospitals above the second class were greatly impacted and couldn't address the rapidly spread epidemic fast enough. On the other hand, community hospitals which should have played the most basic and important role at that time failed to function. Learning from the experience of other countries, we found that, in the case of epidemics and infectious diseases, patients could go to family doctors and community hospitals first for preliminary diagnosis and screening, and might then be sent to higher-level hospitals for further examination and treatment according to the results. Especially in the case of major public health emergencies, community hospitals serve as the first point of contact, and should play the role of a rapid response mechanism, thus realizing early control of the epidemic. However, if the community medical system is weak, and its medical level and credibility are not trustable, or even cannot screen and distribute patients, then people will inevitably swarm to large hospitals for medical treatment, which will inevitably increase the chance of cross-infection and the pressure on the medical system and doctors, thus missing the best window period to control the rapid spread of the epidemic.

A key component of achieving national health coverage is ensuring high-quality healthcare access for all people. As the world's second largest economy, China has made remarkable progress in the healthcare system in recent years. According to a study released in 2018 by The Lancet, an authoritative medical journal, on the healthcare access and quality index for 195 countries and regions from 1990 to 2016, China ranked 48th, and the country has a significant issue of imbalanced development in various regions: the difference between the highest value

(91.5 for Beijing) and the lowest value (48.0 for Tibet) of HAQ is 43.5; the HAQ index of eastern provinces is higher than that of western provinces. We attribute this to the uneven allocation of medical resources. For example, there is still a large gap in medical resource allocation between urban and rural areas, and between coastal and inland areas. The medical systems of Beijing, Shanghai and Guangzhou may reach European and American levels, but those of other provinces and cities and some relatively poverty-stricken areas are not even close. The problems are particularly prominent in healthcare systems at the grassroots level.

For all, we are glad to see that the Communist Party of China (CPC) Central Committee and the State Council published the *Opinions on Intensifying the Reform of Healthcare Security System* on February 25, 2020. Regarding the coordinated advancement of the reform of the supply side of medical services, it clearly requires to improve the modern medical service system featured by division of labor and cooperation of general and specialized medical services, and enhance general medical services at the grassroots level. We believe that this is the most urgent task to make use of system advantages, support the community health service system, reasonably allocate and leverage resources, improve service functions, make full use of modern information technology, establish a big data-based resident health database, conduct online inquiry and remote diagnosis, and develop targeted and personalized services. We propose paying attention to and intensifying the training of talents in community medical institutions including the training of general practitioners, encouraging medical graduates and doctors to work in community health service centers, and effectively improving the treatment capacity and facilities of community hospitals to entitle residents to convenient and high-level community medical services, thus improving people's medical experience and well-being.

3　Focus on malnutrition and hidden hunger

According to the *Healthy China 2030 Planning Outline*, national health is the fundamental purpose of building a healthy China. It is required to focus on the whole population and the entire life cycle, and provide fair, accessible, systematic and continuous health services to achieve a higher level of national health. It is also required to cover the entire life cycle, and identify several priority areas and strengthen intervention based on the main health problems and main influence factors at different stages of life, thus achieving health services and health security covering the entire life circle, and comprehensively maintaining people's health. To achieve this, we believe that prevention of diseases should be more important than treatment, and the most effective way to prevent diseases is to improve people's immunity and nutrition. Therefore, we propose that following:

(1) Focus on nutrition and health intervention in infancy and of preschoolers

Foreign scientific research results show that maternal and infant nutrition during the first 1,000 days of life, i.e. from pregnancy to two years of age, affects the health of a person's whole life. Thus early nutrition intervention is a window period for improving health. Ministry of Health released the *Report on the Nutrition Development of Children Aged between 0 and 6 in China (2012)*, introduced to the public the development status of children's nutrition in China and arouse the attention and concern of the whole society to the problem of children's nutrition. the nutritional status of children is the most sensitive indicator of the measurement of the nutritional status of the whole population, as well as the basis of national health. Internationally, the nutritional status of children under the age of five is usually regarded as an important indicator of the social and economic development of a country, and is emphasized as an important issue related to the survival and development of human beings.

According to the *Implementation Plan for the Three-Year Action on Health and Poverty Alleviation* jointly formulated and issued by the National Health Commission and other units in 2018, China will implement a nutrition improvement program for children in poverty-stricken areas, and provide a nutrition package for each child aged 6-24 months free of charge every day to help infants realize optimal growth, development and health. Besides, with the economic and social development, we also need to pay attention to some nutrition issues for other children. For example, the nutritional status of vulnerable children such as migrant children and left-behind children desperately needs improvement. All these require the attention and support of various departments and the joint efforts of the whole society.

At present, China has a nutrition package intervention policy for children aged 6-24 months in poverty-stricken areas and a nutrition meal program for students receiving compulsory education above six years old in poverty-stricken areas. But China still lacks mature support policies for underprivileged children aged 3-5 years on the problem of malnutrition, and only some charity organizations are helping a limited number of children. We consider poverty alleviation to be important and extremely urgent, because malnutrition will not only lead to reduced GDP, but also cause intergenerational transmission in the population, resulting in a vicious circle from poverty to malnutrition and then to poverty again. Therefore, it is necessary to pay attention to preschoolers aged 3-5 years, and precisely intervene in the situation with better policies. Improving the nutrition and health of children in poverty-stricken areas is related to population quality, economic and social development, and international competitiveness of China in the future, and it is also a concrete action to implement the *Healthy China 2030 Planning Outline* and truly achieve the objectives in it.

(2) Focus on "hidden hunger" and improve national health

The WHO refers to undernutrition or nutritional imbalance as hidden hunger. Modern medicine found that 70% of chronic diseases include cardiovascular disease, diabetes, cancer, obesity and sub-health status are all related to the imbalanced intake of nutrient elements, and hidden hunger poses a great threat to human health. According to the *Report on the Status of Nutrition and Chronic*

Diseases of Chinese Residents prepared by National Health and Family Planning Commission in 2015, Chinese residents take in excessive fat, with the average energy supply ratio of dietary fat exceeding 30%. At the same time, a fairly large number of Chinese residents still lack such nutrients as calcium, iron, vitamin A and vitamin D. According to nutritionists, urban residents eat too much animal food, and some people don't eat staple food and eat less cereals for fear of getting fat. Say dominant hunger is caused by lack of nutrients such as energy, protein and fat, and can be solved by eating one's fill, then hidden hunger arises from imbalanced nutrition and lack of micronutrients, vitamins and minerals, which needs to be solved by eating right and well.

According to the *National Nutrition Plan (2017-2030)*, in recent years Chinese people have experienced continuously increased living standards, significantly enhanced nutrition supply capacity, and obviously improved nutrition and health, but there are still such problems as residents suffering from coexistence of inadequate and excessive nutrition and frequent occurrence of nutrition-related diseases, and non-popularized healthy lifestyles, which have become important factors affecting national health.

In view of this, we propose strengthening healthy diet education, advocating a reasonable and balanced diet and appropriate dietary supplements, comprehensively popularizing dietary nutrition knowledge, and guiding people to develop scientific dietary habits and a reasonable dietary structure. It is necessary to publicize and implement the strategies and actions of the *National Nutrition Plan (2017-2030)*, and advocate the concept of active prevention of diseases instead of passive treatment of them.

The promulgation of the *Healthy China 2030 Planning Outline* and the *National Nutrition Plan (2017-2030)* has made national nutrition and health a national policy. As the world's largest nutrition provider, Royal DSM N.V. , a global purpose-led, science-based company active in Nutrition, Health and Sustainable Living has been working closely with governments, international organizations and industry associations to facilitate nutrition improvement. DSM and The Chinese Nutrition Society jointly established the "Nutrition Research Fund of Chinese Nutrition Society—DSM Special Research Fund" with the sole purpose to advance the development of China's nutrition science and technology, provide scientific basis for the development of nutritious and healthy food, and improve people's health. Since DSM established a strategic partnership with UNWFP in 2007, we have leveraged our expertise in nutrition and food fortification to develop cost-effective, sustainable and nutritious food solutions for those in need, and contributed to the Sustainable Development Goals of the United Nations. DSM actively cooperates with government departments, non-governmental organizations and the private sector in China to implements sustainable nutrition improvement programs for the undernourished populations. For example, DSM has participated in the "Elimination of Infantile Anemia" project jointly conducted by All-China Women's Federation, Ministry of Health, and China Children and Teenagers' Fund, and the pilot project of "Social Equity—Early Childhood Development in Poverty-Stricken Areas" launched by China Development Research Foundation in Qinghai and Yunnan, providing comprehensive technical support and high-quality nutrition packages. DSM has also participated in the "Supporting 'Five'—Nutrition Improvement Program for Preschoolers" conducted by Amway Charity Foundation together with China Development Research Foundation, China Children and Teenagers' Fund and other organizations, which aims to help underprivileged children grow up healthily by distributing children's nutritional chewable tablets to children aged 3-5 years in poverty-stricken areas in China free of charge.

DSM hopes to work with China on nutrition improvement solutions, and safeguard the health and well-being of the Chinese people with our knowledge and expertise!

新冠肺炎疫情对制定企业传染性疾病应急预案的启示

徐　旸　陶氏化学[*]（中国）公共和政府事务总经理

新型冠状病毒肺炎疫情发生后，中国所有省区市立即采取了果断措施冻结人员流动以切断感染途径。其结果是，铁路和高速公路被关闭，或对非执行紧急防控任务的车辆和人员实施禁行；一些国家的边境关闭，对人、车辆、飞机和船舶实施特别检疫措施；春节假期延长；人们被要求在家里多待几周，复工返岗需要得到批准等。

企业主和企业必须在短时间内同时应对多重挑战：追踪员工的行踪以及他们的健康状况，采购防疫用品（例如口罩），为工作场所消毒，持续关注各级及不同地区政府出台的与日常运营相关的政策并及时做出反应，应对原料供应的突然中断、产品运输的中断和仓库爆仓，筹措慈善捐赠，接听员工、供应商和客户的电话咨询，确保 IT 设施能够容纳大量的远程工作，并保持公司的财务健康。

疫情发生时适逢春节长假，很多企业的管理人员身处不同的城市，甚至不同的时区。中小企业固然感受到经营中断的阵阵寒意，大型企业，尤其是那些在全国甚至跨国运营的企业，应对这些状况也并不轻松。

17 年前的"非典"给社会和经济造成重大损失。现在的许多企业在当时甚至还没有成立，加上当时中国经济结构没有今天这么复杂，全球供应

＊　陶氏化学是一家研制及生产系列化工产品的化学公司，成立于 1897 年，总部位于美国密歇根州米特兰。

特别感谢俞昕、蔡行益对本文的贡献。

链的相互依存度也远没有今天这么高。

疫情还未结束，许多企业家和企业已经开始复盘反思，是否原本可在疫情发生之前和期间做得更好。

危机的教训绝不应被浪费！如果企业以前没有传染性疾病疫情的应急预案，那么今后最好要制定一个。

一 为什么要制定企业传染性疾病应急预案

《中华人民共和国传染病防治法》第三十一条规定，"任何单位和个人发现感染或者疑似感染病例，应当向所在地的疾病预防控制中心或者医疗机构报告"。

该法律第四十二条规定："传染病发生或者流行时，当地政府应当立即组织力量控制，切断传播途径；必要时，可以采取下列紧急措施，但须报请上一级地方政府决定。

（一）限制或者停止集市、集会、影展、文艺演出等群众性集会活动。

（二）停工、停业、停课。

（三）……

（四）……

（五）关闭可能传播感染的场所。"

显然，公司在疫情发生时需承担一定的法律义务，并面临业务中断的风险。

疫情发生时公司会面临什么样的情况？

人力短缺：员工可能无法上班，他们可能被限制及时返岗、生病、必须照顾生病的家人和因为学校关闭而在家的孩子，甚至只是因为害怕。

商业模式的改变：在传染性病疫情发生期间，与防控相关的产品需求可能会大幅增加，而消费者对其他商品的需求可能会减少，消费者更倾向送货上门，而不是出门购物。

供应链中断：全球供应链的相互依赖很容易牵一发而动全身；武汉的一家零部件供应商因疫情停产可以导致韩国的整车厂不得不停下生产线；富士康的工人不能及时复工会导致苹果没有足够的产品销售。原材料和产品的运输可能会受到限制。

资产无法使用：办公室和工厂可能会因为员工感染被迫关闭，更不用说众多因为疫情而中断营业几周的餐馆、电影院、体育馆、商场和公园了。

新冠肺炎疫情也许只是个偶发事件，但流感和禽流感几乎每年都在世界不同地区发生，它们也可导致严重的疾病或死亡。据美国疾病控制与预防中心（Center for Disease Control and Prevention of the United States）的数据，自 2019 年下半年以来，美国至少有 1900 万人感染，1 万人死于流感。中国每年也有数以百万计的人感染流感，影响企业的生产力和医疗费用。做好传染性疾病的应急预案不仅可以帮助公司应对不确定性、保护员工、降低成本，使企业在疫情暴发时保持运转，而且还可以使它们比竞争对手更快摆脱疫情干扰，开展业务重建。

制定应急预案的思考过程本身也能帮助企业提升应对自然灾害和重大安全事故的能力。

案例（1）分享

陶氏公司的卫生服务团队负责监测全球的季节性和传染性疾病信息。2020 年 1 月 20 日，中央电视台报道称一种新型冠状病毒引发的肺炎能够在人与人之间传播，该团队立即向亚太危机管理团队发出了警报。

1 月 21 日，亚太地区和大中华区危机管理团队开会讨论形势。

1 月 22 日，公司要求所有的员工向主管和公司医生报告他们最近是否去过武汉，是否发烧。全球发布了禁止到武汉出差的通知（第二天禁止范围又扩大到湖北省全境）。公司内网开辟了新冠肺炎疫情的专栏，每天更新有关的科学知识和疫情发展状况。要求中国的所有分支机构和工厂复习传染病应急预案并检查准备情况。开放医疗热线回答员工的问题。

1月26日，亚太应急管理团队和大中华区应急管理团队开始每天召开联席电话会议，因为中国面临非常复杂的情况，需要更多内部支持。

由于整个组织的迅速和有效的反应，陶氏中国3200多名员工和他们的家人无一感染，包括在疫情期间身处湖北省的34名员工和他们的家人。

2月8日和9日，陶氏化学在中国的7家工厂均在所在地区第一批获得批准恢复生产，大部分工厂的复工方案兼顾生产和员工安全，获得地方政府的高度评价，成为"抄作业"的对象。

二 什么是企业传染性疾病应急预案

当一种新的流感病毒在人群中几乎或根本没有免疫力并开始引起严重疾病，然后在全世界范围内轻易地展开人际传播时，就会发生传染性疾病大暴发。传染性疾病大暴发可能对全球经济产生重大影响，包括差旅、贸易、旅游、食品、消费，并最终影响投资和金融市场。企业和行业对传染性疾病大暴发的应急预案对于最大限度地减轻传染性疾病大暴发影响至关重要。提供关键基础设施服务（如电力和电信）的企业还负有在危机中持续运营的特殊责任，并应据此制定方案。与任何灾难一样，制定应急预案至关重要。

在传染性疾病大暴发的情况下，雇主将在保护雇员健康和安全及减少对经济和社会影响方面发挥关键作用。雇主可能会经历员工缺勤、商业模式改变以及供应和交付计划中断等情况。适当的方案可使公共和私营部门雇主更好地保护其雇员，并减轻传染性疾病大暴发对社会和经济造成的影响。正如美国总统在《国家流感战略》所述，所有利益攸关方都必须做好计划和准备。①

"制定传染性疾病大暴发应急预案（PRCM）的目的是了解风险和可

---

① 美国职业安全与健康管理局：《工作场所应对流感大流行指南》。

能性，充分预测和降低潜在风险，并在传染性疾病大暴发时采取相应措施做出最佳反应。"①

虽然格式和具体内容可能因公司而异，但 PRCM 需要注意以下几点。

- 预案通常以准备、响应和缓解为核心
- 预案应该包括治理结构和决策树
- 应规定企业如何在员工不能到岗的持续期间内继续提供基本服务
- 该预案应详细说明如何将疾病在员工中传染风险最小化
- 该预案需要考虑对公司资产的潜在影响，包括有形资产和财务资产，以及来源、客户、供应商、股东和声誉
- 该预案应着眼于其价值链在极端压力下的可持续性
- 随着越来越多的业务操作是云计算或基于网络的，该方案应该涵盖 IT 基础设施的容量和远程服务功能
- 预案应评估防护装备的库存
- 预案应安排定期演习，使管理层和员工熟悉计划
- 预案应定期检讨和更新
- 预案应考虑其对社区影响

三 如何制定企业传染性疾病应急预案

制定企业传染性疾病应急预案应当首先收集当地政府和社区的应对方案，尤其当某个公司的业务是关键基础设施或关键资源的一部分的时候（如政府机关、电厂、市政水和废物处理、食品和农业、医药、银行、电信、交通、物流、快递服务等）。这些是公司在暴发疫情时所必须采取措施的最低要求，并可以为公司区分警示级别提供参考。与地方政府就当地规定和社区以对社会负责的态度进行对话是非常有必要的。

---

① 陶氏化学：《企业传染性疾病应急预案》。

强烈建议拥有国际办事处和分支机构的企业在制定预案时，阅读并熟悉对其业务有重大影响的国家和市场的传染病应急预案，并将合规要求体现在企业预案中。

中小企业的业务可能没有那么复杂，员工数量也没有大企业那么多，可能没有资源或必要制定一个庞大的预案，尽管如此，我们仍建议企业关注风险并定期检视其业务在极端情况下的耐受性。

外部信息收集齐备后，公司相关部门的决策者就可以开始实际撰写方案。这些部门通常包括人力资源、法律、信息技术、安全健康环保、物流、采购、财务和对外沟通。

对新冠肺炎疫情深刻记忆可以作为制定预案的假想场景。

根据有关政府机构和企业最佳实践，在此谨对具体编写提一些建议。

（一）分阶段方法

中国的突发事件应对体系有四个警示级别，其中最高级别为一级，世界卫生组织也有四个阶段的体系，包括传染性疾病暴发间隔、预警、大暴发和过渡阶段，这是根据世界面临的疾病类型和风险来定义的。

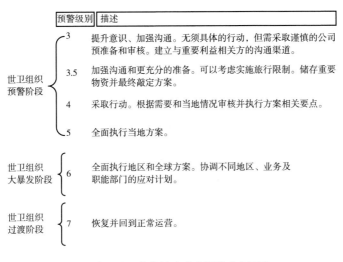

图　陶氏公司传染性疾病大暴发应急预案

公司的应急预案不一定一一对应中国国家的规定或世界卫生组织的级别定义。然而，使用该方案的经理人员需要清楚地了解公司自身的定义具体对应到政府和世卫组织的警示系统的哪一级别，以确保在情况发生变化时能够采取适当的行动。

（二）通过战略性提问方式决定在疫情每个阶段需要采取的行动

1. 与管理相关的问题

- 在疫情发生时期，企业的价值取向是什么？
- 谁应该是应急管理团队（CMT）的成员？
- 公司内部是否有卫生健康专业人员？如果没有，我们可以从哪里得到专业指导？
- 什么时候应该启动CMT？
- 在这个警示级别上，CMT应该多久召开一次会议并做出决定？
- 我们有在极端情况下保持CMT运转的技术方案吗？
- CMT如何了解最新发布的政府指令？

2. 与人员有关的问题

- 在当前情况下，员工面临的风险有多大？哪些工作有较高的暴露风险，可能需要加强防护？
- 我们应该为个人提供哪些培训？
- 在当前级别，我们需要改变差旅政策吗？
- 考虑到公司的日常运营，公司可以采取什么措施来保护工作场所的员工？
- 如果员工在工作中被发现感染，我们需要做什么？如果多名员工被感染呢？维持基本服务所需的最少人数是多少？基本服务包括哪些？
- 公司的关键岗位是哪些？如果主要人员不能履行职责，还能有什么替代方案？我们需要为外籍人士或关键岗位提供额外的保护吗？
- 每个员工的联系方式都是最新的吗？在疫情暴发期间，我们如何与每位员工保持联系？

- 我们需要对人力资源政策做出哪些调整，尤其是薪酬和休假政策？我们需要采用激励措施来鼓励人们冒险来上班吗？
- 我们还可以为员工提供哪些额外的支持？

3. 与工作场所和个人防护装备的供应相关的问题

- 政府的要求是什么？
- 我们是否需要在这个阶段重新安排办公室／工厂的功能？
- 我们应该考虑或限制哪些设施操作？
- 在当前级别，我们对于接待外部访客的规定是什么？
- 我们是否需要储存个人防护用品、装备、物料、食物或水？
- 我们知道这些物资是哪里生产的吗？ 如果我们的库存用完了，他们多快能发货给我们？ 我们附近有生产商吗？ 我们认识他们吗？

4. 与财务相关的问题

- 我们需要买灾害保险作为预防措施吗？
- 如果业务中断数周甚至数月，我们能做哪些来确保公司的财务健康？
- 在疫情暴发期间，我们如何有效地处理紧急支出？我们需要特殊的审批和付款流程吗？
- 我们往来的银行有应急预案吗？如果暴发大规模疫情，我们可以从他们那里得到哪些帮助？

5. 与信息技术相关的问题

- 可以容纳多少名员工进行远程办公？
- 我们需要增加额外的容量吗？如果是，在暴发期间是否可以使用？
- 如果没有，有哪些替代方案？
- 是否有必须在办公室处理的业务程序？我们可以将其数字化以进行远程操作吗？

6. 与供应链和物流相关的问题

- 我们对重要原材料的依赖程度有多大？

- 如果主要供应商受到疫情影响，他们是否制定了继续开展业务的应急计划？

- 我们还有其他选择吗？有供应商在我们附近吗？我们认识他们吗？

- 在什么情况下，我们需要开始加大库存以维持对客户的服务？

- 如果我们不能按正常水平生产，哪些客户需要优先服务？

- 我们有什么方法继续为客户提供产品和服务？

- 政府对物流运输有何限制？我们应如何应对？

7. 与沟通相关的问题

- 我们是否知道哪些外部信息对于 CMT 做出决定很重要？

- 我们是否有针对内部和外部利益相关者在不同情况下的沟通计划？

- 我们如何增强归属感和保持员工士气？

8. 与慈善和捐赠相关

- 我们需要在当前阶段捐款吗？现金还是物资？

- 我们和那些活跃的慈善组织有日常联系吗？

特别注意以下几点。

（1）草案完成后，请所有 CMT 成员审查方案以确保一致性，并进行律师审查，以确保企业的应对举措符合适用的法律和法规。

（2）在关键岗位上，至少需要准备三名或以上员工组成梯队，以维持业务运营，并确保每个人都了解在重大疫情暴发期间他们的责任。

（3）储备物资，例如肥皂、纸巾、洗手液、消毒剂、口罩、护目镜、手套和工业用防护服。"存储物资时，请注意每种产品的保质期和存储条件（例如避免放置在潮湿或温度极端的区域），并将物资定期更新（例如首先消耗保存时间最久的耗材）纳入库存管理程序。"[①]

（4）协助员工应对与疫情有关的额外压力，例如个人或家庭疾病，生活中断，失去家人、朋友或同事的悲伤以及生活脱离日常轨道。在疫情暴发期间，确保及时准确的沟通对于减少恐惧和担忧十分重要。

---

① 美国职业安全与健康管理局：《工作场所应对流感大流行指南》。

案例（2）分享

当整个湖北省被封闭时，陶氏化学（中国）投资有限公司的34名员工都在该省。

公司立刻成立了一个微信群，成员包括所有这些员工和陶氏亚太区总裁、大中华区总裁、人力资源总监、中国责任关怀负责人（也是中国CMT协调员）和企业卫生服务负责人。员工使用此微信群寻求有关公司政策和个人安全的问题答案，并建立一个临时的互助小组。

在公司层面，卫生服务部为员工组织了两次网络研讨会，帮助他们了解有关冠状病毒的最新可靠信息，并在困难时期管理压力。

很多公司会进行慈善捐赠。捐赠在回馈社会的同时也可以极大地鼓舞员工士气。除了现金和物资外，也可以考虑其他的捐赠方式，例如提供免费服务和志愿者服务等。由于疫情通常会持续较长时间，因此也可以考虑根据在不同阶段对遭受疫情影响的不同人群进行多批次捐赠。尽管医院和医务人员一般是关注的焦点，但面向当地社区和志愿者的援助也会产生很好的社会效益。

案例（3）分享

在COVID-19暴发期间，陶氏化学（中国）投资有限公司进行了三批捐赠，其中一笔是现金，两笔是实物。

1月29日，陶氏化学通过壹基金捐款100万元用于购买医疗用品。之所以选择壹基金，是因为它与湖北省当地的志愿者团体有着密切的联系，可以确保在交通运输面临巨大挑战的时候准时将物品运送到医院。

2月19日，在得知咸宁市确诊病例突增后，陶氏第二批捐赠的60吨消毒剂被运往鲜有人关注的咸宁市。

第三批捐赠的2000瓶洗手液被捐赠给了武汉和孝感的8个志愿者团

体以及 1 家医院。这些志愿者战斗在第一线，他们用自己的汽车和电瓶车为老年人和病人购买物资，运载医务人员上下班，并维持社区的运转。他们只能依靠私人捐助者提供所需的大部分物资。

目前，我们正在考虑第四批捐赠，将优先考虑与恢复和重建相关的项目。

（三）培训，演练和定期更新

预案完成后，需要针对 CMT、公司职能部门和企业分支机构进行培训，使相关人员熟悉预案并在疫情暴发时能够采取相应的行动。公司对每个员工的要求也应分发给每个人，并组织培训，增强意识。

针对 CMT 或关键领导者的定期沙盘演练也是一种有效的工具，可以帮助人们加深记忆、内化方案并发现预案中的缺漏。

沙盘演练通常根据预案中不同的警示级别来设定场景，并要求参加人员讨论在各场景下公司需要采取什么措施以应对形势的升级。记录是演练的重要一环，它将帮助 CMT 利用讨论中出现的好想法来进一步完善方案。

还可以按照方案中一小部分场景进行临时检查，以测试响应能力。以下是在临时检查中可以测试的一些项目（不仅限于此）。

①验证关键岗位。

②测试关键岗位人员远程办公的网络和设备。

③测试并确认应对工具、设备的维护情况，例如体温测量设备和个人防护设备。

④检查现有卫生防疫措施，建议至少每年对方案进行检讨和更新。

俗话说，未雨绸缪。在艰难的 2020 年春季，中国公司表现出非凡的应变能力和创造力。通过回顾、反思和展望，一家优秀的公司才有可能成为一家伟大的公司。

What COVID-19 Tells about Corporate Pandemic Preparedness

By Gloria Xu, General Manager of Publice Government Affairs of Dow Chemical (China) Co., Ltd.

The outbreak of COVID-19 starting December 2019 caught the business world by whirl winds.

Within less than a week, the government in all provinces of China elevated the response to Level 1 and imposed immediate and resolute measures to cut off the routes of infection by freezing the movement of people.

As a result, railroads and highways were totally shut down or partially denied access to passengers and vehicles not on relief duties; borders were closed and travels were restricted; quarantine requirements were announced applying to people, vehicles, airplanes and ships; the Chinese New Year holiday was extended; people were asked to stay at home for extra weeks and returning to work required permission.

Business owners and companies had to grapple with many challenges all at once within a very short window: tracking the whereabout of employees and their health conditions, sourcing protective gears (i.e. masks) for employees, disinfecting the work place, monitoring the policy announcements of government at different levels and different geographies relevant to daily operations while reacting to them, navigating the sudden outage of feedstock supplies, disruption of product shipment and shortage of warehouse, making decisions on relief donations, answering calls of employees, suppliers and customers, ensuring IT capacity can host large portion of employees working remotely, and maintaining the financial strength of the company.

And bigger portion of those actions needed to be taken during holiday when management might be in different locations and even different time zones. While SMEs felt the chill of business continuity, large enterprises, especially those with national or even global footprints, did not trudge through easily as well.

It was 17 years ago when the last epidemic claimed its tolls. Many companies were not even existing at the time, not to mention the economy of China and its interconnectedness with the global supply chain were not as sophisticated.

Many business owners and companies will be reflecting, hopefully, whether they could have done better and more before and during the crisis.

A crisis should never be wasted! It is time for company to think about keeping a Pandemic Plan if you have not got one.

1   Why to develop a corporate pandemic plan

Article 31 of the "The Law of the People's Republic of China on the Treatment of Diseases" stipulates that "any unit or individual should report to local Center for Disease Control or medical institutions when they identify an infection or suspected infection case".

Article 42 of the same law says that "in the event of an outbreak or a prevalence of an infectious disease, the local government shall immediately get people organized to control them and cut off the route of transmission; when necessary, it may take the following emergency measures, subject to reporting to and decision by the local government at the next higher level:

(1) restricting or suspending fairs, assemblies, cinema shows, theatrical performances and other types of mass congregation;

(2) suspension of work, business and school classes;

(3) …

(4) ...

(5) close down premises which may spread the infection

Clearly, there are both legal obligations and business continuity risks if a company does not do the right thing when an outbreak happens.

Companies may experience

- Manpower shortage - Employees may not come to work because they are restricted to return to work locations in time, sick, must care for sick family members or for children if schools are closed, are just afraid.
- Change in patterns of commerce - During a pandemic, consumer demand for items related to infection control is likely to increase dramatically, while consumer interest in other goods may decline. Consumers will prefer home delivery services to going shopping in person.
- Supply Chain disruption - The interconnectedness of global supply chain easily makes the pain of others felt by all players. A car factory in South Korea had to suspend production because a component supplier's factory is Wuhan. Apple did not have enough to sell because Foxconn did not have enough people on the production lines. Shipment of raw materials and products may be restricted.
- Asset shut-down – Offices and factories may be forced to be closed because people are infected, not to mention the closure of numerous restaurants, cinemas, gyms, retail stores and parks for months.

COVID-19 may be a rare incidence, but influenza and avian flu, which can also cause severe illness to fatality, happen almost every year in different parts of the world. At least 10000 people died from influenza since second half in the US in 2019 while 19 million people were infected, according to the Center for Disease Control and Prevention of the United States. Millions of people in China contract flu every year, which result in loss of productivity and spike of healthcare bills in the minimum. Being better in pandemic preparedness not only can help companies deal with the uncertainties, protect employees, minimize costs and keep businesses going in an outbreak but also enable them to come out faster than competition and be stronger moving forward.

The exercise is also an excellent thinking process useful at times of natural disasters and major operational accidents.

Case Sharing I

The Health Services team of Dow Inc. has responsibilities to monitor seasonal and contagious disease information around the world. Upon CCTV report that a new type of pneumonia was able to transmit from people to people on Jan 20th, the team alerted Asia Pacific Crisis Management Team immediately.

On Jan 21st, the Asia Pacific and Greater China Crisis Management teams met to discuss situation.

On Jan 22nd, all employees were asked to report to their supervisors and medical focal point if they had recently travelled to Wuhan or if they were having fever. A global travel ban to Wuhan was announced, which was expanded to Hubei in the following day. All available information about the virus and scientific advice was published on intranet. All offices and plants in China were asked to review their respective pandemic plans and check preparedness. Medical hotline was open to answer questions of employees.

On Jan 26th, AP CMT and Greater China CMT started to have daily conference calls as the scale of response in China needed many resources to support.

Thanks to the immediate and effective response of the whole organization, all the over 3200 Dow China employees and their family members are safe from the virus, including 34 people and their families who were in Hubei Province during the outbreak.

Dow's 7 factories in China returned to work on Feb 8th and 9th with many of them praised by local governments as example in maintaining productivity while keeping employees safe.

2 What is corporate pandemic plan

"A pandemic is a global disease outbreak. A pandemic occurs when a new influenza virus emerges for which there is little or no immunity in the human population, begins to cause serious illness and then spreads easily person-to-person worldwide. A worldwide pandemic could have a major effect on the global economy, including travel, trade, tourism, food, consumption and eventually, investment and financial markets. Planning for pandemic by business and industry is essential to minimize a pandemic's impact. Companies that provide critical infrastructure services, such as power and telecommunications, also have a special responsibility to plan for continued operation in a crisis and should plan accordingly. As with any catastrophe, having a contingency plan is essential.

In the event of a pandemic, employers will play a key role in protecting employees' health and safety as well as in limiting the impact on the economy and society. Employers will likely experience employee absences, changes in patterns of commerce and interrupted supply and delivery schedules. Proper planning will allow employers in the public and private sectors to better protect their employees and lessen the impact of a pandemic on society and the economy. As stated in the President's *National Strategy for Pandemic Influenza*, all stakeholders must plan and be prepared". [1]

"A Corporate Pandemic Response Crisis Management (PRCM) Plan is developed to understand the risks and possible scenarios, adequately anticipate and mitigate potential risk, and if a pandemic occurs; to be prepared to react optimally." [2]

While the format and the exact content might vary from company to

---

[1] OSHA, *Guidance on Preparing Workplaces for an Influenza Pandemic*.

[2] Dow Corporate Pandemic Response Crisis Management Plan.

company, here are a few things a PRCM needs to take care of:

- The plan usually is centered on preparedness, response and mitigation.
- The plan should include governance structure and decision tree
- A pandemic plan should lay out how a business will continue to provide essential services through a sustained period with significant employee absenteeism.
- The plan should specify measures how the business will minimize the risk of contagion among employees.
- The plan needs to look at the potential to impact the company's assets including physical and financial assets and sources, customers, suppliers, stockholders and reputation.
- The plan should look at the sustainability of its value chain under extreme pressure
- As more and more business operations are now cloud or web-based, the plan should cover capacity of IT infrastructure and remote capability
- The plan should evaluate the stockpile of protective gears
- Regular drills should be arranged to familiarize management and employees with the plan
- The plan should be reviewed and updated regularly
- The plan should consider its impact on the community

3   How to develop a corporate pandemic plan

A Corporate Pandemic Plan should always start by collecting information on the plans of the local government and communities, particularly when a company's business is part of critical infrastructure or key resources *(government offices, power plants, municipal water and waste treatment, food and agriculture, pharmaceuticals, banks, telecommunications, transportation and logistics, delivery services),* which provides an understanding of the minimum a company needs to do in the event of an outbreak and good reference measures a company needs to take at different levels of alert.

Conversations with local authorities on requirements and the community in a socially responsible manner are always helpful.

It is highly recommended that companies with international offices/branches to review the pandemic plans of countries and markets where they have big stakes and take those into account when developing an integrated corporate plan which meets different regulatory requirements.

Small and medium-sized enterprises with much less sophisticated operations and amount of employees than big corporations may not have the resources or need to have a complicated pan, though it is recommended for business owners to be mindful of the risks and periodically review the resilience of the business under difficult circumstances.

With the external information ready, the actual writing of the plan can be kicked off by decision-makers from relevant parts of the company, which typically should include human resources, legal, IT, SHE, logistics, sourcing, finance and communications.

Vivid memories of COVID-19 may serve as a hypothetical scenario to craft the plan.

The following is a playbook based on recommendations of government agencies and industry best practice.

- Phased approach

The Chinese emergency response system has 4 alert levels with 1 as the highest while the World Health Organization also has a 4-phase system, including interpandemic, alert, pandemic and transition, which are defined based on disease type and risks the world faces.

A Corporate Pandemic Plan does not have to exactly follow the level protocols in the Chinese regulation or WHO's system. However, managers who will be using the plan need to have a clear picture how the company's own structure fits into the government and WHO systems so as to ensure proper

	Alert Level	Description
WHO Alert Phase	3	Heightened awareness and communications.Specific actions are not necessary, but prudent company preplanning and reviews should occur. Regular communications between key stakeholders should be established.
	3.5	Increased communications and advanced preparations. Travel restrictions may be considered. Assemble critical supplies and finalize plans.
	4	Actions are required. Review and implement elements of the plan as appropriate and as the local situation dictates.
	5	Full implementation of the local plans.
WHO Pandemic Phase	6	Full implementation of regional and global plans.Coordination of response plans across geographies,businesses,functions.
WHO Transition Phase	7	Recovery and return to normal operations.

Figure   Dow Corporate Pandemic Plan

actions can be taken when situations change.

- Using these strategic questions to identify the actions needed at each phase of the outbreak

  ○ Management-related

    What are the corporate core values to adhere during time of crisis?

    Who should be members of the Crisis Management Team (CMT)?

    Do we have expertise within the company to provide professional advice on human health? If not, where can we get the expertise?

    When should the CMT be activated?

    How frequently should the CMT meet and make decisions at this level?

    Do we have the technology keep the CMT functioning under extreme circumstances?

    How CMT is kept updated about newly released gov't requirement?

  ○ People-related

    How much risk are employees exposed to at this level? Which are some of the work with higher risk of exposure and may need enhanced protection?

    What trainings shall we provide to individuals?

Do we need to change travel policy at this level?

What are the measures the company can take to protect the work force in the workplace, taking into consideration all the routine activities every day?

What do we need to do if an employee is found infected at work? What about multiple employees? What is the minimum number of people we need to maintain basic services? What are the basic services?

Which are the key roles in the company? What is the alternative if a key person cannot perform the duty? Do we need to provide extra protection to the expats or key people?

Is the contact information of each employee up-to-dated? How do we keep each employee connected during an outbreak?

What adjustments might we need to make to the Human Resources policy at this level, particularly pay and leave? Do we need incentives to encourage people to take the risk of coming to work?

What extra support can we provide to employees?

○ Facility and PPE (Personal Protective Equipment) supply-related

What are the requirements of government?

Do we need to re-arrange functions of office/plant at this stage?

What facility operations shall we consider or restrict?

What is our policy about external visitors at this level?

Do we need to stockpile PPEs, equipment, materials, food or water?

Do we know who the producers are and how fast can they ship the products to us if we run out of inventory? Is there anyone who is in our neighborhood? Do we know them?

○ Finance related

Shall we buy a disaster insurance as a pre-emptive measure?

What can we do to ensure the financial health of the company if businesses are cut off for weeks or even months?

How efficient can we handle urgent expenditures during an outbreak? Do we need a special approval and payment process?

What are the emergency response plans of the banks we deal with? What kind of help can we get from them if there is a major outbreak?

- ○ IT related

  How many office employees can we accommodate to work remotely?

  Do we need extra capacity? If yes, is that available during an outbreak? If not, what are the alternatives?

  Are there essential business procedures which need to be performed physically in office? Can we digitize it for remote access?

- ○ Supply chain and logistics related

  What is the dependency level of important raw materials?

  Do our key suppliers have a contingency plan to continue business if they are affected by the outbreak?

  Do we have alternatives? Are there suppliers close to us? Do we know them?

  What are the key indicators for us to start to build inventory to continue to serve customers?

  Do we have proper prioritization of customers if we cannot produce at normal levels?

  What means do we have to be able to deliver products and services to customers?

  What are the government's restrictions affecting logistics capabilities?

- ○ Communications related

  Do we know what external information is important for the CMT to make decisions?

  Do we have a crisis communication plan for internal and external stakeholders on different scenarios things go wrong?

  How do we strengthen the sense of belonging and keep the morale of employees?

○ Charity related

Shall we make a charity donation at this level? Cash or products?

Do we know the charity organizations which usually are active at a time like this?

- Useful tips
  ○ Once the draft is completed, have all CMT members review the details to ensure consistency and have Legal review whether the measures are compliant with the applicable laws and regulations.
  ○ On critical roles, prepare to three or more employees to be able to sustain business-necessary functions and operations, and communicate the expectation for available employees to perform these functions if needed during a pandemic.
  ○ Stockpile items such as soap, tissue, hand sanitizer, disinfectants, masks, goggles, gloves and industrial coveralls. "When stockpiling items, be aware of each product's shelf life and storage conditions (e.g., avoid areas that are damp or have temperature extremes) and incorporate product rotation (e.g., consume oldest supplies first) into your stockpile management program." [1]
  ○ Assist employees in managing additional stress related to the pandemic, such as personal or family illness, life disruption, grief related to loss of family, friends or coworkers and loss of routine support systems. Assuring timely and accurate communication will also be important throughout the duration of the pandemic in decreasing fear or worry.

Case Sharing II

When the whole of Hubei Province was locked down 34 employees of the Dow Chemical (China) Investment Ltd were in the province.

---

[1]　OSHA, *Guidance on Preparing Workplaces for an Influenza Pandemic*.

A WeChat group was formed, which included all these employees, the Dow Asia Pacific President, Greater China President, HR Director, China Responsible Care Leader (also China CMT coordinator) and the corporate Health Service Leader. Employees used this WeChat group to seek answers to their questions about company policies and personal safety tips, as well as building a temporary community of mutual support.

At the corporate level, the Health Services organized two webinars for employees on the latest credible information on Coronavirus and managing stress during difficult times.

- Many companies will make donations to relief efforts to return to the society. These donations can also enormously energize the employees. In addition to cash and products, there are other ways to contribute, such as services and volunteering. And as a pandemic is always prolonged, companies many think of making multiple batches of donations according to the needs of different group of people hit by the outbreak at different stages. While hospitals and medical workers are at the center of attention, allocation of some aids to local communities and volunteers can also make a big difference.

Case Sharing III

During the COVID-19 outbreak, Dow Chemical (China) Investment Ltd has made three batches of donations, 1 in cash and 2 in products.

The initial cash donation of RMB1 million was made via One Foundation on Jan 29th to buy medical supplies. One Foundation was chosen because of their strong connection with local volunteer groups in Hubei Province, which can make sure the goods could be delivered to the hospitals on time at a time when transportation was a huge challenge.

The 2nd batch of donation of 60 tons of disinfectants was given to Xianing, a less well-known city out of the radar of many donors on Feb 19th, after knowing that the city just had a spike of confirmed cases.

The 3rd batch of donation of 2,000 bottles of hand sanitizers was mainly sent to 8 volunteer groups plus 1 hospital in Wuhan and Xiaogan. Those volunteers were the people in the front line who used their own cars and scooters to buy supplies for elderly and sick people, drive medical staff to and from work and keep communities running. They relied on private donors to supply most of what they needed.

A 4th batch of donation is being considered now and very likely will be invested in recovery related projects.

Training, drills and regular updates

Once the Plan is completed, there need to be training sessions for the CMT, functions and local branches of the company to familiarize them with the plan and what actions different people in the organization are supposed to take when there is an outbreak. Requirements for individual employees should also be disseminated to everyone and awareness trainings organized.

Regular table-top drill with CMT or key leaders is an effective tool to refresh memory, and help people internalize the plan and identify the gaps in the plan.

A table-top drill typically unfolds scenarios based on the different alert levels in the Corporate Pandemic Plan and asks people to discuss what the actions the company needs to take in response as situation escalates. Note-taking is an important part of the drill, which will help the CMT update the plan with the good ideas emerged in the discussions.

A Field test can be a simple hypothetical run through of a small part of the plan to test response. Following are some activities (but not limited to) that can be done during a field test:

- Verify the critical roles
- Test connectivity of critical workers who will be assigned to work from home/

remotely

- Test and confirm the readiness of tools/equipment for Pandemic response such as body temperature measurement equipment and PPE
- Check the existing hygiene practices of the facility

It is recommended that the Plan at least should be reviewed and updated annually.

As the old saying goes, do not have thy cloak to make when it begins to rain. Chinese companies have demonstrated extraordinary resilience and creativity in the difficult Spring of 2020. There is chance for a good company to become a great company by looking forward via looking back.

应急响应机制与经验及对中国企业的借鉴意义

力拓集团*（中国）投资有限公司

新型冠状病毒肺炎疫情暴发以来，数百万人的生命和健康受到了严重威胁。在中国政府的坚强领导、中国人民的团结一致，以及国际社会的慷慨支持下，中国采取了前所未有的公共卫生应对措施。中国－世界卫生组织联合专家组认为，这些措施在阻断病毒的人际传播方面取得了显著成效，为保护国际社会发挥了至关重要的作用，并为各国采取积极的防控措施争取了宝贵时间，也提供了值得借鉴的经验。习近平总书记已经指出，当前已初步呈现疫情防控形势持续向好、生产生活秩序加快恢复的态势；加强疫情防控必须慎终如始，对疫情的警惕性不能降低，防控要求不能降低；同时，要抓紧推进经济社会发展各项工作，精准有序扎实推动复工复产，把疫情造成的损失降到最低。

力拓集团作为国际领先的矿业公司，一直是采矿及金属领域的开拓者，目前在 6 大洲超过 35 个国家和地区拥有 47500 名员工。疫情发生后，力拓在第一时间向中国合作伙伴致以深切慰问，并向中国红十字基金会捐赠 100 万美元，以支持中国抗击新型冠状病毒肺炎疫情。捐赠款项将用于采购负压救护车、口罩、防护服等急需的医疗物资。力拓也与中国合作伙伴保持密切沟通，希望能发挥全球资源网络优势，提供其他切实可行的支援。力拓还拥有独特且经过实践多次检验的应急响应机制和抗击疫情

＊　力拓集团（Rio Tinto Group），西班牙文"Rio Tinto"意思是红色的河流。1873 年成立于西班牙，集团总部在英国，全球最具影响力的矿业公司之一，也被称为铁矿石三巨头之一。

的丰富经验，可以为正在努力防控疫情和积极复工复产两线作战的中国企业提供一定的借鉴。

一　力拓集团的应急响应机制

力拓集团位于世界各地的办事处和运营项目每天都会面临各种各样的风险，这些风险对日常经营构成一定威胁。力拓应急准备工作的基础，是名为"企业应急和恢复方案"（Business Resilience and Recovery Programme，以下简称"应急恢复方案"）的集团治理框架。它是我们健康、安全与环境管理体系的重要组成部分，覆盖力拓的每一个运营项目和办事处。

实施该"应急恢复方案"将涉及若干关键环节。首先，运营单位必须了解自身风险状况，制定简单而有针对性的"企业应急管理计划"（Business Resilience Management Plan，以下简称"应急管理计划"）。"应急管理计划"涵盖应急响应、企业应急（或危机）响应、业务连续性、复工安排等事宜。规划控制和实施的规模要参考运营单位的具体情况和风险状况。

应急管理计划主要包括以下内容。

①目的或背景说明（以管理可能影响力拓特定地区业务的事件）。

②应急恢复方案涉及的范围（方案将覆盖哪些运营单位）。

③应急管理计划中的术语定义和简称。

④应急响应小组（Business Resilience Team，BRT）的启动和管理（如何通知小组成员启动应急响应工作，在哪里启动响应，以及在哪里设立应急响应中心）。

⑤报告（应急响应小组工作启动后，发送企业内部通知）。

⑥事件分类（重大事故或灾难事件升级，或移交另一支应急响应小组管理）。

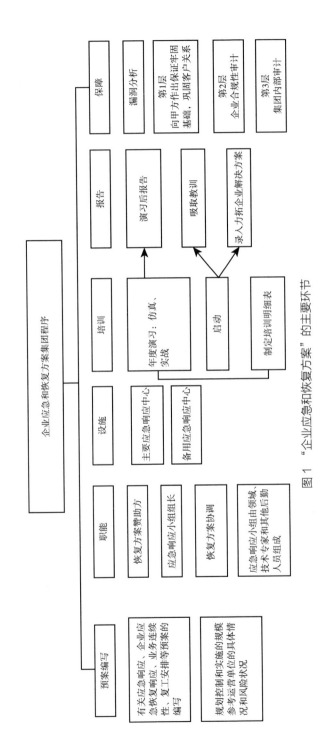

图 1 "企业应急和恢复方案"的主要环节

⑦突发情况设想（可能会对运营单位造成影响的事件类型），主要包括违规行为、与主要利益相关方的关系恶化、人员被合法拘留、人员失踪、人员受到暴力／人质劫持威胁、恐怖主义／炸弹威胁、火灾／爆炸、建筑物人员疏散、建筑物出入口封闭或阻断、商务旅行、医疗紧急事件／死亡、大流行病、自然灾害、恶劣天气／台风／洪水，以及关键信息技术基础设施故障。

⑧应急响应小组的职能和责任。

⑨业务影响评估和业务连续性安排。

⑩实用文档（例如事件日志、情况报告、利益相关方分析图等）。

⑪版本控制。

通常而言，所在地办公室的应急响应小组设有以下几类主要和辅助职能。

（1）应急响应小组组长：总体责任人，负责提供并接收简报，提供战

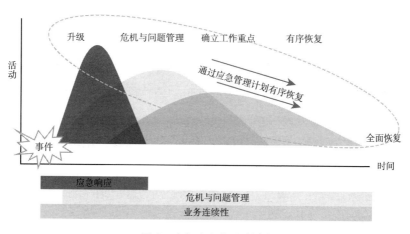

图2　应急响应典型时间线

略指导，管理与利益相关方的关系，授权内部和外部沟通。

（2）应急恢复方案协调员：根据应急响应小组组长的要求快速调动组员，管理工作流程、资源配置和各方协调；为应急响应中心提供物资装备；安排培训和演习，支持保障工作，报告应急响应小组的启动情况，并要及时更新应急管理计划。

（3）财务协调员：管理财务和保险事宜，与客户和供应商保持适当联络。

（4）外部事务和沟通协调员：发现支持应急响应工作所需的沟通渠道，提供清晰一致的即时信息，就内部和外部信息与应急响应小组组长保持沟通，确保员工了解最新情况。

（5）人力资源协调员：通过人力资源和紧急联络信息寻找并查明员工的下落；监测伤亡和失踪人员的详细情况；与对外事务和法律部门保持联络；协助员工家属，包括安排相关出行等；为员工及其家属心理援助服务做好安排。

（6）法律协调员：发现法律问题并为企业提供法律咨询：①确立调查的法律保密特权；②聘用外部律师；③收集并保留证据，如证人证词等；④就民事和刑事风险提供法律咨询；⑤应对监管机构要求我方提供文件、约谈我方人员的事宜。

（7）健康、安全与环境协调员：确保员工安全与保障；发现并管理各项设施面临的任何健康、安全与环境隐患或风险；提供事件和响应工作对健康、安全与环境领域影响的战略概述；与法务等相关部门合作，配合进行全面调查。

（8）设施协调员：负责根据需要寻找外部安置场所，在事件发生期间与该建筑的物业管理部门联络。

（9）业务连续性协调员：一旦建筑物遭损毁，总结产品／辅助集团业务的关键职能和依存关系。

（10）信息技术协调员：负责尽量减轻事件对信息网络硬件、应用软件、系统存储的信息所造成的冲击。

（11）信息系统和技术支持：在启动应急响应期间为应急响应中心提供技术支持。

（12）应急响应支持小组组长：发现并培养可以在突发事件中担任助手、通信员、勤务员的员工；在启动应急响应期间领导支助小组；协助建立应急响应中心；支持应急恢复方案协调员启动应急响应小组。

（13）应急响应支持小组：在启动应急响应期间提供支持。其人员和职能包括：日志管理员、助理日志管理员、更新 3IA 动态板、提交情况报告、计时员、汇总伤亡情况、绘制利益相关方分析图。

各小组不应该低估所需支持的规模。虽然应急响应很大程度上被认为是高管和技术专家的专长，但具备行政、组织或业务优化技能并熟悉业务本身的人才，其实非常适合在企业应急响应团队中担任关键的协调角色。正是这些角色为企业增加了真正的价值。

为提升应急团队的能力，培训是不可或缺的。培训可以有多种形式，例如展开课堂教学、个人辅导或在线培训。力拓集团应急响应小组每年至少举行一次应急响应演习。演习的目的是演练应急响应小组对于某个预先设定的突发事件的反应能力。例如：

①预演应急响应小组的响应情况。

②验证应急响应小组结构的有效性。

③在模拟环境下启动应急响应支持小组。

④测试应急响应中心的功能完备性。

⑤满足企业对一年开展一次演习的要求。

在实战压力下定期进行小组和系统演习，是演练实践和内化流程的最佳方式。这些流程包括确立常设议程、简报周期、事件日志、行动记录，绘制利益相关方分析图，制定内部和外部沟通策略等。

应急响应小组组长负责决定是否需要启动应急响应机制。应急响应小组可以借助"3IA"评估程序，来做出明智的决定。首先，要确定、组织、鉴别现有的信息（information）。然后查明并分析从所得信息中发现或剔除的问题（issue）。其次，要根据以往的经验、技巧和判断，集思广益（idea），克服或解决问题。最后，小组根据切实可行的目标展开行动（action）。所有行动都必须指定负责人和最后完成期限。

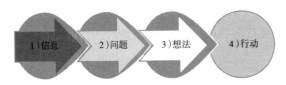

在应急响应中心设立 3IA 动态板（活页挂图），并由应急响应支持小组补充/更新相关信息。

图 3　力拓集团 31A 动态板

"PEAR"排序法，或可译作"梨式排序法"，是应急响应小组判定工作优先次序的基本指导原则。实际上"PEAR"一词是由四个单词的首字母组成的缩略词。

①人员（People）：人员的安全和福祉是重中之重。

②环境（Environment）：保护、维护并恢复环境。

③资产（Assets）：保护所有资产和财产。

④声誉（Reputation）：保护声誉，并在可能的情况下提高声誉。

二　力拓集团防控新冠肺炎疫情的做法和经验

2020 年 1 月中旬，中国感染新冠肺炎病毒的人数不断攀升，中国国内和国际社会都对此表示高度关切。力拓中国管理团队及时了解相关信息，开始密切监测疫情发展，同时要求应急响应小组成员随时待命，准备视情启动应急响应机制。力拓中国于 1 月 20 日开始正式建立疫情日报制度，与集团健康安全环保（HSE）团队和应急响应团队保持密切沟通，评估疫情发展趋势及影响，春节假期期间亦未暂停。中国管理团队还在第一时间向全球采购团队寻求支持并在全球范围内寻找可靠的防护用品采购渠道。由于日常的规划、培训和演习，应急响应小组分工明确，责任落实到位，关键利益相关方的联系信息也已更新至最新，已做好了随时启动的准备。

随着中国感染人数急剧增加，中国政府对湖北、武汉人员流动实行了管制措施。力拓进一步意识到疫情的严峻性，集团和全球各地区办公室相继成立应急响应小组，启动紧急情况响应机制。力拓中国在春节假期后第一天，即2月3日正式启动力拓中国应急响应小组。力拓始终秉持将员工的健康与安全放在首位的原则。应急响应小组迅速展开工作，定期举行应急响应小组会议，制定了强有力的对内对外沟通策略，包括向集团执行委员会和全球其他已启动的应急响应小组发送情况报告（Situation Report），部署办公室全面防控措施。北京和上海办公室实行了严格的出入筛查制度，并积极响应中国政府号召，鼓励员工远程办公，启动弹性工作模式；暂停所有不必要的国际、国内差旅；强化办公室消毒杀菌工作，加强员工卫生防护，减少社交接触；保持与员工的定期沟通，了解员工所关注的核心问题并予以及时解答，定期向员工通报疫情防控最新情况，并要求员工及时反馈健康状况和所在地；充分体现人文关怀，倾听员工的真实关切，为员工提供在线心理及健康咨询，聘请驻场医生提供办公室现场医疗服务；并制定全面的复工保障措施等。此外，我们也积极与当地公共卫生部门及写字楼物业管理部门协调，为可能出现确诊或疑似病例的情况做好应对预案。

在梳理防控工作所面临的关键问题和挑战时，应急响应小组发现公司口罩储备不足，员工复工时缺乏必要的防护。由于中国国内口罩库存告急，应急响应小组在采购团队的协助下，充分发挥其资源网络优势在全球范围内采购口罩，并确保口罩及时从海外各地寄到中国，使口罩短缺问题得到有效缓解。收到口罩后，应急响应小组及时将口罩分批快递至员工家中，解决其燃眉之急，确保员工的健康及安全得到保障，减轻员工对复工的思想压力，帮助员工顺利返岗。

总之，力拓中国通过每年培训和实战演习，定期审核并更新应急管理计划，并与力拓集团安全与企业应急响应专家保持紧密联系，力拓中国应急响应小组迅速而有序地开展行动，有效应对新冠肺炎疫情给公司员工和业务所带来的挑战。截至目前，力拓上海和北京办公室已经重新开放，尚未发生员工感染。应急响应小组将继续密切关注疫情动向，一旦疫情出现反复，将采取进一步的防控措施，例如，调整工作安排，提高办公场地消毒杀菌的频率，延长"避免非必要差旅"政策，以及加强对员工的人文关怀等。

三 对中国企业防控疫情的建议

疫情期间，力拓集团还积极为中方合作伙伴提供力所能及的帮助，比如向位于疫区核心的企业捐赠口罩用于生产防护、提供海外防护装备供应商联系方式等。同时，通过总结自身应急响应机制的实践以及之前成功应对埃博拉疫情的经验，力拓提出以下建议供中国企业借鉴或参考。

（1）中国企业应在集团层面上建立或更新一套全面、可操作、可报告、可衡量的应急响应机制，这其中应该包括应对疫情等多种突发情况的计划，并将责任落实到具体个人。为了做出合理的应急响应，每个地区分支机构都应该制定独立的应急管理计划，以符合当地政府或风险防控要求，并将地方触发信号和应对行动灵活纳入其中。集团还应支持和组织每个地区分支机构开展年度应急响应演习，并将演习成绩纳入对分支机构的业绩考核当中。

（2）应对疫情的计划应该作为应急响应机制的重要组成部分。在制定过程中，应该遵循预防、准备、应对和恢复的原则，并树立"合理响应"和"沟通协商"两大核心。

（3）中国公司在制定疫情应急响应计划时，应该提前纳入企业的战略目标。

①将传染率、发病率和死亡率降到最低。

②将医疗团队和系统的负担降到最低。

③通知员工最新进展情况，让员工参与进来，并为他们赋权。

（4）应急响应计划制定完成后，应该开展实战演习。通过不断演习，公司可以找出计划的漏洞，提高响应能力，并确保应急响应小组成员深入了解应急响应流程、熟练掌握计划的最新变化。为保证应急响应计划与时俱进，最好的办法就是演习，演习，再演习！

（5）中国企业应考虑建立并执行内部的旅行限制和隔离措施，以便先人一步掌握防控疫情的主动权。制定相关政策时，应严格依照风险水平进行管理，同时考虑到科学证据、道德和人文关怀、国际权利、国际机构的建议以及当地政府的建议（仅限地方分支机构）。

（6）中国企业应在疫情防控期间，随时关注国内外可靠的官方信源，从而更客观、准确、全面地及时掌握疫情发展趋势，并视情况及时调整必要的防控行动和措施，封堵防控漏洞。例如，在目前的新冠肺炎疫情期间，可关注并参考以下信息渠道。

①世卫组织官方报告／中国政府（数据）／约翰·霍普金斯大学病例报告。

②世卫组织、疾控中心以及各国政府（中国、英国、加拿大、澳大利亚、新加坡、韩国、日本等）公共卫生和相关工作部门。

③国际 SOS 和 WorldAware 等与公司建立合作伙伴关系的机构。

（7）最后也是最重要的一个原则，即以人为本，尊重生命，始终将员工的健康与安全放在首位，尊重和爱护每一位员工，了解其真实关切，并提供及时支持。同时，不歧视任何来自特定地区的人员。

中国采取的强有力抗疫措施令人由衷敬佩，中国人民战胜疫情的坚定决心让人动容。在中国政府的领导下，相信勇敢、智慧、坚韧的中华民族一定能够战胜疫情！力拓集团愿意就应急响应机制及应对疫情的经验与中国企业进行更深入的沟通与交流，力拓全球员工为中国加油！

Rio Tinto's Emergency Responding Mechanism

By Rio Tinto

In December 2019, COVID-19 outbreak occurred in Wuhan, Hubei Province of China, quickly turning to a major threat to the lives of millions of people. Under the strong leadership of the Chinese government along with the unity of Chinese people, and generous support from international society, China has been taking unprecedented public health measures in response to the COVID-19 outbreak, which, according to the China-WHO Joint Commission, "have yielded notable results in blocking human-to-human transmission of the virus, and have also played a critical role in protecting the international community, buying precious time for countries to adopt active prevention and control measures and providing them with valuable experience."

After the outbreak, Rio Tinto immediately reached out to its Chinese partners to offer support and donated US$ 1 million to China Red Cross Foundation in support of China's fighting against COVID-19. The funds will be used for purchasing negative pressure ambulances, face masks, protective suits and other medical supplies in urgent needs. Besides, Rio Tinto has been in close contact with its Chinese partners, identifying other practical ways to offer support by leveraging its strength in global resource networking.

Rio Tinto, as pioneers in mining and metals, is a global leading mining company with 46,000 employees in more than 35 countries across six continents. Its unique emergency responding mechanism and experience of fighting against pandemic outbreak could provide best practices for Chinese companies, which are making great efforts to prevent and control the COVID-19 while actively promoting production resumption.

1   Rio Tinto's emergency responding mechanism

Every day our offices and operations around the world face a range of potential situations that may threaten our business. The foundation of Rio Tinto's preparedness is the Group-wide governance framework known as the Business Resilience and Recovery Programme (BRRP). It is an essential part of our Health, Safety and Environment Management System and each site and office across every part of Rio Tinto must be covered by a BRRP.

There are a number of key components involved in the implementation of the BRRP. Firstly, locations must understand their risk profile and develop simple, fit-for-purpose plans. The Business Resilience Management Plan (BRMP) comprises emergency response, business resilience (or crisis) response, and business continuity and recovery arrangements. The scale of planning controls and implementation is contingent upon the characteristics of the site and its risk profile.

The structure of the BRMP covers:

- Statement of Purpose or context (to manage incidents that may impact R`io Tinto operations in a specific location)
- Scope of the BRRP (which locations are covered under the programme)
- Definitions and acronyms used within the plan
- Business Resilience Team (BRT) Activation and ongoing management (how the team will be notified of an activation, and where the team will activate including the location of the business resilience centre)
- Reporting (notifications within the business when the BRT is activated)
- Incident triage (escalation of major or catastrophic incidents; or handover to another BRT to manage)

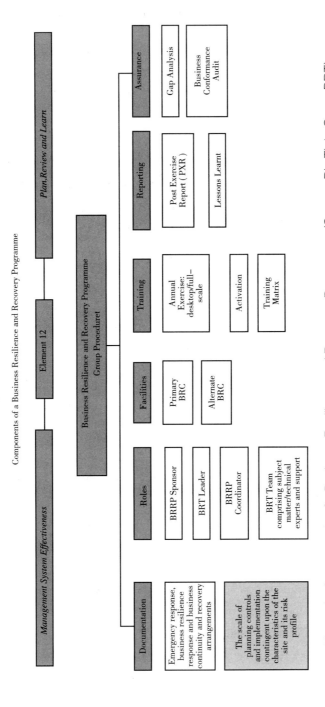

Figure 1 Components of a Business Resilience and Recovery Programme (Source: Rio Tinto Group BRT)

- Incident scenarios (types of incidents with the potential to impact the location), mainly including misconduct, deteriorating relationship with a key stakeholder, legal detention of personnel, missing persons, threat of violence/hostage taking, terrorism/bomb threat, fire/explosion, building evacuation, loss of building access, business travel, medical emergency/fatality, pandemic, natural disaster, severe weather/typhoon/flood, and failure of critical IT.
- Roles and Responsibilities of the Business Resilience Team
- Business Impact Assessment and business continuity arrangements
- Useful documents (e.g. incident log, situation report, stakeholder map)
- Version Control

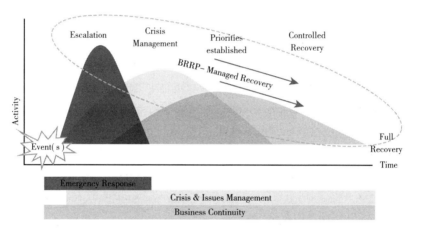

Figure 2　Typical Timeline of the Response (Source: Rio Tinto Group BRT)

Typically, office based BRT comprise the following primary and alternate roles:
- BRT Leader: Overall responsibility for BRT; provide and receive briefings; provide strategic direction; manage relationships with stakeholders; authorise internal and external communications.
- BRRP Coordinator: Mobilises the BRT as required by the BRT Leader and manages process, resourcing and coordination; equip the business resilience

centre; schedule training and exercises, support assurance activities, report BRT activations, and update the BRMP.

- Finance Coordinator: Managing financial and insurance issues, liaison with customers and suppliers as appropriate.

- External Affairs and Communications Coordinator: Identify communications channels needed to support the incident response; provide clear consistent and timely messages; liaise with BRT leader regarding internal and external messaging. Ensure personnel are kept well informed.

- Human Resources Coordinator: Support efforts to locate and account for personnel via HR and emergency contact information; monitor casualties, fatalities and missing person details; liaise with External Affairs and Legal; support family members/next of kin, including travel arrangements; coordinate EAP for employees and next of kin.

- Legal Coordinator: Identify and advise the business on legal issues: (i) establish legal privilege over an investigation, (ii) engagement of external counsel, (iii) secure and collect evidence, including witness statements, (iv) advise on civil and criminal exposure, (v) manage regulators seeking documents and to interview our personnel.

- HSE Coordinator: Ensure the safety & security of personnel; identify and manage any HSE hazards or risks to facilities; provide a strategic overview of the HSE implications of the event and response; work with Legal and other involved departments to ensure a cohesive and comprehensive investigation is conducted.

- Facilities Coordinator: Responsible for sourcing external accommodation as required; liaison with building management during an event.

- Business Continuity Coordinator: Summarise PG/Functional Group business critical roles and dependencies in the event that a loss of building event occurs.

- Information Technology Coordinator: Responsible for minimising impact of an incident on information networks hardware, applications software and the information stored within the system data.

- IS&T Support: Provision of technical support within the BRC during an activation.

- Business Resilience Support Lead: Identify and train personnel capable of acting as assistants, messengers and runners in an incident; lead the support team during an activation of the BRT; assist in set-up of BRC; support BRRP Coordinator to activate the BRT.
- Business Resilience Support Team: Provide support during an activation of the BRT. Roles include: log keeper, assistant log keeper, 3IA status boards, Situation Report, Timekeeper, casualty status, stakeholder mapping.

Teams should not under-estimate the number of support resources required. Whilst Business Resilience is largely seen as the domain of senior leaders and technical specialists; individuals with administrative, organisational or business improvement skills and who know the business well, are ideally positioned to take on vital coordination roles on business resilience teams – roles that add genuine value to the business.

Training of business resilience team members is delivered in a number for formats: class room style, individual sessions and online. Rio Tinto Business Resilience Teams are required to conduct a BRT exercise at least once per annum. The purpose of exercises is to rehearse the team's response to a scenario with pre-determined objectives, for example:
- Rehearse the response of the BRT
- Validate the structure of the BRT
- Activate the support team in an exercise environment
- Test the functionality of the Business Resilience Centre
- Satisfy the business requirement for an annual exercise

Regularly rehearsing the team and systems under realistic stressed conditions is the best way to exercise and embed processes such as the standing agenda, cycle of briefings, incident log, action register, stakeholder mapper and communications strategy (internal and external).

The decision to activate the BRT rests with the BRT Leader. A recommended appraisal process known as '3IA' assists the BRT to make informed decisions. Available *information* at the time is identified, structured and qualified. *Issues* arising or deducted from the information received are identified and analysed. Using past experience, skill and judgement, *ideas* are brainstormed to overcome or resolve issues. *Actions* are based on what the team can realistically achieve. Actions must have an owner and a deadline.

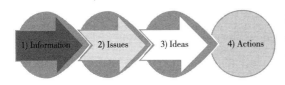

3IA status board (flip charts) are positioned in the BRC, and populated with information by the business resilience support team.

Figure 3　Rio Tinto 3IA Flip Charts

Source: Rio Tinto Group BRT.

PEAR is an acronym to assist BRTs in their response prioritisation:

- People: the safety and wellbeing of people is the highest priority
- Environment: protection, preservation and restoration of the environment
- Assets: protection of all assets and property
- Reputation: protection, and where possible, enhancement of our reputation

2　Rio Tinto's experience in responding to COVID-19

By mid-January 2020, it became evident that the number of people infected with COVID-19 was rapidly increasing and concerns were expressed in China and internationally. The Rio Tinto Group and China management team commenced monitoring the situation and members of the BRT were requested to remain on standby in the event the BRT was activated. Starting from January 20, Rio Tinto China started to prepare epidemic daily report. The team maintained close communication with the group's HSE team and BRT team to access the pandemic situation and its impact, even during the Chinese Spring Festival break.

The management team in China reached out to global procurement team for support to look for reliable sourcing channel for protection supplies. Benefiting from regular planning, training and exercising, the China BRT has clear understanding of accountability and responsibility, the contact details for key stakeholders are up-to-date and is ready to activate at any time.

With sharp increase in the number of people infected in China, the Chinese Government imposed control measures on the movement of people in Wuhan and Hubei province. Rio Tinto further realised the severity of the epidemic, the group and regional offices set up BRTs, and activated emergency responding mechanism. Rio Tinto China officially activated BRT on February 3, the first working day after the extended Spring Festival holiday. Rio Tinto always adheres to the core value of putting the safety and wellbeing of employee first. The BRT acted quickly, held regular BRT meetings, established effective internal and external communication strategy, including sending situation report to Group Executive Committee and other global BRTs, and implemented comprehensive prevention and control measures in offices. Our Beijing and Shanghai offices have imposed strict entry screening system, actively responded to the call of the Chinese government to encourage employee to work from home, activate flexible working arrangement; suspend all unnecessary international and domestic business travels; strengthen office disinfection, enhance employee's healthy protection and social distancing practices; maintain regular communications with employees, understand and address employee's key questions and concerns, regularly update latest epidemic situation, request employees to report health condition and location in time; demonstrate humanistic care by listening to real concerns of employees, providing online mental and health consultation, and retaining doctors to provide on-site medic services; and establish comprehensive prevention and control measures for returning to work. In addition, the BRT also actively coordinated with the local public health department and office property management department to make a response plan for the situation of possible confirmed or suspected cases.

When sorting out the key problems and challenges faced by the prevention and control work, the BRT realized a large amount of masks would be required to support the employees to return to work. Due to the shortage of mask inventory in China, the BRT, with assistance of the global procurement team, made full use of sourcing network advantage to purchase masks worldwide, and ensured that masks were sent to China from overseas in a timely manner, so as to effectively alleviate the shortage of masks. After receiving the masks, the BRT promptly expressed the masks to the employees' home in batches to solve their urgent needs and ensure the health and safety of the employees, reduced the ideological pressure of the employees for returning to work, and helped the employees to return to work smoothly.

The solid foundation, which Rio Tinto has built through annual training and exercises, regularly reviewing and updating plans, and maintaining strong relationships with Rio Tinto Group Security and Business Resilience specialists, has contributed to the BRT's timely and orderly response to effectively cope with the challenges posed by COVID-19 to employees and businesses. So far, Rio Tinto's offices in Shanghai and Beijing have been reopened with no employee being infected. China BRT has been closely monitoring the situation. If the pandemic continuously deteriorates, additional prevention and control measures will be taken accordingly, including but not limited to adjusting working arrangement, increasing the frequency of disinfection in office, extending the policy of "avoiding unnecessary business trip", and strengthening the humanistic care for employees.

3 Suggestions to Chinese companies

During the pandemic, Rio Tinto proactively offered help to our Chinese partners in a timely manner, such as donating masks to the company at the epicenter and sharing Rio Tinto's oversea vendor contacts for supplying protective equipment. Based on past best practices, including our experiences in fighting against Ebola, Rio Tinto would like to share the following suggestions with Chinese companies for reference:

- Companies should, at group level, establish/update a comprehensive, operable, reportable, and measurable emergency responding mechanism, with pandemic plan and other risk scenarios included. In alignment with proportionate response, each regional branch should create an individual plan that includes local government requirements or risk-based features, and flexibility to embed local triggers and actions. Each regional branch should have an annual simulation exercise, with the support and guidance from the group level.
- The pandemic plan, as an important part of the emergency responding mechanism, should follow the principles of prevention, preparedness, response and recovery and is supported in two pillars: proportionate response, and communication and consultation.
- Companies should pre-establish business strategic objectives in the plan
    - Minimise transmissibility, morbidity and mortality;
    - Minimise the burden on the health teams / systems; and
    - Inform, engage and empower the workforce.
- Once the plan is developed, and then exercise. Through continuous exercising, company could identify gaps in the plan, increase response readiness and ensure the team remains abreast of change. Do ensure the plan is always up-to-date and … exercise, exercise, exercise!
- Companies should consider implementing internal travel restrictions and quarantine policies, which are put in place in strict alignment with risk, taking into account scientific evidence, ethical/human principles, international right, recommendations from international bodies, and (only at local level) local government recommendations.
- During the pandemic outbreak, companies should timely update necessary actions based on the latest reliable information from official reliable sources, domestic and international, such as (in the present COVID-19 outbreak):
    - WHO official reports / John Hopkins for cases / China government (statistics)

- WHO, CDC and multiple governments (China, UK, Canada, Australia, Singapore, Korea, Japan, etc) public health and work authorities
- Company partners, such as International SOS and WorldAware
- The last and the most important principle is to be people-oriented. Respect life and put employee's wellbeing and safety at the first place. Respecting and protecting every one of them, listening to their concerns and offering timely support. In the meantime, do not discriminate the employees who are from any specific country or region.

Strong measures taken by China to fight again COVID-19 is remarkable and impressive, and the determination of the Chinese people to combat the pandemic is inspirational. Under leadership of the Chinese government, we believe the brave, wise and resilient Chinese nation will win this battle. Rio Tinto is honored to have in-depth communication and discussion with Chinese companies to share our emergency responding mechanism and experiences in response to a pandemic, and learn from each other. On behalf of Rio Tinto's global employees, we would like to say, "Stay strong, China!"

从新冠肺炎疫情看制造业供应链的应对与启示

施耐德电气 *（中国）有限公司

新冠肺炎疫情对中国社会经济造成了很大的冲击，无论是社会公众还是企业，经济的运转尤其是生产制造环节似乎被按下了暂停键。中国作为全球供应链的重要参与者，疫情导致长时间停工停产致使一部分产业链、供应链中断，对依赖中国供应链的企业和国家也形成了巨大冲击。

施耐德电气也经历了这场毫无预演的大考。值得一提的是，我们交出了较为令人满意的答卷，不仅保证企业自身在允许的第一时间内复工复产，并与上下游供应链通力合作，确保生产资料和物流的迅速畅通以实现产能的全面恢复。截至 2020 年 2 月 21 日，施耐德电气自身 23 家工厂的复工率达到 90%，遍布全国千家上游供应商也实现了近 90% 的复工率，其中未复工的主要是位于湖北地区的企业。同期，在 23 个已经公布复工率（以当地规模以上工业企业的复工率计）的省份中，仅 5 个沿海地区省份和上海市复工率超过 70%。[①] 能够"跑赢大盘"，自然和各地政府对我们的支持分不开，而我们在抗击疫情中所采取的积极应对措施，也赢得了不少认可。

---

* 施耐德电气是一家全球能效管理专家，为 100 多个国家的能源及基础设施、工业、数据中心及网络、楼宇和住宅市场提供整体解决方案。成立于 1836 年，一直是法国的工业先锋之一，总部位于法国巴黎。

特别感谢夏学英和张寒对本文的贡献。

① 《全国复工地图：24 城规上企业复工率超 80%，广东浙江成人口迁入主要地区》，21 财 经，http://m.21jingji.com/article/20200221/herald/2c1508a2b810a8c211b6e6704112f9de.html 2020。

本文将通过分享我们在应对突发公共事件时有效的应急管理、供应链的灵敏反应、全球协同、全方位合作、智能化手段等方面的相关做法和经验，希望对一些企业和政府提供借鉴。从更长期来看，希望与更多企业和政府共同加强能力建设，构建更加灵敏、稳健的供应链应急反应机制和城市治理机制，防御此类重大突发公共事件给实体经济运行造成的冲击和伤害。

一　新冠肺炎疫情对制造业的影响

从经济和供应链来看，疫情对制造业造成的影响主要有以下几方面。

（1）物料：来自受灾地区的物流枢纽运输的物料或半成品的供应短缺，供应商复工缓慢，产能跟不上。

（2）劳力：由于城市间的隔离政策差异，或封城封乡，员工无法及时复工。

（3）采购：由于地区出行限制，公司无法进行新业务或计划业务的开展。

（4）物流：已经建立的物流网络会受到各国禁航禁运、各地物流限制政策的影响而无法顺利开展，寻找替代路线和运输方式将变得更加困难。

（5）客户：同样受疫情影响，下游的客户需求处于停滞或缩减的状态，比如房地产、商业建筑、工业、基础设施建设、数据中心等。客户面临销售停滞、订单延迟、供应链中断、工人返岗各地政策差异，复工复产进度缓慢。

供应链以及生态圈中断所带来的冲击比贸易摩擦要大得多，并且一旦中断形成转移替代，就会对部分行业 30 年来打下的制造业基础造成冲击。黄奇帆建议[1]，"我们必须像是重视疫情自身一样，高度重视保护产业生态、保护产业链和供应链、保护中小企业，只有这样我们才真正能够渡过难关"。

---

[1]　《黄奇帆：新冠肺炎疫情下对经济发展和制造业复工的几点建议》，《第一财经》2020年2月11日，https://www.yicai.com/news/100499981.html?from=groupmessage。

中央政府针对疫情对制造业供应链可能造成的危害有充分的认识，并多次做出指示。2月23日召开的统筹推进新冠肺炎疫情防控和经济社会发展工作部署会议特别提到，[①] 要推动企业复工复产。要落实分区分级精准防控策略，打通人流、物流堵点，放开货运物流限制，推动产业链各环节协同复工复产。随着疫情形势不断出现积极变化，各地复工复产的脚步也开始加快，到2月24日，6个省份的复工率已超过80%。[②]

二 高效的应急管理体系，全力保障复工复产的顺利进行

应急预案属于施耐德电气供应链日常管理的一部分。在疫情发布的第一时间，中国区立即成立了疫情防控工作领导小组，同时在全球成立特别行动组。每日召开各部门碰头会，从安全、采购、生产、运输、人员、订单、资金等各方面随时更新，敏捷反应，制定了公司级别的安全防护计划，严格落实疫情防控工作；除此之外，中国供应链每日与海外供应链团队以及中国销售市场团队联动，并召开应急管理会议，做到横向、纵向的高度协同，高效决策，敏捷响应。

在执行层面，各地工厂根据统一发布的指导手册，结合当地政府具体要求制定了特定的防疫方案，精细管理，确保员工身体健康安全。防疫方案层层落实到部门，责任到人。具体包括：对人员较密集的生产场所、仓库团队及岗位进行专项细则管理；对办公室人员密度、分散办公的可行性等进行评估规划，利用线上线下结合、线上为主的方式展开工作沟通和协作；针对可能的风险点如食堂、更衣室等，实施分批次管理，采取设定人数上限、增加执勤人员等多种形式及方案，以降低人员密集度，确保员工

---

① 《习近平：在统筹推进新冠肺炎疫情防控和经济社会发展工作部署会议上的讲话》，新华网，2020年2月23日，http://www.xinhuanet.com/politics/2020-02/23/c_1125616016.htm。

② 《全国复工地图最新版来了！广东等6省规上企业复工率超80%》，凤凰网，2020年2月24日，http://finance.ifeng.com/c/7uKrR4311fc。

安全。由于具有全面性、针对性并且可操作性，我们的防疫方案和复工手册得到了各地政府的认可，成为其他企业借鉴和参考的样板，也为政府快速审批我们的复工申请提供了保证。

通过实践和观察，我们认为，企业层面（尤其是中小型企业）未来应着力加强应急管理能力建设，并寻求应急管理协同效应；应将应急管理预案提上日程，将其制度化；加强应急管理计划，做好情景演习。在此方面，政府的助力和敦促不可或缺，比如搭建平台，将重点企业的应急管理经验推广到更多的中小企业，鼓励企业在日常管理中制定自己的"应急预案"，以积极敏捷应对突发事件。未来，施耐德电气也将更加主动、积极地向我们的业务合作伙伴分享并传授实际经验，提供相关的咨询服务。

三 灵敏的供应链响应，全球联动，上下游全面协同

施耐德电气全球供应链覆盖 46 个国家 200 家工厂和 98 个物流中心，每天管理超过 26 万份条目，处理超过 15 万笔订单。在中国，施耐德电气供应链覆盖 23 家工厂和 7 个物流中心，近 1 万名员工。我们位于全球各个区域的工厂的生产流程、职位设置、生产语言、管理层架构都是一致的，因此具备很强的替换性。当任何一个地区出现重大突发性公共事件，我们能够无缝衔接平衡全球资源，而不是由某一区域单独承担生产或者供应链断裂所导致的损失。在此次疫情处理中，供应链的应急响应主要体现出以下几点特征。

1.全球联动，共同应对疫情导致的区域性影响

坚持全球一盘棋的思路，特殊时期进行集中管理。成立了特别行动组，每天更新情况汇报给公司管理层，定期召开高级别会议。对生产资料、产能进行全球调度，通过确定受封锁影响地区工厂的替代资源并增加库存水平；通过确定受影响的关键供应商并迅速做出判断，动态调整产品供应产地。比如，施耐德电气在疫情暴发地的武汉拥有 1 家分公司、1 家工厂、1

个物流中心，以及各职能部门约 1500 名员工，基于武汉复工具备极大不确定性，公司即刻全球统一分配，调用法国、印度尼西业等兄弟工厂资源，确保武汉工厂的订单交付。此外，调动全球采购团队，为公司锁定生产资料以外的资源，比如防疫装备，公司 80% 的防护口罩是在春节期间从国外进口（迪拜、中东、欧洲、印度、新加坡）。管理层授权间接采购团队，全球摸底，锁定需求，即刻下单。同时，面对禁运（印度）、停航等重重障碍，利用全球统一的物流体系，物流团队寻找周转的解决方案。

2. 积极推动上下游全面协同，打通产业链

现代产业链上下游企业密切关联，牵一发而动全身。受疫情影响，如果链条上的某一环卡住，其上下游的生产都会出现问题。调查显示，生产性、跨区域物流供应链保障不足是企业复工复产的主要痛点之一。征集的 1852 家企业中，有 229 家提及因供应链、物流问题导致无法复工。总体来看，生产性和跨区域的物流问题更加凸显，而且这些问题不仅影响物流业行业本身，还将进一步导致相关产业原材料供应不足、制成品交付延迟、物流成本增加等问题，从而影响整体经济的恢复进程。[①]

复工第一周，施耐德电气也遇到了同样的困境，由于供应商的复工率低，缺乏生产资料而难以恢复产能。我们迅速协助各级供应商复工，积极分享复工指南，并向各地政府出具协助复工公函。同时，与各级政府积极沟通，通过聚焦主要矛盾，厘清思路，探索解决路径。让我们非常钦佩的是，2020 年 2 月 19 日，天津市委书记李鸿忠在考察施耐德万高（天津）电气设备有限公司时，针对工厂提出的上下游供应商的情况，提出了采取一个企业复工牵引恢复一整条产业链的思路方法，即对已开工重点企业的供货链、物流链进行全面梳理，按照供需关系检索排查尚未开工企业，协调督导相关配套企业在做好防疫工作的前提下加紧复工，

---

① 《调查：仍有 34.8% 的企业未复工 集成电路行业难度最高》，新浪财经，2020 年 2 月 21 日，http://finance.sina.com.cn/review/jcgc/2020-02-21/doc-iimxyqvz4603862.shtml。

由点到面、稳步有序地实现产业链、企业群复产达产。在这一思路指导下，施耐德万高（天津）电气设备有限公司供应商复工率从 2 月 10 日的 24% 上升到 2 月 21 号的 70%。2020 年 2 月 24 日，国家发展和改革委员会在国务院新闻办公室举行新闻发布会上表示，大型企业相对中小企业复工复产进度快，上游行业和资本技术密集型企业相对下游行业和劳动密集型企业进度更快。[①] 我们认为天津的做法，由规模以上企业 / 上游龙头企业的复工带动整条产业链的做法非常有成效，可以为各地政府作为参考。

此次疫情也提醒我们，企业未来应注重平衡供需和建立缓冲库存。评估供应商生态系统多样化的机会，审查或创建组织的总体风险管理办法。与内部利益相关者、战略部门和关键供应商合作，建立一致的风险管理方法，以监控和准备潜在的材料，避免出现制造能力短缺情况。同时，企业在发展的大路上要有大局观，在应对危机时要抱团取暖。对于与自己企业紧密相关的企业，不管上游、下游，一定要相互支持促进，构建良好的商业生态圈。呆板地只关注个体，容易导致唇亡齿寒。

政府在物资和生产方面的灾备能力建设也尤为重要，不仅有助于对突发事件的迅速响应，保护人民生命财产安全，也能更有效、精准地协助产业链整体疏通和恢复，重启社会经济活动。根据不同灾情类型，建议政府拟定灾备物资供应计划和重点企业名录（尤其是上游关键零件供应的企业），这样在面对譬如医疗物资的生产恢复，临时医院建设的物资准备等突发情况时，有能力与时间赛跑，将应急关口前移。此外，政府在助力企业以及产业链整体复工的时候，强调搭建上下游产能供需平台，助力平衡供需关系，灵活调节产能，针对实际困难挑战精准施策，成为企业的主心骨。

---

① 《发改委：全国规模以上工业企业复工率逐步提高 浙江已超 90%》，《北京商报》2020 年 2 月 24 日，https://baijiahao.baidu.com/s?id=1659384035330198660&wfr=spider&for=pc。

四 智能化手段凸显优势，应加大应用力度，助力产业升级、城市治理

中国人的危机观向来强调危中有机，在解决问题的过程中实现自我转变。北京大学国家发展研究院商学院院长陈春花认为，这次疫情是面向数字化、面向未来和面向智能化的一个转型契机，"那些与数字化、与人工智能、与我们讲的共生和协同模式发展的企业，应该是恢复和快速反弹比较快的企业"。[1] 在中金公司发布的《百家企业调研——疫情渐稳 复工进展几何？》[2] 中，就"突如其来的疫情，对企业经营管理可能会产生哪些中长期的深远影响"部分，大部分企业表示，未来将重点加大数字化和智能化的快速推进，比如"建立企业信息化管理体系""重视远程办公的实现""工厂生产自动化"等。我们对此深表认同。

1. 数字化手段保证业务连续性

特殊时期不能见面，但商业行为不能断。施耐德电气的前端销售人员通过数字化平台与客户、合作伙伴保持沟通和互动，确保订单持续不受影响。同时，为了更好地支持外部合作伙伴的发展，我们在专业领先智能化企业学习云平台上火速开通了 3000 个学习账号，专门定制了各种安全培训、产品培训等课程提供给客户与合作伙伴，一起共建学习生态圈，共同成长，共克时艰。此外，面对人才招聘的挑战，施耐德电气开启云招聘，空中宣讲，在线投递，智能推荐，视频面试，测评集成，前置培训的数字化招聘模式，以确保企业人才供应储备。

---

[1] 《全球产业链上的中国制造：少一个零部件都没法生产，疫情后将发生两大变化》，新浪财经，2020 年 2 月 25 日，http://finance.sina.com.cn/roll/2020-02-25/doc-iimxxstf4215007.shtml。

[2] 中金公司:《百家企业调研——疫情渐稳 复工进展几何？》，金融界，2020 年 2 月 12 日，https://baijiahao.baidu.com/s?id=1658301627838628342&wfr=spider&for=pc。

2. 智能供应链体系在应急响应中彰显独特优势

供应链的智能化、可视化有助于更客观地看到各个节点的状况，能够使供应链管理者更清晰地进行规划设计，使物资更合理地进行调配。并对扰乱供应链的时间进行实时监控，及时地做出调整方案。施耐德电气的智能物流体系，又称端到端物流控制系统，以多年精心构建覆盖全供应链运输控制体系为基础，依托物联网、数据连接与数据融合、机器人流程自动化等技术，以及商务智能解决方案，从计划、采购、生产、仓储、运输五大领域，全方位赋能，显著提高订单与收货的可预测性及可靠性，改善客户体验，提升施耐德电气供应链的核心竞争力。在这次疫情期间，因为物流中断、各地应急措施各异，很多物资无法快速送达最需要的地方。端到端控制塔台系统的可视化平台，基于不同城市的疫情管制和复工现状，针对订单各个流通节点进行实时监控，每天更新疫情对关键物料、生产产能、国内和国际运输的影响，并对异常情况进行评估、预测和沟通，提前预警，同时协调供应链各环节指定跨部门应急预案，基于订单紧急程度优化现有资源，最大限度地规避风险，达成急单交付周期，大大解决了疫情给供应链物流带来的挑战。

3. 制造业的数字化、智能化转型至关重要

就施耐德电气而言，尽管具备全球灵活调配产能、应急响应灵敏、复工率高等优势，由于东南沿海制造业劳动力几乎都是靠内陆省份输送，各地的交通管制以及人员隔离措施使得员工到岗率偏低，公司仍然遭遇了生产能力上不去的瓶颈。例如，疫情发生之前招聘的116名技术实习生被困武汉，疫情后既无法返校，也无法调用至人力短缺的上海等地支援复工。又如，某地复工政策规定，外地员工需核酸检测呈阴性、企业出具复工证明、专车接送，才给予复工批准。从短期来看，随着整个产业链的重启，提高一线员工返岗率、提升产能成为制造企业的迫切需求。从长远来看，制造企业要更加务实推进智能制造，构建智能工厂，通过新一代信息技术与生产制造深度融合，提高生产运营的透明度和效率，推进柔性生产，减

少对人工的依赖，从而能够更好地应对劳动力的波动。同时，通过数字化手段实现企业内部多部门、跨区域的产能优化配置、智能优化排产，以及企业与供应商、客户的多地、远程业务协同等。这将有助于最终实现工业部门整体有效产能的高效配置，提升工业部门抗风险能力。

4. 作为企业公民，我们也希望积极为城市治理应急响应出谋划策

除了在工业中的具体运用外，智能化的技术手段同样能在城市管理过程中大显身手，甚至能从根本上改变城市治理，以及此类危机事件暴发时应急处理的模式。

首先，在最前端的医疗诊断、救治阶段，包括无人技术的智能技术可以发挥更大的作用。新型冠状病毒传染性极强，疫情暴发期间，人与人面对面的接触感染风险高，必须要尽量减少面对面的接触。智能技术可以将面对面的接触转变成人与机器的接触，这种优势不止于疫情防控与应对工作中，也能演变成公共医疗体系中的一种常态，比如医院门诊智能筛查、辅助医学诊疗工作，AI 帮助 CT 进行初步医学判断，甚至少量的医学机器人手术应用等。

其次，疫情暴发后，信息瞬息万变，各种需求呈暴发式增长，各单位、区域之间的协调也千丝万缕，在人员紧、任务重、速度快的情况下很容易形成失控的局面。我们看到在很多街道和社区的一线工作中，人员管控基本上靠登记填表、高音喇叭等"人海"技术，生活和防护物资的统计和分派也是靠表格，耗费大量人力，效果甚微。建议未来社区管理中引进智能化的工具和手段，将会更加高效、精准。值得一提的是，杭州上线"健康码"对全市人口进行分级和监控，浙江长兴县通过智能门锁收集住户居住信息，表明在疫情危机时期，智能技术可以在防疫隔离和卫生安全工作中有所作为。比如机场、火车站和公共场所等无人测温、人脸识别和摄像监控等的信息，如果能与街道社区共享，将会减少许多重复的上门核查工作。又如，无人机、无人车如果能在"封城"和禁行的空旷城市中，分发口罩、酒精和常见预防药物等防疫物资，运送基本生活物资，接送病

人，承担有限公共交通职能，也能减轻基层工作人员的负担，同时降低接触风险。

同样重要的是城市 IT 基础设施的建设。我们观察到，此次救急紧缺物资的运输、分配缺乏有效的 IT 系统支持，在供给端、需求端以及运输端均存在很多盲点，物资调配一度陷入混乱，由于信息不对称，相关物资产能提升也十分不及时。其实智能技术的运用在我国的消费领域已经非常成熟，此次疫情期间各商业机构也积极与政府合作，比如，京东承建湖北省政府应急物资供应链管理平台，美团启动"无人配送防疫助力计划"。这让我们不禁期待未来的城市建设中能加大 IT 基础设施的分量，以及着力开发智能技术在公共管理上的应用。比如，基于物联网、大数据分析等技术构建智能化的城市供应链管理体系，有助于指挥部随时掌握包括采购、生产、仓储、运输、配送等在内的所有环节的情况，精准传递信息，配置资源。特别是，依托物流大数据分析的可预见性，能够为城市实时提供风险预测和预警，包括对不可抗力因素（洪水、地震、突发公共卫生事件等）造成的风险进行预测，第一时间评估影响，提出应急管理措施，并通过主动干预的方式减小风险，最大限度上确保货物的稳定交付；或者通过对异常数据的收集，进行贸易风险预测，为精准施策提供依据。

五　结语

经此一役，我们的心得是。危机管理一定要过硬，平时多练兵急时方能战。制造型企业要有组织和整体思维，要通过全球、全产业链协同，辅之以数字化、智能化的技术手段。我们一定能打赢中国制造保卫战，打赢中国经济保卫战。

Response of Supply Chain in Manufacturing Sector to COVID-19 and Revelations

By Schneider Electric (China) Co., Ltd.

COVID-19 has greatly impacted China for its society and economy. From social life to business operation, and to the whole Chinese economy, in particular, the manufacturing sector, all seemed to have hit the pause button. As an important part in the global supply chain, China suffered long period of work and production stoppage, which in turn disrupted the industry chain and supply chain, bringing tremendous shock to those enterprises and countries that rely on China's supply chain.

Schneider Electric was put to this unprepared test too. What is worth mentioning is that we have come out of the test with some initial success. The company not only resumed its production at the first allowable time, but also worked with the upstream and downstream enterprises, ensuring smooth delivery of capital goods and logistics and full recovery of the production capacity. As of February 21st, 2020, 90 percent of 23 Schneider Electric China plants have resumed production. Nearly 90 percent of its 1000 upstream suppliers throughout the country have returned to work. Most of the suppliers who fail to go back to work are from Hubei province. During the same period, among 23 provinces which announced work resumption, calculated by the resumption ratio for industrial enterprise above designated size, only 5 coastal provinces and Shanghai achieved 70 percent of work resumption. [1] Schneider Electric's outperformance

---

[1]   21jingji.com: *Map for Work Resumption in China* on February 21, 2020; 24 cities above designated size achieve more than 80% of work resumption. Guangdong Province and Zhejiang Province become the major destinations of migrate workers http://m.21jingji. com/article/20200221/herald/2c1508a2b810a8c211b6e6704112f9de.html 2020.

couldn't have been achieved without support of the local governments. But our proactive response measures in combating the pandemic also helped win some good recognition.

This paper shares the practices and experiences about Schneider Electric's response to the emergencies, including its quick reaction from supply chain, global synergy, all-around cooperation and intelligent technologies adopted to deal with the public emergencies, with the purpose of providing some references to the government and other enterprises. In the long run, we wish to build capacity with more enterprises and local governments to develop more agile and prudent supply chain response system and city management, to guard against the shock and damages brought by major public incidents to the real economy.

1 COVID-19 impact on manufacturing sector

From the perspective of economy and supply chain, COVID-19 has the following impacts on the manufacturing sector.

- Materials: Due to supply shortage of materials or semi-finished products transported from the logistics hub in the hardest hit regions, suppliers are slow to resume production and suffer insufficient production capacity.
- Labor: Employees are unable to go back to work on time due to different quarantine or lockdown policies in various cities.
- Procurement: New business or planned business cannot proceed due to travel restrictions.
- Logistics: Established logistics network could not function well due to flight or shipping embargo in countries and logistics restrictions in regions. Finding alternative routes and ways of transportation become more difficult.
- Customer: Demand from downstream customers, such as sectors as real estate, commercial buildings, industry, infrastructure construction and data center, is either stagnant or shrinking under COVID-19. Customers are slow in resuming

work or production in face of sluggish sales, delayed orders, interrupted supply chain and varied policies for workers to resume production.

Disruption of supply chain and ecosphere bring more shock than trade frictions do. If trade diversion and substitution appear due to interruption, it will shake the manufacturing foundation that China has laid down in the past three decades. Mr. Huang Qifan[1] in his article suggests that we must place high importance to protecting the industry ecosphere, industry chain and supply chain and SMEs, at the same level as we fight against the pandemic, to withstand this hard time.

The central government has sufficient understanding about how the pandemic may damage the manufacturing supply chain, so has given instructions on multiple occasions. In the Work Arrangement Conference on COVID-19 Prevention & Control and Economic & Social Development on February 23,[2] the central government pointed out that it is important to boost production resumption, implement tiered and precise control measures for various regions, break bottlenecks for people and logistics flow, relax restrictions on freight logistics and promote aligned work resumption in every link of the industry chain. As anti-pandemic situation turns better, enterprises in different areas speed up going back to work. By February 24th, more than 80 percent of enterprises[3] in 6 provinces have resumed production.

---

[1] Yicai, February 11, 2020: Huang Qifan: *Suggestions on Economic Development and Manufacturing Resumption under COVID-19* https://www.yicai.com/news/100499981.html?from=groupmessage.

[2] XinhuaNet, February 23, 2020: Xi Jinping: *Speech on Work Arrangement Conference for Coordinated Promotion of COVID-19 Control & Treatment and Economic & Social Development.* http://www.xinhuanet.com/politics/2020-02/23/c_1125616016.htm.

[3] Ifeng.com, February 24, 2020, Updated Version of *Map of Work Resumption in China*, Work resumption ratio in Guangdong and other 5 provinces exceed 80% http://finance.ifeng.com/c/7uKrR4311fc.

2 Efficient emergency management system to ensure production resumption

Contingency plan is part of the routine management for supply chain at Schneider Electric. We have set up, in the first time since outbreak, a COVID-19 Control and Treatment Command Center and a global Special Action Team. Cross functional meetings were organized on a daily basis, to deliver updates on security, procurement, production, transportation, people, order and funds, which helped agile responses. Corporate-level safety protection plan was put in place. Besides, internal cooperation, both along the industry chain and across different functions, played an important role. Global Supply Chain (GSC) China team, working closely with global team, and China sales and marketing team, organized emergency meetings to make timely decisions and quick response.

In terms of execution, local plants prepared specific prevention plans based on the distributed instruction manual and the requirements of local governments, to ensure health and safety of employees with refined management. Accountable departments and individuals were assigned in the plan. Detailed rules and regulations were followed in the staff-intensive areas as production and warehousing etc. Feasibility of decentralized workspace was assessed where office staff were encouraged to work both online and offline, mostly online. In risky areas such as the canteen or changeroom, measures were taken as setting maximum allowable visitors, and arranging more on-duty guards, to reduce people density and ensure staff security. Our control plan and work resumption manual, being praised as comprehensive, targeted and operable by local governments, have become the reference book for other enterprises. They also warranted quick approval from the local governments for our production resumption.

From our observations in practice, we believe that enterprises, in particular SMEs, shall put more effort to build their capability on emergency handling and seek synergy effect. Contingency plan shall be put on the agenda and become a routine system. Enterprises shall strengthen contingency plan and play the drill regularly. In this respect, the local government plays an indispensable role, such as building platform to introduce good practices and experiences of emergency handling to more SMEs and encouraging enterprises to develop their own Contingency Plan as part of their routine management, so that they can quickly respond to the unexpected incidents. Schneider Electric will be more proactive in the future to share and impart our practical experiences, and provide relevant consulting services to our business partners.

3 Agile response of supply chain with global collaboration and upstream and downstream alignment

The Global Supply Chain of Schneider Electric covers 200 plants and 98 logistics centers in 46 countries, which manages more than 260,000 entries and process over 150,000 orders daily. In China, Schneider Electric employs nearly 10,000 supply chain staff in 23 plants and 7 logistics centers. In various plants all over the world, we have standardized production process, job settings, production languages and management structures. This makes it possible to seamlessly leverage global resources when sudden public events hit one region, instead of leaving a single site to bear all the losses and damages from disruption of production or supply chain. In this pandemic outbreak, emergency response of the supply chain shows the following features.

(1) Global alignment to address regional impact caused by COVID-19

With the mindset of unified management, centralized control measures were taken in this special period. Schneider Electric China has set up a special action team and organized regular high-level meetings to update the corporate executives daily, schedule means of production and capacity globally, increase level of inventory by identifying alternative resources for the affected plants in the lockdown areas. We also adjusted the supplying place of origin by identifying affected critical suppliers. For example, Schneider Electric has one branch, one plant, one logistics center and about 1500 employees in the city of Wuhan, where COVID-19 broke out. Considering the great uncertainty of timing for Wuhan to resume production, Schneider Electric decided to leverage the production capacity from France and Indonesia to guarantee on time delivery of orders of Wuhan plants. Schneider Electric also mobilized its GSC team to lock in resources besides production materials, i.e. protective outfits. 80 percent of the protective facial masks were imported from countries as Middle East (Dubai), Europe, India, and Singapore. Corporate executives granted authorization to the GSC team to find resources globally and place orders as soon as demand was determined. In face of obstacles as embargo from countries like India and suspended air or shipping services, Schneider Electric employed its global unified logistics system and team to find out the turnaround solutions.

(2) Promote upstream and downstream collaboration and ensure an unobstructed supply chain.

Modern industry chain is featured with interconnectedness of the upstream and downstream enterprises, in which any changes of one may affect the others. If one enterprise along the chain gets stuck, as affected by the pandemic, all the other upstream and downstream enterprises will be affected. According to the survey, one of the major pains for work resumption came from insufficient supply of production-intensive and trans-regional logistics supply chain. 229 out of 1852 surveyed enterprises mentioned supply chain and logistics as an obstacle for their back to work. Trans-regional logistics for production was a more prominent issue. These problems not only affected the logistics industry itself but also led to insufficient supply of raw materials, delayed delivery of finished products, and increased logistics costs, therefore affecting recovery of the whole economy. [1]

Schneider Electric encountered the same dilemma in the first week of coming back to work. We found it hard to recover production capacity due to low level of work resumption at the suppliers and lack of raw materials. To solve the problem, we quickly assisted suppliers to resume work by sharing our Work Resumption Guide and issued official letters to the local governments. We also communicated with the local governments, working out possible solutions for major issues. Mr. Li Hongzhong, the CPC party secretary in Tianjin, proposed a good suggestion in his visit to Schneider Wingoal (Tianjin) Electric Equipment Co Ltd. The idea aims at recovering a whole industry through restoring production of one leading upstream enterprise first. That requires us to look at the supply chain and logistics chain for major in-service enterprises, screen out the suppliers who have not yet started production. The local government then coordinates and urges those enterprises to resume production as soon as possible under the premise of good pandemic control. In this way, we can resume production of the whole industry chain and enterprise clusters in a steady and orderly way.

Guided by this thought, the resumption ratio of suppliers to Schneider Wingoal Tianjin Plants increased from 24 percent on February 10 to 70 percent on February 21. China National Development and Reform Commission shared at the press conference held by the State Council Information Office on February 24, 2020, that large enterprises resume work faster than SMEs, upstream companies and capital intensive or technology intensive enterprises faster than the downstream and labor-intensive enterprises. [2] We believe that the

---

[1] finance sina.com, February 21, 2020, Survey: 34.8 Percent of Enterprises are yet to Resume Production. Integrated Circuit Industry is Facing the Toughest Situation. http://finance.sina.com.cn/review/jcgc/2020-02-21/doc-iimxyqvz4603862.shtml.

[2] Beijing Business Today, February 24, 2020, NDRC: Work Resumption for Industrial Enterprises above Designated Size Gradually Increase, more than 90 Percent in Zhejiang Province. https://baijiahao.baidu.com/s?id=1659384035330198660&wfr=spider&for=pc.

Tianjin practice, where enterprises above designated size and leading upstream enterprises driving the whole industry chain, work efficiently. It can be taken as a reference for other local governments.

This pandemic outbreak also reminds us that enterprises shall pay more attention to demand and supply balance and develop a buffer inventory, assess the possibility of diversified supplier's ecology, and review or create the master risk assessment methodology. Enterprises shall work with the internal stakeholders, strategic departments and critical suppliers, to establish a consistent method of risk management, monitor and prepare materials to avoid shortage of manufacturing capacity. Also, enterprises shall have a broader insight for business growth. They shall work together in crisis response. Enterprises with critical stakes, either in the upstream or downstream, must support each other to build a good commercial ecosphere. Neglecting others and caring oneself only may put everyone in danger.

It is of critical importance for local government to build capacity in disaster recovery for materials and production. Such capacity not only helps us respond quickly to the emergencies, protect people for the safety of their life and property, but also assists the circulation and recovery of the industry chain more efficiently and precisely, so as to reboot the social and economic activities. We suggest local governments prepare the Disaster Discovery Plan for Goods Supply and List of Critical Enterprises for different types of disasters, in particular, for upstream critical components providers, so that when we face unexpected incidents which require us to recover production of medical supplies, prepare materials for constructing makeshift hospitals, we are able to race against the time and move emergency handling time forward. Besides, local governments could become the mainstay for enterprises. They shall stress the importance of building demand and supply platform for upstream and downstream enterprises, help balancing demand and supply, adjust production capacity as needed and make targeted policies to address the real difficulties faced by enterprises as they help enterprises and the industry resume production.

4 Intelligent technologies, with prominent advantages, shall be applied more to assist industry upgrading and city management

The Chinese always has a crisis view that opportunities arise from crisis. People may change in the process of problem solving. Mrs. Chen Chunhua, president of the business school from National School of Development, Peking University, believes that this pandemic will become a chance for enterprises to shift towards digital, future-oriented and intelligent. Enterprises that adopt digitalization, AI, symbiosis and synergy pattern are the ones that recover and rebound more quickly. [1] In the Survey on 100 Enterprises- About Work Resumption as the Pandemic Mitigates [2] - an article released by CICC, the writer asked what far-reaching impact the pandemic outbreak may have on business management in the mid and long term? Most enterprises say that they will speed up digitalization and application of intelligent technologies in the future, for example, developing the business IT system, allowing telecommuting and automating production in plants. We fully agree with these ideas.

① Digital technologies are adopted to ensure business continuity. During this special time, people are not allowed to meet each other, but business activities must continue. The front-end sales of Schneider Electric keep communication and interaction with customers and partners via digital platforms, ensuring that the orders are unaffected. In order to better support external partners, Schneider Electric established a learning community by opening 3000 accounts in the

---

[1] finance sina.com, February 25, 2020: *Made in China in Global Industry Chain: Production Impossible with a Single Component Missing, Two Changes after COVID-19.* http://finance.sina.com.cn/roll/2020-02-25/doc-iimxxstf4215007.shtml.

[2] February 12, 2020, CICC: *Survey on 100 Enterprises- About Work Resumption as the Pandemic Mitigates.* https://baijiahao.baidu.com/s?id=1658301627 838628342&wfr=spider&for=pc.

leading cloud platform of advanced learning, developing and providing various training courses on safety and products to customers and partners, so that we can make progress together during this hard time. Schneider Electric also kicked off "Cloud Recruitment" to address the talent challenge. We encourage digital recruitment model such as online training, online CV posting, smart recommendation, video interviewing, integrated appraisal and lead training, to ensure sufficient talent supply for enterprises.

② Intelligent supply chain has shown its unique strength in responding to emergencies. An intelligent and visualized supply chain may help us see what is happening in each part of the chain, and allow supply chain managers to plan more accurately, allocate materials more reasonably. It enables real time monitoring to any disruptions in the supply chain, so that people can make timely adjustment. The intelligent logistics system of Schneider Electric, or end-to-end logistics control system, is based on the supply chain transport control system which we build with years of efforts, and the technologies as IOT, data link and data fusion, robot process automation, and business intelligence solutions. It empowers enterprises from five areas as planning, procurement, production, warehousing and transportation, which significantly increase the predictability and reliability for the order and goods receipt, improve customer experiences and boost the core competitiveness of the supply chain of Schneider Electric. During this COVID-19 outbreak, many materials could not get to places that need them most due to interrupted logistics and varied handling policies in different regions. A visualization platform equipped with the end-to-end control tower may allow real time monitoring to each circulation gates for the order based on the current level of pandemic control and work resumption in different cities. This system updates daily the COVID-19 impact on critical materials, production capacity, domestic and international transportation, and assess, predict and communicate abnormal conditions, send early warnings, coordinate different parts of the supply chain, and develop trans-department contingency plans. It uses available resources based on the level of order urgency. Such system helps minimize risks, ensures timely delivery for urgent orders, which greatly mitigate the challenges to the supply chain caused by the outbreak.

③ Digital and intelligent transformation in the manufacturing sector is of critical importance. Although Schneider Electric has advantages as flexible allocation of global production capacity, quick response to emergencies and high level of work resumption, it still encountered bottleneck of production capacity due to work force availability, as most labors in the coastal manufacturing base come from inner land provinces, who were blocked by the traffic control and quarantine measures. For example, 116 technical interns recruited before the outbreak could not leave Wuhan for neither their school nor cities as Shanghai, where shortage of labors was a big issue. Another example is that some work resumption policies stipulate that employees from other cities may not get approval of back to work unless they can demonstrate that they are negative in the nucleic acid test, present evidence of employer's work resumption, and prove that these employees are transported by chartered cars. In the short term, with restart of the whole industry, encouraging more front-line workers to go back to work and improving capacity have become a pressing request from manufacturers. But in the long run, manufacturers shall push forward smart manufacturing more pragmatically through building smart plants, promoting transparency and efficiency in business operation through deep integration of new generation of IT technology with manufacturing. Enterprises shall encourage flexible manufacturing, relying less on human labors to better deal with labor force changes. They shall also adopt digital technologies to optimize allocation of production capacity among internal departments or across regions, schedule production intelligently and coordinate multi-site businesses remotely with suppliers and customers. This may be helpful for the whole industry as enterprises can allocate their production capacity more efficiently and build their capacity to fight against risks.

④ As a responsible corporate citizen, we would also like to contribute ideas on emergency response in city management. In addition to industrial use, intelligent technologies can play their role in city management. It may even fundamentally change city management and the way of dealing with emergencies in future crisis outbreak.

First, intelligent technologies such as drones can play a bigger role in the front-end medical diagnosis and treatment. COVID-19 is highly contagious. As people may easily get infected during the outbreak period, we must minimize face to face contact. Intelligent technologies may help turn human-to-human contact into human-to-machine contact. This is not only helpful for pandemic control and treatment, but also can become a new normal in the public health system. For example, it can be used for smart patient screening at the outpatient service in hospitals and assist with medical diagnosis. AI can also be used to make preliminary medical judgement in combination with CT. We can even use a small number of medical robots for surgical operations.

Second, the pandemic outbreak comes with rapid changing information and explosive growth of incoming demands. It requires numerous interactions among different enterprises and regions. In this case, things may easily get out of control with shortage of manpower, pressing tasks and quickly changing situation. Among front line work at streets and community level, personnel control mainly rely on registration, form completion and loudspeakers. That's also the case for calculation and distribution of living supplies and protective materials. Such practices cost large amount of manpower but with undesirable effect.

Schneider Electric suggests introducing intelligent tools and technologies to future community management, to make it more efficient and accurate. It is worth mentioning that the Health Code launched first by Hangzhou city helps classify and monitor Hangzhou population. In Changxing County in Zhejiang Province, residents' information is collected through smart door locks. These have shown that intelligent technologies can play a role in pandemic control and quarantine as well as in sanitation and safety. If the information collected in the airport, railway station and public places from unmanned body temperature measurement, facial recognition and camera surveillance can be shared by the street-level communities, repeated door to door visits could be greatly reduced. If drones and unmanned vehicles can travel and distribute facial masks, alcohol and other common prophylactic drugs in the empty lockdown or forbidden cities, transport basic living supplies or patients, or serve as public transport vehicles, they can both alleviate the work burdens of frontline staff and reduce the risks for virus contact.

Equally important is the urban IT infrastructure construction. From our observation, many cities were short of a well-performing IT system for transporting and distributing the badly needed goods and materials. There were many blind spots on part of supply and demand and transportation. Materials allocation easily fell into chaos. Production capacity increase was not timely, due to asymmetrical information. In fact, AI has been widely applied for consumer business in China. We have seen many commercial businesses actively collaborate with local governments during the outbreak. For example, JD.com committed to building a disaster relief supply chain management platform for Hubei Province. Meituan.com launched the Pandemic Control Plan with Drone Delivery. This reminded us to give IT infrastructure more weight in future city management, and to put more efforts in developing intelligent technologies and their applications for public management. Technologies as IOT and big data analytics used in building a smart urban supply chain management system, for example, may help the command center get timely updates about information on procurement, production, warehousing, transportation and distribution, which enables accurate information sharing and resources allocation. In particular, big data analytics for logistics, with its predictability, can make real time risk forecasts and send early warnings, including forecast for potential risks caused by any force majeure events, such as flooding, earthquake or public health emergencies, assess possible impact and propose emergency handling measures as early as possible, so that we can minimize risks with proactive intervention, maximize steady delivery of supplies, predict trade risks by collecting abnormal information and providing basis for targeted policy making.

5 Conclusion

Some learnings from this battle tell us that we shall keep calm and act quickly in face of the pandemic outbreak. We need to have a robust crisis management system in place, and to conduct drills regularly in dealing with emergencies. As a manufacturer, we shall think and act with an integrated mindset and approach. Through collaboration with global and full industry chain players, and assisted with digital and intelligent technologies, we will surely win the battle, to protect China's economy and its manufacturing sector.

5G 应用赋能疫情常态化下经济转型

高通公司 *

中国政府在动员全社会力量有效阻击新冠肺炎疫情蔓延的同时，积极出台各种政策，鼓励企业复工复产，并将 5G 网络建设、5G 应用场景和 5G 手机等终端视为促进消费增长和经济发展的主要推动力之一。作为一项实现万物互联和赋能颠覆性创新的通用技术，5G 在疫情防控期间得到大规模使用，为疫情常态化下赋能创新应用、经济转型、产业升级和社会治理等积累了难得的实战经验和变革动力。

5G 因其高带宽、低时延和广覆盖的技术特点，在远程会诊、远程指挥、防疫机器人、红外线测温仪、大数据管理等疫情防控和社会治理领域发挥了显著作用。中国的重大疫情防控体系、应急物资保障体系、公共卫生体系（尤其是医院）的信息化水平也将在此次疫情防控的推动下得到提升，5G 将发挥非常重要的赋能作用。

尽管疫情给中国经济发展带来短期挑战，然而"有危就有机"，一些新经济、新业态和新模式在移动通信技术尤其是 5G 的赋能下得到超出预期的推动和升级发展，为中国新旧经济模式的转换提供了一个范式。由疫情防控催生的新型消费习惯，如"宅经济"、便捷式消费、非人际接触式消费、"云"生活和办公方式，以及相关支撑性应用，既给在家中的人们创造了生活消费便利，又有效缓解了疫情对经济的冲击，还培育了企业线上业务的竞争

---

* 高通（Qualcomm）是一家无线电通信技术和芯片研发公司，于 1985 年 7 月由美国加州大学圣地亚哥分校教授厄文·马克·雅各布和安德鲁·维特比创建，总部位于美国加利福尼亚圣迭戈市。

特别感谢谭晓龙对本文的贡献。

力和国家社会治理的数字能力，激发了许多行业就如何与5G技术融合进行深度思考和长远布局。据中国信息通信研究院（以下简称"信通院"）截至2020年3月8日的不完全统计，自疫情暴发以来，共有55家企业开发了225个5G应用，涵盖了智慧教育、智慧医疗、智慧城市、智慧社区、智慧平台和媒体娱乐等领域。信通院与5G应用产业联盟（5G AIA）联合开发的"5G应用仓库平台"则征集了300余款App助力疫情防控和企业复工复产，涵盖研发设计、生产制造、经营管理、运维服务和疫情防控等领域。

关于5G应用对中国经济转型和产业升级的推动作用，中共中央领导有着清晰的战略判断。习近平主席在2月3日中共中央政治局常委会关于疫情防控工作会议上强调，扩大消费是对冲疫情影响的重要着力点之一，要求加快释放新兴消费潜力，积极丰富5G技术应用场景，带动5G手机等终端消费，推动增加电子商务、电子政务、网络教育、网络娱乐等方面消费。3月5日，在中共中央政治局常务委员会会议上又提出，加快5G网络、数据中心等"新基建"建设进度。工业和信息化部2月22日召开关于加快推进5G发展、做好信息通信业复工复产工作电视电话会议，强调要加快5G商用步伐，发挥5G建设对"稳投资"、带动产业链发展的积极作用，推动信息通信业高质量发展。同时，要求推动融合发展，研究出台5G跨行业应用指导政策和融合标准，进一步深化5G与工业、医疗、教育、车联网等垂直行业的融合发展。加快推动"5G+工业互联网"融合应用，促进传统产业数字化、网络化、智能化转型。此外，强调丰富应用场景，梳理总结5G在疫情防控中发挥的作用，加快推广新业务、新模式、新应用。抓住5G在远程教育、在线医疗、远程办公等业务发展机遇，释放新兴消费潜力，扩大网络消费，促进信息消费。

《中国5G经济报告2020》发现[①]，5G将催生工业数据分析、智能算法开发、5G行业应用解决方案等新型信息服务岗位，并预测到2030年，

---

① 该报告由美国高通公司于2019年委托中国国际经济交流中心、国经咨询有限公司和中国信息通信研究院联合完成。

信息服务商将创造约 320 万个就业岗位。信通院 5G 经济社会影响白皮书预测，在 5G 商用中后期，互联网企业与 5G 相关的信息服务收入增长显著，成为直接产出的主要来源，预计 2030 年，互联网信息服务收入达到 2.6 万亿元，占 5G 直接经济总产出的 42%。

随着 5G 在疫情防控中作用的凸显，业界对国内 5G 的商用部署在短期内实现高速成长已达成共识。根据全球移动通信系统协会（GSMA）的最新研究预测数据，2020 年中国在全球 5G 连接中的占比将达到 70%；而到 2025 年 5G 在中国的渗透率将增至近 50%。[①]

基于对疫情防控与 5G 关键应用相互促进的观察，高通公司认为，此次疫情并不会影响中国 5G 的商用进程，相反，由疫情防控推动的 5G 关键应用以及激发的新经济、新业态和新模式将会赋能中国经济转型和产业升级的提升。我们认为疫情常态化下经济下 5G 关键应用主要由五大先锋行业推动，即泛娱乐（包括在线娱乐、高清直播等业态）、工业互联网（以物联网和人工智能大数据为支撑）、医疗健康、新业态商务（以移动电商和无人零售为代表）以及远程教育及办公。我们建议中国政府积极推动建设 5G 关键应用发展的创新生态，抓住此次疫情带来的经济转型和产业升级的"二次改革"机遇。我们基于 5G 和垂直行业必须融合发展的认知，梳理总结了疫情防控推动的 5G 关键应用所带来的发展机遇，并在培育丰富的 5G 应用场景，建设 5G 应用产业生态对接平台，打通 5G 应用中小微企业资金链、产业链、创新链，加强知识产权保护和推动相关行业进一步对外开放等方面提出了政策建议。

一 疫情防控促进的 5G 关键应用

高通公司认为疫情防控推动了五大产业加速发展，主要表现在以下几方面。

---

① GSMA 官方网站 5G 资源信息库，https://www.gsma.com/futurenetworks/technology/understanding-5G/5g-resources/。

1. 泛娱乐

疫情防控时期，居家隔离导致民众对泛娱乐业需求大幅增多。泛娱乐是基于 IP，涉及文学、影视、音乐、动漫，延伸至游戏、演出和衍生品多元化融合的产业。在对泛娱乐需求增多的同时，对泛娱乐的种类内容、互动形式、网络承载能力也提出了更高的要求。在疫情防控时期，消费习惯的培养将使泛娱乐产业迎来更大的发展。

依据赢利能力、信息化水平、对 5G 的刚性需求、市场竞争地位等指标，5G 在泛娱乐领域应用最突出的将是云游戏和高清视频。本次疫情与春节假期叠加，因人们大幅减少出游旅行和线下消费娱乐，导致网民对手机游戏和移动终端观影的热度大幅超过此前同期相关统计。不少云游戏公司预计其 2020 年第一季度将取得业绩增长。[1] 同时，基于 5G 传输的高清视频直播也扮演了十分重要的角色。据央视新闻报道，武汉雷神山医院和火神山医院投建之始，采用中国联通 5Gn live 超高清视频直播平台，开启两座医院项目建设现场 5G 全景直播。两座医院的近景、远景四大直播间最高同时在线观看人数超过 4000 万人。[2]

2. 工业互联网

工业互联网是应用于数字时代的先进生产模式，依托 5G 网络、云服务平台，面向工业客户，融合云计算、大数据、人工智能，通过对工业数据深度感知、实时传输、快速计算及高级建模分析，实现生产及运营组织方式的变革，助力传统工业企业转型。在智能制造时代，工厂车间中将出现更多的无线连接，促使车间网络架构不断优化，网络化协同制造与管理水平有效提升，保持对整个产品生命周期的全连接。未来工厂中所有智能单元均可基于 5G 无线组网，生产流程和智能装备的组合可快速、灵活调

---

[1] 《疫情加速云游戏的崛起》，淘股吧，2020 年 3 月 2 日，https://www.taoguba.com.cn/Article/2738391/1。

[2] 《海南电视新闻网 2020 年 1 月 30 官方网站登载央视网等媒体 24 小时高清直播报道》，http://www.hnwtv.com/zb/CCTV12/2020-01-31/181481.html。

整，适应市场的变化和客户需求个性化、定制化的趋势。5G 将升级智能制造流程，赋能柔性生产线，帮助制造业降本增效，深度挖掘设备和用户价值并提升大数据分析能力。

在疫情防控期间，严控疫情蔓延与经济增长、企业复工之间存在难以调和的矛盾，在人力密集型制造领域表现得尤为明显。而一些企业利用工业互联网优势在关键阶段解决了企业生产制造、服务加工的难题。例如，三一重工、徐工集团等企业基于工业互联网对设备远程调度能力合理安排工业机械机群作业，支撑了火神山医院的快速建成；海尔卡奥斯工业互联网平台上线医疗物资信息共享资源汇聚平台，对接物资供需，连接 600 余家医院和 20 多家企业，发布超过 20 万只口罩和防护服等物资。①

3. 医疗健康

5G 为远程医疗提供了技术上的支持，促进医疗资源的线上流动，不同地区、不同级别的医院之间互联互通，打破医患的空间限制，大幅提升医疗效率，有助于偏远地区获取优质医疗资源，改善医疗资源供给不足、分布不均的现状。

中国由人口众多，医疗资源供给不足、分布不均导致的"看病难、看病贵"问题长期存在。这些难点在疫情防控期间也被放大和关注。此外，人口老龄化在中国已经呈现明显的加速趋势，先进的远程医疗水平在老龄化社会将成为重要保障。近年来，远程医疗虽备受关注，但在 4G 网络环境下，受画面和语音延迟、画面清晰度较低等诸多限制而未能大范围应用。5G 网络的技术优势可有效改善以上问题，促进远程医疗的进一步推广实施。对高质量远程医疗的需求在疫情防控中更是得到充分体现。在疫情高发期，湖北和武汉曾经一度聚集了来自占全国总数 1/10 的胸科、呼吸科的医疗专业人员。即便如此，在医疗资源挤兑的情况下医患比例依然严重失衡。据报道，浙江大学医学院附属二院等新冠肺炎重症隔离病区通

---

① 《工业互联网：制造业的疫情应对之策》，中国产业经济信息网，2020 年 2 月 28 日，http://www.cinic.org.cn/xw/cjfx/745829.html。

过中国移动推出的"5G+VR 重症监护室远程观察及指导"系统有效助力病患医治与抢救工作，同时家属也可利用该系统对隔离区病患进行实时探视。利用 5G 的大带宽、低时延特性，该系统使异地专家医生可通过系统进行 360 度全方位高清远程诊疗指导。[①]

此外，在健康检测预警方面，上海、广州、杭州等全国主要大城市在疫情期间针对公共场所，部署了 5G 无感红外体温探测解决方案，运用 AI 摄像机、热成像摄像机等设备，对流动人群进行口罩佩戴和体温实时检测，对未戴口罩人员进行平台告警声光联动报警，如遇体温异常，系统自动告警，提醒管理人员对体温异常人员采取进一步疫情检测措施，实现高效、可靠、无接触的安全检测，助力一站式疫情防控，提升了公共卫生数字化治理能力。

可以预期，由于 5G 的赋能，未来基于移动化、泛在化、智能化的包括远程医疗、智能机器人辅助诊疗在内的医疗健康将会获得空前的重视和发展。

4. 新业态商务

疫情防控期间，依托电子商务的线上消费模式展现出绝对优势。

根据商务部的相关简报，电商行业充分发挥了自身平台和网络优势，力保疫情防控期间商品价格稳定、防疫物资供应、严格平台价格管控、配送高效安全、退改政策落实到位，尤其是突出重点地区保障。这反映出电商行业在防疫物资和生活必需品应急保供、出行票务服务、用户权益保障等方面无可比拟的优势。[②]

疫情防控培养了人们诸多新型消费习惯，譬如线上化消费（在线售房售车）、便捷化消费（远程办公、生鲜电商）、非人际接触式消费（无人零售）等。根据微信小程序官方数据，春节假期期间因与疫情叠加，小程

---

① 《登载全民战"疫"，VR 等高科技是防疫坚实后盾》，搜狐网，2020 年 2 月 4 日，https://www.sohu.com/a/370481131_100133504。

② 《抗击疫情 电商企业在行动》，国家商务部网站，2020 年 1 月 31 日，http://www.mofcom.gov.cn/article/jiguanzx/202001/20200102933029.shtml。

序生鲜果蔬业态交易笔数增长149%，社区电商业态交易笔数增长322%；每日优鲜春节期间平台交易额同比增长超300%。而苏宁菜场的"到店模式"在疫情期间全国销售增长已达到650%。[①] 电商直播成为疫情下传统行业转型与自救的一场"及时雨"。直播主厨、美妆、菜农、健身，甚至直播卖房、卖车，为"全民直播"摁下加速键。危机之下，开拓新渠道、探索数字化转型成为很多线下商企的重要课题。在"人"的方面，直播电商和短视频的社交属性和娱乐属性激发了人群的购物欲望；"货"的层面，相较于传统网购的图文展示，直播式的商品展示形式变得更加直接且更生动；"场"的层面，5G推动的网络技术升级，网速和视频清晰度的提升给直播电商提供了重要加持，也让消费者观看直播越来越方便。相关市场分析机构认为，社交网络加网红电商的应用场景刚好和下沉市场用户匹配，激发下沉消费市场的巨大潜力，电商服务业有望持续收益。随着5G、虚拟等新技术的不断成熟和发展，直播形式将进一步演进，未来"云逛街""云购物"的模式将在不远的将来成为普遍现实。餐饮、生鲜、服装、家居等行业都在迅速布局线上经营，传统行业依靠5G高速连接的新业态商务将成为新增长级。

同时，无人零售也逐渐受关注。根据光明网报道，武汉火神山医院投入使用伊始，其无人值守的疫区超市即开始营业。超市内没有收银员和店员，顾客购买商品通过扫码付款即可完成。据了解，该无人超市整个建筑过程仅使用24小时，超市营业首日已接待200多位客人。[②] 而在整个抗疫一线，无人超市仅是无人零售中的一环。因疫情原因，甚至出现自动生鲜售货机入驻社区，且使用频率也十分可观。无人超市和售货机进入疫情防控一线和社区使得民众对于无人售货的接受程度大大增加，新业态商务

---

① 《生鲜电商疫情突围：业务量激增，但缺货也缺人》，新浪科技网站，2020年2月14日，https://tech.sina.com.cn/roll/2020-02-14-doc-iimxxstf1423875.shtml。

② 《24小时！火神山院区无人超市火速开张》，光明网，2020年2月4日，http://it.gmw.cn/2020-02/04/content_33524083.htm。

在精细数字化管理、品控、运营等方面普遍面对的技术门槛也在 5G 赋能下得到解决。

5. 远程教育及办公

在疫情防控期间，远程办公成为一种潮流。中央电视台《新闻联播》2020 年 2 月 6 日报道，疫情期间全国上千万企业近 2 亿人在家办公。在远程办公带来便利的同时，也对网络连接质量及稳定性（尤其是在海量网络连接的峰值需求下）特别是网络信息传输的安全性提出了更高的要求。未来基于 5G 的高连接将使远程会议和办公场景向移动化、个性化的趋势发展，使多方在线沟通的方式更加灵活，效果更有保证。同时，基于 5G 新空口的安全优势，信息传输的安全性相对于传统方式的网络连接更加可靠。

此外，针对学生的各式远程教育应用在疫情环境下也得到大范围的使用。该部分应用需求激增，对远程教育的网络连接质量和稳定性以及远程教学内容有了更加迫切的要求。基于 5G 超高速连接的优势，未来的远程教育和培训将与 VR/AR 技术进行更紧密的结合。5G 数字平台相较于传统在线平台具有功能性强、成本低和可支持对培训应用的扩展等优势。VR 技术是文字、图像、视频等传统授课手段与技术实训之间的桥梁，不仅可以打破地理空间限制，还能通过体验式、游戏化教学激发受训者的学习兴趣，让技能学习更加简单有趣。

基于 5G 技术，VR 教育还能扩展至更多应用场景，尤其是在职业教育领域，从而助力疫情常态化下教育水平的提升：一是创造出许多此前难以实现的场景教学，比如地震、消防等灾害场景的模拟演习；二是模拟诸多高成本、高风险的教学培训，比如车辆拆装、飞机驾驶、手术模拟等；三是还原历史或其他三维场景，如博物馆展览、史前时代、深海、太空等进行科普教学；四是模拟真人陪练，如英语培训中的语言环境植入，一对一或一对多的远程教学，实现学生与模拟真人的对话。

二 促进疫情常态化下 5G 关键应用发展的政策建议

当前，5G 关键应用发展仍面临诸多挑战，主要问题包括通信技术供给和相关行业相互沟通磨合不足、消费者和行业用户较难看到 5G 的长期裨益与回报、市场亟须培养 5G 复合型高端人才、5G 网络建设和运营成本高、政策环境供给尚显不足等。5G 正处于技术标准形成和产业化培育的关键时期，中国要紧抓这一历史性新机遇，加大统筹推进力度，加快 5G 商用化进程，超前部署网络基础设施，营造产业生态环境，深化各领域融合应用，开创 5G 发展新局面，为全球 5G 应用落地提供"中国方案"和"中国经验"。

（一）培育丰富的 5G 应用场景，促进 5G 网络建设

网络需求与应用水平协同发展，只有发展出更丰富的应用场景，才能更好地牵引网络性能的提升。从运营的角度来看，只有发展出更丰富的 5G 应用业务，才能让运营商在 5G 上的投入得到更好的回报，推动 5G 商业进入良性的正循环。要通过疫情常态化下经济下 5G 关键应用牵引，依托以科技为主线的"新基建"密集部署与推进，结合 5G 商用部署，针对 5G 应用进行顶层设计，规划 5G 应用与网络协同推进路线图，统筹把握重点应用发展关键节点。从国家层面，建立跨行业、跨部门协调推进机制，明确 5G 关键应用的发展规划和具体行动计划，营造良好的 5G 应用创新环境，并同时推进支持 5G 融合应用发展的政策、法规、监管、金融措施，完善电信、工业、医疗等行业管理法规。

2020 年 3 月，国家发展和改革委员会、工业和信息化部联合下发了《关于组织实施 2020 年新型基础设施建设工程（宽带网络和 5G 领域）的通知》，发起 5G 创新应用提升工程，加快建设 5G 赋能的智慧医疗、"互联网 + 协同制造"、智能电网、车联网、智慧教育、智慧港口、5G+4K/8K 超高清制播系统等领域。

（二）建立 5G 应用产业生态

1.建设应用产业生态对接平台

统筹重点行业，围绕业务需求、技术服务、应用孵化、资金扶持等 5G 应用发展的关键环节，建立产业生态对接平台，促进相关主体间的交流和深度合作，对接供需各方需求，寻找关键行业痛点与 5G 结合的突破口，深度挖掘行业需求，从技术角度提出解决方案，并通过合作探索找到相关行业共赢的全新商业模式，全面促进 5G 应用创新，并加强应用推广，有效推进 5G 产业发展。

2.建设国家级 5G 应用示范区，开展应用培育

推进国家级 5G 协同创新示范区建设，统筹行业应用相关单位围绕终端、网络、数据处理、应用等方面，协同开展 5G 跨行业应用创新，支持针对 5G 关键行业开展应用培育，打造相关行业示范应用标杆，形成一批可复制性成果并加快推广。加强 5G 产业支撑平台建设，加快建设 5G 产品技术验证、质量检测、入网检测等公共平台。

3.打通 5G 应用中小微企业资金链、产业链、创新链

中小微企业是受此次疫情冲击最厉害的群体，但是疫情防控中涌现出的新经济、新业态和新模式也为中小微企业进行线上创新创业提供了机遇。相关政府部门可以梳理此次疫情防控中的典型应用，搭建 5G 应用相关中小微企业与创新中心、孵化器、实验室、投融资机构的沟通与合作平台，提供技术支持、资金对接、业务咨询等多方面的服务，促进资金链、产业链、创新链融合发展，开展 5G 应用联合孵化，培育一批主营业务突出、竞争力强、成长性好的 5G 融合应用专精特新的"小巨人"企业。

（三）支持 5G 应用产业发展

1.加快出台 5G 应用产业规划，引导商业应用有序发展

目前，在国家层面，《信息通信行业发展规划（2016-2020 年）》《信

息产业发展指南》等文件从战略上对 5G 的发展方向和重点任务进行了明确；在省级层面，北京、浙江等省份出台 5G 产业发展指导意见或行动方案。为了保障 5G 产业全方位有序发展，国家应出台更广泛、多层次、更具针对性、更有利于产业生态整体发展的国家级 5G 应用产业发展规划。为了推动经济持续发展，中国政府强调 5G 网络建设作为"新基建"的主要组成是一项积极的举措。但同时也应注意到各地 5G 网络积极部署和推进需要结合那些符合民众切实需求和社会治理需要的 5G 实际应用，避免资源的浪费和不切实际的投入。

2. 推动试点示范成熟和推广，深度挖掘商业模式，探索相关行业进一步对外开放

第一，集中资源推动试点示范。认定一批产业带动作用明显的中外 5G 新技术、新产品、新业态、新模式示范项目，中央财政和地方财政给予项目奖励。集中财力精选和开展几个政府 5G 应用示范重大工程，围绕疫情常态化下经济 5G 关键应用，发挥先行先试引领作用。

第二，深度挖掘新型商业模式。出台相关行业 5G 新产品和服务的定价制度，建立产业链合作相关方的利益分配机制。运营商与产业链合作伙伴和客户开展深入的合作，为客户提供行业应用的整体化解决方案。开始按照应用免费单点试用，让相关行业了解 5G 网络的益处之后再付费订阅，基于试点应用倒逼 5G 网络部署，推动应用场景的丰富，助推商业模式的深刻变革。

第三，探索相关行业进一步对外开放。5G 应用的真正落地需要相关先进技术的融合，以及国际先进商业模式的带动，包括数据中心、在线医疗、远程教育等领域。中国近年来在相关行业进一步对外开放方面做出的举措已有目共睹。为了把握住新经济、新业态所推动的经济转型的机遇，使中国 5G 关键应用和相关行业与国际标准和实践充分融合、更好地融入全球 5G 产业链，建议可以适当放宽相关增值电信业务的外资市场准入，进一步开放网络教育、在线医疗等 5G 关键应用行业，或以试点方式对相

关行业进行有限度开放，并辅以相对灵活宽松的金融服务，通过试点效果将相关准入和开放政策在更大范围内进一步推广。

3. 实施严格的知识产权保护制度，促进应用产业创新能力提升

加大知识产权保护力度，激励企业增加 5G 研发投入，促进 5G 应用产业技术创新和研发能力提升。

第一，加快完善移动通信和相关行业应用领域的知识产权保护，对专利侵权行为要严厉打击，营造鼓励科研创新的良好氛围。中国已经将创新驱动作为一项核心国策，将其视为经济高质量发展的途径，而知识产权制度是保护、激励创新投入的重要制度。

第二，重视专利质量，有效加强专利布局。各国在 5G 技术创新领域不断发力，不断加强专利布局。根据德国专利数据公司 IPlytics 关于 5G 标准必要专利排名的统计，中国声明的 5G 相关标准必要专利数量占比超过 30%。这体现了中国在 5G 相关领域研发实力的提升和整体专利布局的增强。但是专利价值不能仅从数量上进行衡量。首先，每一件专利的技术内容不同，每一件专利的价值都有非常大的差别。其次，标准必要专利披露数据的准确性有待检验。标准化组织对于标准必要专利的披露仅凭借自觉性，即企业自己认为这个专利有可能是标准必要的，就可以披露，其中没有第三方权威机构或者法律流程去核实。最后，专利价值是在市场上得到体现的。例如，专利的价值不仅体现在授权许可谈判中，也体现在专利侵权诉讼和专利无效程序中。因此，业界在评价通信领域专利价值时，仅从数量上进行衡量并不全面，专利价值应通过市场来体现。

第三，建立与 5G 相关的市场驱动型专利交易和许可平台，为 5G 技术的转让和许可提供便利。对核心技术的授权许可对移动通信技术获得快速和高性价比发展起到了关键性的作用，通过技术授权等有效激励手段，可以挖掘移动通信领域技术创新者最大创新潜能，提升先进技术引进吸收消化再创新能力，保障消费者和商业用户及时获得最先进的技术应用。

4. 政府营造创新环境，促进产业融合发展

第一，探索包容创新的审慎监管制度。加快融合应用领域法规制度建设，进一步强化科技、金融、财政、税收、人才、定价、知识产权等政策支持，深化放管服改革，消除行业政策壁垒，鼓励支持多元市场主体平等进入，促进5G产业生态加快壮大。

第二，扩大先进成果宣传，提高5G行业应用的社会感知度。先进科技成果和应用模式应获得较高的社会认同以体现其社会价值。多举办高水平的行业创新应用大赛能够充分集思广益、孵化应用、挖掘商机，也能够提高先进成果的社会感知度。疫情期间，相关行业联盟和组织积极动员相关单位将疫情期典型案例和应用进行汇总梳理并向社会进行及时发布，推动和鼓励相关关键应用平台共享，使应用价值最大化并减少信息闭塞和重复开发。这种做法值得充分肯定，并应进一步在行业内宣传和提倡。

Key 5G Applications: Enablers of Economic Transformation & Industry Upgrading under the Regular Epidemic Prevention and Control Measures

By Qualcomm Technologies, Inc.

The Chinese government has actively introduced policies to encourage enterprises to resume work while mobilizing all social forces to effectively prevent the spread of COVID-19 epidemic. It regards 5G network construction, 5G application scenarios and 5G terminals including mobile phones as some of the major driving forces to bolster consumption growth and economic development. As a general-purpose technology (GPT) making interconnection of all things and disruptive innovations possible, 5G has been employed on a large scale during the epidemic prevention and control, thus accumulating precious practical experience and revolutionary impetus for enabling innovative applications, economic transformation, industry upgrading and social governance under the regular epidemic prevention and control measures.

The ultrahigh bandwidth, ultra reliable low latency and wide coverage of the 5G network have ensured its remarkable role in epidemic prevention and control and social governance, including remote consultation, remote command, epidemic prevention robots, infrared thermometer and big data management. 5G will further play a vital role in improving the IT maturity of China's major epidemic prevention and control system, emergency material support system and public health system (especially hospitals).

Although the COVID-19 epidemic has posed short-term challenges to China's economic growth, it carries with opportunities – some new economies, business forms and models have been upgraded beyond expectations by mobile communication technologies, especially 5G. These upgradings provide a paradigm for China to shift from an old economic model to a new one. The epidemic prevention and control have hastened new consumption habits, including "otaku economy", convenient consumption, contactless consumption, "cloud-based" lifestyles and work models, and related supporting applications. All of these elements have not only facilitated the life of people grounded at home, but effectively alleviated the epidemic's impact on the economy. Meanwhile, they have boosted competitiveness of enterprises' online business, improved China's capabilities to perform social governance by using digital tools, and stimulated industries to ponder over and make long-term arrangements in integrating 5G technology with their development.

According to the incomplete statistics released by the China Academy of Information and Communications Technology (CAICT) as of March 8, 2020, since the outbreak of the epidemic, 55 companies have developed a total of 225 5G applications, covering smart education and healthcare, smart cities and communities, smart platforms, media and entertainment. The "5G Application Warehouse Platform", co-launched by CAICT and the 5G Application Industry Alliance (5G AIA), has collected over 300 apps that are dedicated to helping prevent and control COVID-19 and assisting firms to resume work, covering R&D, production and manufacturing, operation and management, operation and maintenance services, as well as epidemic prevention and control.

China's central leadership has a clear strategic judgment on the role of 5G applications in promoting the country's economic transformation and industry upgrading. As stressed by General Secretary Xi Jinping at a meeting of the Standing Committee of the Political Bureau of the Communist Party of

China (CPC) Central Committee on epidemic prevention and control convened on February 3, 2020, increasing consumption is one of the important focuses to offset the epidemic's impact, and efforts should be made to accelerate the unleashing of emerging consumption potentials, enrich 5G technology application scenarios to drive consumption of 5G terminals such as 5G mobile phones, and boost consumption in e-commerce, e-government, online education and online entertainment. At another meeting of the aforementioned Committee held on March 5, it was proposed to speed up the construction of "New Infrastructure" such as 5G networks and data centers.

At a teleconference on speeding up the development of 5G and resuming production in the information and communication industry held by the Ministry of Industry and Information Technology (MIIT) of China on February 22, it was emphasized that the pace of the 5G commercialization should be accelerated, the positive role of 5G construction in "stabilizing investment" and promoting the development of the industry value chain be given full play, and the quality development of the information and telecommunications industry be enhanced. At the same time, it was proposed to foster integrated development, study and promulgate guidelines and integration standards on 5G cross-industry applications, and further strengthen integrated development of 5G with vertical industries, such as industrial manufacturing, healthcare, education, and connected vehicles. Focused efforts are demanded to expedite the integration and application of "5G+Industrial Internet" and boost the digital, networked and intelligent transformation of traditional industries. In addition, it is essential to enrich application scenarios, summarize the role 5G played in epidemic prevention and control, and quicken the promotion of new businesses, models and applications. Enterprises are encouraged to seize 5G development opportunities in distance education, online healthcare and telecommuting, unlock potential of emerging consumption, and stimulate online consumption and information consumption.

As per the *China 5G Economy Report 2020* [1], 5G will bring new types of jobs in information services such as industrial data analytics, intelligence algorithm development and 5G application solutions. It is predicted that information service providers will create about 3.2 million jobs by 2030. According to the estimation of the White Paper on 5G's Economic and Social Impact prepared by CAICT, in the middle and later stages of 5G commercialization, internet companies' revenue from 5G-related information services will grow dramatically to be the main source of their direct outputs; it is forecasted that the income from internet information services will reach RMB 2.6 trillion in 2030, accounting for 42% of 5G's total direct economic outputs.

As 5G is playing a prominent role in China's epidemic prevention and control, the industry has reached a consensus that the 5G rollout in China will achieve rapid growth in the short term. According to the latest research and forecast data from the Global System for Mobile Communications Association (GSMA), China's 5G connections will account for 70% of the world's total in 2020; the penetration rate of 5G in China will rise to nearly 50% by 2025. [2]

Based on the observation on the reciprocal enhancement between epidemic prevention and control and key 5G applications, Qualcomm believes that the epidemic will not affect the process of 5G rollout in China. On the contrary, key 5G applications as well as new economies, business forms and models stimulated by disease prevention and control will empower China's economic transformation and industry upgrading. We deem that key 5G applications under the regular epidemic prevention and control measures will be primarily driven by five pioneer industries, namely, pan-entertainment (including online entertainment and HD live broadcasting), Industrial Internet (supported by the industry internet,

---

[1] This Report was prepared by China Center for International Economic Exchanges, China Economic Consulting Corporation and CAICT, under the commission of Qualcomm Technologies. Inc. in 2019.

[2] 5G Resource Information base on the Official Website of GSMA. https://www.gsma.com/futurenetworks/technology/understanding-5G/5g-resources/.

AI and big data), healthcare, new forms of commerce (represented by mobile e-commerce and unmanned retail), and distance education and telecommuting. We suggest that the Chinese government actively foster an innovation ecosystem for the development of key 5G applications, and seize "second reform" opportunities created by the epidemic to carry out economic transformation and industry upgrading. In view of the conviction that 5G and vertical industries must develop as a whole, we have summarized development opportunities brought by key 5G applications propelled by epidemic prevention and control. We have also proposed policy suggestions on nurturing ample 5G application scenarios, building platforms for 5G application eco-system, resolving capital, industry and innovation problems hindering growth of micro, small and medium-sized enterprises (MSMEs) involved in 5G applications, strengthening protection of Intellectual Property Rights (IPR), and pushing forward further opening-up of relevant industries.

1 Key 5G applications propelled by epidemic prevention and control

Qualcomm regards that the epidemic prevention and control has driven the accelerated expansion of the following five industries:

(1) Pan-entertainment

The pan-entertainment industry is an IP-based sector comprising of literature, film and television, music, animation, games, performances and various derivatives. During the COVID-19 outbreak, home quarantine has given rise to a substantial increase in demand for pan-entertainment. The increased need for pan-entertainment set out higher requirements for diverse content, interactive forms and network bandwidth. The consumption habits cultivated during the outbreak will usher in greater development of the industry in the post-epidemic era.

According to the five traits of 5G pioneer industries – profitability, IT maturity, rigid demand for 5G, competitive threats and competitive opportunities, cloud gaming and HD video streaming will enjoy steady development. Since the outbreak of COIVID 19 coincided with the Chinese Spring Festival holiday, which led to sharply reduced travels and offline consumption of entertainment, the number of internet users, who played mobile games and watched videos on portable terminals, became significantly higher than the statistics of the same period in previous years. As a result, many cloud gaming companies expected their performance to grow in Q1 2020.[1] 5G HD video broadcasting also produced a marked effect. According to CCTV news reports, at the beginning of the construction of the Leishenshan Hospital and Huoshenshan Hospital in Wuhan, China Unicom's 5Gn live ultra-HD video broadcasting platform was employed to realize panoramic broadcasting of activities on the two hospitals' construction sites. The four live broadcasting rooms, including close view and distant view, attracted over 40 million concurrent online viewers.[2]

(2) Industrial internet

As an advanced production mode for industrial enterprises in the digital age, industrial internet is based on 5G networks and cloud service platforms, and integrates cloud computing, big data and AI. It can help upgrade traditional industrial enterprises by transforming their production and operation modes through depth perception, real-time transmission, fast computing and advanced modeling analysis of industrial data. In the era of smart manufacturing, there will be more wireless connections on the factory floor, which will help optimize workshops' network structure, improve network-based collaborative

---

[1] Outbreak of COVID-19 Accelerates the Rise of Cloud Games, published on Taoguba.com.cn, March 2, 2020. https://www.taoguba.com.cn/Article/2738391/1.

[2] 24-Hour HD Live Reports by CCTV and Other Media, published on the official website of Hainan TV News Network, January 30, 2020. http://www.hnwtv.com/zb/CCTV12/2020-01-31/181481.html.

manufacturing and management, and ensure full connections across the entire product life cycle. All the smart units of a future factory will be able to form a network based on 5G wireless connection. Production processes and smart equipment can be quickly and flexibly regrouped in response to the changing market and customers' personalized demands. 5G will upgrade smart manufacturing processes and make production lines more flexible, enabling the manufacturing industry to lower costs and increase efficiency, deeply explore value from products and customers, and enhance big data analytics capability.

During the epidemic, the irreconcilable contradictions between strictly containing the spread of COVID-19 and economic growth and enterprises' resumption of work are particularly evident in the labor-intensive manufacturing industry. However, some companies have leveraged advantages of industry internet to solve their problems of production, manufacturing, services and processing in this special period. For example, corporations including SANY and XCMG exercised remote control over industrial machinery fleets through IIoT to orderly arrange their operations to support the speedy construction of Huoshenshan Hospital. Haier COSMOPlat launched a platform for collecting and sharing information on medical materials resources to connect 22 enterprises and over 600 hospitals to coordinate their supplies and demands, securing the delivery of over 200,000 face masks and protective suits. [1]

(3) Healthcare

5G will facilitate the sharing of medical resources online, enhance interconnectivity between hospitals in different regions and of different ratings, and connect patients with medical professionals regardless of geographic barriers, significantly improving the efficiency in the provision of healthcare.

---

[1] IIoT: A Tool for the Manufacturing Industry to Deal with COVID-2019, published on the CINIC.com.cn, February 28, 2020. http://www.cinic.org.cn/xw/cjfx/745829.html.

China's large population and insufficient supply and uneven distribution of medical resources have resulted in the long-standing issue of medical services being unaffordable and inadequate, which has been magnified during the epidemic. In addition, the population aging is accelerating in China. Against such backdrops, advanced telehealth technology will rise as strong support for an older China. In recent years, although telehealth has attracted great attention, 4G has prevented its wide adoption with limitations such as picture and sound delay and low resolution. However, 5G's technological advantages can solve the problems and promote further development and deployment of telehealth.

The demand for quality telehealth has surged in the epidemic prevention and control period. At the height of the epidemic, one-tenth of China's medical professionals from the departments of thoracic medicine and respiratory medicine gathered in Hubei Province and its capital Wuhan to treat local patients. Even so, the doctor-patient ratio was still seriously unbalanced when patients thronged the hospitals. It was reported that the "5G+VR Remote Monitoring and Guidance System for ICUs", introduced by China Mobile, facilitated the treatment and rescue of pneumonia victims in ICUs at the Second Affiliated Hospital of Medical College of Zhejiang University. Family members could also use the system to visit patients in quarantine in real time. Empowered by the 5G network featuring high bandwidth and low latency, the system enables experts and doctors to remotely conduct 360-degree omni-directional HD instruction on diagnosis and treatment. [1]

In addition, major cities such as Shanghai, Guangzhou and Hangzhou have deployed the 5G non-contact infrared temperature detection system in public places during the epidemic to perform health detection and issue early warnings. Equipment including AI cameras and thermal imaging cameras is used

---

[1] High Technologies such as VR Are Solid Props for China to Prevent the Spread of the Coronavirus Disease 2019, published on Sohu.com, February 4, 2020. https://www.sohu.com/a/370481131_100133504.

to carry out real-time detection of mask-wearing status and body temperature of the mobile population. If a person is spotted without wearing a mask, alarms will be sounded. In case of people with abnormal temperature, the system will automatically remind personnel in charge to take further measures. Therefore, efficient, reliable, contactless and safe detection is realized to reinforce one-stop epidemic prevention and control, thus improving digital management capabilities of these cities in public health.

It can be expected that the mobile, ubiquitous and intelligent healthcare services empowered by 5G, including those of telehealth and smart robot-assisted diagnosis and treatment, will receive unprecedented attention and achieve remarkable development.

(4) New forms of commerce

During the prevention and control of the COVID-19 epidemic, the online consumption pattern based on e-commerce reigns supreme.

According to the Ministry of Commerce of China (MOFCOM), the e-commerce industry has leveraged its platforms and networks to ensure, in the combat against the epidemic, price stability, sufficient supply of epidemic prevention materials, efficient and safe distribution, honest implementation of booking cancellation and change policies, and particularly provision of sufficient supplies for the worst-hit areas. This reflects the incomparable advantages of the e-commerce industry in terms of emergency supply of epidemic prevention materials and daily necessities, travel ticketing services, and protection of user rights and interests.[1]

Public response to the epidemic includes development of such new habits as online consumption (e.g. online sale of houses and cars), convenience consumption (e.g. fresh food e-commerce), and non-contact transaction (e.g. self-

---

[1] E-commerce Industry in Combat Against the Epidemic, published on the official website of MOFCOM, January 31, 2020. http://www.mofcom.gov.cn/article/jiguanzx/202001/20200102933029.shtml.

service retail). According to the official data that WeChat Mini Program collected from its applet users, after the coronavirus outbreak during the Spring Festival holiday, the number of fresh food transactions increased by 149% and that of community-based e-commerce transactions increased by 322%; the volume of transactions completed through the applet named "MissFresh" saw a year-on-year growth of 300%; Suning's online grocery business, which offers self-pickup service, increased by 650% nationwide. [1]

In the context of the epidemic, livestreaming e-commerce becomes a lifesaver for traditional industries to restructure and rescue themselves. Livestreaming of cooking, makeup, growing vegetables, workout, and even sales of houses and cars has swept across the country. Under the menace of the coronavirus, exploring new channels and digital transformation has become a life-and-death issue for many offline businesses.

Livestreaming e-commerce has three major advantages. First, by virtue of meeting the audience's social and entertainment needs, e-commerce livestreams and short videos stimulate their desire to shop. Second, compared with traditional online marketing featuring picture display and text description, live product demonstration is more attention-grabbing and vivid. Third, thanks to the 5G-based network technology upgrade, the improved connection speed and video definition provide a boon for livestreaming e-commerce, while making it more convenient for consumers to watch livestreams.

Some market analysts believe that social network plus cyber celebrity e-commerce can be a favored combination for small town and rural markets; by tapping these markets in an effective manner, the e-commerce service industry is expected to remain profitable. With the maturity and development of 5G,

---

[1] The Thriving of Fresh Food E-commerce During the Epidemic: Surge in Business and Short Supply of Goods and Workforce, published on tech.sina.com.cn, February 14, 2020. https://tech.sina.com.cn/roll/2020-02-14/doc-iimxxstf1423875.shtml.

virtualization and other new technologies, livestreaming will further evolve to make "cloud window shopping" and "cloud shopping" commonplace in the near future. Various industries, including catering, fresh food, clothing and home furnishing, are rapidly going online. In the post-epidemic economy, traditional industries reinvented by 5G high speed connection are set to become a brand-new growth pole.

Meanwhile, self-service retail is getting increasing attention. According to Guangming Online, at Huoshenshan Hospital in Wuhan, an unattended self-service supermarket opened for business as soon as the hospital started to operate. Without cashiers or shop assistants, the supermarket allows customers to buy goods by scanning codes. It's learnt that the supermarket was built within just 24 hours and was visited by more than 200 customers on its first day of business.[1] Nevertheless, on the frontline of the battle against coronavirus, unattended supermarkets merely play a part in self-service retail. Fresh food vending machines make their debut in residential communities and are used with considerable frequency. Self-service retail has gained great public acceptance through the introduction of unattended supermarkets and vending machines to hospitals and residential communities. Furthermore, the technological barriers commonly faced in promoting new business forms in terms offline digital management, quality control and business operation will be tackled with the aid of 5G.

(5) Distance education and teleworking

During the fight against COVID-19, teleworking has become a fashion. As reported by the CCTV News on February 6, nearly 200 million workers from tens of millions of firms worked from home across the country. While

---

[1] In Just 24 Hours! The Unattended Supermarket at Huoshenshan Hospital Opens for Business, by Guangming Online, February 4, 2020. http://it.gmw.cn/2020-02/04/content_33524083.htm.

teleworking brings convenience, it also puts forward higher requirements for the quality and stability of network connection (particularly when the mass network connection reaches its full capacity), especially the security of network information transmission. In the future, 5G-based high connectivity will enable more mobility-oriented and personalized teleconferences and work locations and will make multi-party online communication more flexible and effective. In the meantime, thanks to the security advantages of 5G New Radio (5G NR), the security of information transmission will become more reliable than that of traditional network connection.

In addition, during the epidemic, various distance education applications developed for students are extensively used. Demand for these applications has soared, presenting more urgent and higher requirements on the quality and stability of network connection for distance education, as well as on the content of courses. By virtue of 5G ultra-high-speed connection, future distance education and training will be more closely integrated with VR/AR technologies. Compared with traditional online education platforms, 5G platforms boasts more powerful functions and lower cost, and are able to expand training applications. VR technology bridges technical training with traditional teaching methods like text, images and videos. Location will no longer be a problem when VR comes, which stimulates trainees' passion through unique experience and gamification, making skill learning easier and more interesting.

Powered by 5G technology, VR education can be applied in more scenarios, especially vocational education, thus contributing to the improvement of post-epidemic education. First, training scenarios that are considered impossible before, e.g. disaster simulation like earthquake, fire, etc. Second, costly and risky training processes, e.g. vehicle disassembly, aircraft piloting, and medical surgery. Third, 3D restoration of history or other scenarios such as museum exhibitions, prehistoric times, deep sea or outer space for popular science. Fourth, training partner simulation. For instance, students are able to be immersed in English-speaking environments with a simulated English tutor.

2   Policy suggestions on promoting development of key 5G applications under the regular epidemic prevention and control measures

Currently, the development of key 5G applications is beset by multitude challenges: ineffective cooperation and communication between telecommunications technology providers and other industries, long-term rewards inexplicit to customers and businesses, a dearth of competent, versatile 5G experts, high costs of network construction and operation, and insufficient policy support. Despite the obstacles, 5G is undergoing a critical period of technical standards establishment and industry development. Seizing this historic opportunity, China has made greater coordinated efforts to promote the rollout of 5G technology, plan ahead network infrastructure construction, create a favorable industry ecosystem, and deepen integration of various industry applications, thus opening up new possibilities of 5G development, and offering the world "Chinese solutions and knowhow".

(1) Diversifying application scenarios to push forward network construction

Only by developing more applications can network performance be better improved and carriers get better returns on their 5G investment. In face of a pandemic-stricken economy, policy makers need to forge ahead with the application of core 5G-based technologies, by taking advantage of the rapid deployment of "New Infrastructure". To this end, policy makers should carry out top-level design, and create a road map for collaborative efforts, and conduct overall planning of key nodes for core applications development.

Measures to be taken at the national level include:

① establishing coordinated promotion mechanisms between different industries and departments to define development plans and specific action plans for key 5G applications in connected vehicles, pan-entertainment, healthcare, industrial internet, etc.;

② developing favorable policies for 5G application innovations;

③ studying and creating policies, laws, regulations, and financial measures to support the integrated application of 5G in related industries; and

④ improving management regulations on telecommunications, industry, transportation, healthcare, etc.

As stated in the *Notice on Organizing the Implementation of the 2020 New Infrastructure Construction Project*, jointly issued by the National Development and Reform Commission and the MIIT in March 2020, China plans to initiate a 5G innovation enhancement program in support of developing a range of sectors, including 5G-powered smart healthcare, electrical grids, education and ports, along with Internet + collaborative manufacturing, connected vehicles, and 5G + 4K/8K ultra-HD broadcasting.

(2) Building a 5G ecosystem for vertical industries

① Setting up a platform to facilitate industry communication and cooperation.

Based on the key steps of a 5G application development process, a platform should be built accordingly to increase communication and in-depth cooperation between these different enterprises and institutions, with a view to addressing pain points through 5G-enabled solutions and identifying needs across industries. As part of the effort to boost the development of the 5G industry, the platform is set to offer technological solutions, explore a new win-win business model for relevant industries through cooperation, and promote wider application of 5G.

② Launching national demonstration projects to develop 5G applications.

National demonstration projects aimed at promoting coordinated 5G innovation to be launched to:

• enlist all related organizations to make cross-industry innovations in terminals, networks, data processing and applications;

• support developing 5G applications in priority industries;

• establish a benchmark for applications in related industries; and

• identify replicable use cases that can be quickly spread across industries.

These projects will enhance the platforms that support the 5G industry and accelerate the development of public platforms dedicated to technology certification, as well as quality and network access tests.

③ Coordinating related capital，industries and innovation for MSMEs surrounding 5G applications.

Amid the fight against the epidemic, which has hit MSMEs hard, new economies and business models have cropped up, presenting new opportunities of making innovations in online business activities. Relevant authorities are suggested to scale up effective applications in disease prevention and control by:

① setting up communication and cooperation platforms that connect MSMEs involved in 5G applications with innovation centers, business incubators, labs and institutional investors and financing institutions;

② providing technical support, financial services, business consultation, and other types of services; and

③ launching a coordinated 5G application business incubation to nurture a group of emerging "giants" in 5G application that have outstanding business capabilities, strong competitive advantages and good growth potential.

(3) Supporting 5G application development

① Promoting the issue of vertical industry plans to guide the commercialization of 5G

At present, at the national level, China has defined development directions and key tasks of the 5G industry in strategic documents such as *Information and Communication Industry Development Plan (2016-2020)* and *Guidelines on Development of the Information Industry*. At the provincial level, municipalities and provinces such as Beijing and Zhejiang have issued guidelines or action plans on 5G industry development. In order to ensure all-round and orderly development of the 5G industry, it should be encouraged to make multi-level plans that are more extensive, targeted and conducive to the overall development of the 5G industry ecosystem.

In driving sustainable economic growth, China has proactively fueled the development of 5G networks as part of its "New Infrastructure" program. Meanwhile, when deploying 5G networks, the country focuses on creating 5G applications for the better benefits of Chinese people and social governance to avoid resource squander and unreasonable input.

② Facilitating pilot projects' development, discovering new possibilities in business models and exploring approaches to make relevant industries more international

First, pooling resources to promote development of model pilot projects. Governments should designate a number of model projects involving new home-grown and imported 5G technologies and products, new business forms and models, which will push forward expansion of the 5G industry noticeably. Rewards should be given to each of those projects introduced by central and local governments. Financial resources should be concentrated to carry out selected model government-supported 5G applications in support of the post-epidemic economic development, so as to lead and boost the 5G industry development.

Second, striving to discover new business models. Pricing systems for 5G new products and services in relevant industries should be introduced, and benefit distribution mechanisms for stakeholders along the industry value chain should be set up. Carriers will be encouraged to carry out extensive cooperation with partners and clients, enabling partners in the industry ecosystem and providing clients with overall solutions specifically designed for their industries. At the beginning, free single-point trial of applications can be offered to clients in related industries, which will help them understand benefits of 5G networks. After that, they may pay for subscription. Those pilot applications will in turn drive the wider deployment of 5G networks, create more application scenarios and promote profound changes in business models.

Third, exploring approaches to make relevant industries more international. Putting 5G applications in place means an integration of advanced technologies and positive changes brought by up-to-date international business models in areas such as data centers, online healthcare, and distance education. In recent years, China has made impressive strides in opening up relevant industries. To capitalize on the benefits of new economies and business models, China should expand telecommunications service market access, and further open up online education and healthcare and other key 5G application-related industries, better aligning the country's 5G applications and related industries with international standards and practices. For this to happen, China should launch pilot programs to open related industries to the world step by step, while offering flexible, accessible financial services. Continued efforts will be made to increase market access and policy support in light of pilot program achievements.

③ Implementing strict IPR protection rules to strengthen innovation capacities of industries

Strengthened IPR protection will encourage enterprises to increase their investment in 5G R&D, subsequently improving technological innovation and R&D capabilities in 5G related industries.

First, it is recommended to step up IPR protection in telecommunications and other related industries. Patent infringement must be cracked down on to create an enabling environment for technological innovation. China has already put innovation at the center of its national strategy and seen it as a way to improve the quality of its economic growth, while IPR protection laws have been in place to protect and encourage investment in innovation.

Second, it is also crucial to improve the quality and distribution of patents. As national governments continue to double down on 5G innovation, they have also improved 5G patent distribution. According to statistics released by IPlytics, a German company that collects patent data and publishes on a regular basis a ranking list of 5G standard-essential patent owners, China accounts for more than 30% of all 5G related standard-essential patents (SEPs), which shows how China has improved its R&D capabilities and its overall patent distribution in 5G related areas.

But the value of patents should not be judged only by their quantity. Firstly, each patent has different technical details, and the value is also different from each other. Secondly, the accuracy of data disclosed by SEPs have yet to be verified. Standardization bodies have no compulsory requirements on data disclosure of SEPs, which fully relies on companies' discretion. This means companies can choose to disclose a patent as standard-essential if they think it is so, and there is no need to have it confirmed by any third party verification or legal procedure. Thirdly, the value of patents is reflected by the market. For example, a patent's value is not only presented during license negotiation, but also reflated in the process of infringement lawsuits or invalidation procedures. We should keep in mind that measuring the value of patents leadership only by quantity is not a comprehensive approach. The patents' value should be judged by the market.

Third, a market-driven patent trading and licensing platform should be established to facilitate the transfer and licensing of 5G technology. Licensing of core technologies plays a key role in the rapid and cost-effective development of mobile communication technologies. Through incentives such as technology licensing, the maximum potential of technological innovators in mobile communications can be tapped, the ability to import, absorb, internalize and re-innovate advanced technologies can be enhanced, and consumers and commercial users can be guaranteed timely access to the most advanced technology applications.

④ Creating an innovation-friendly environment to promote integrated industry development

First, the government should explore the establishment of an inclusive and innovative prudential supervision system. Measures to be taken:

• speeding up the formulation and improvement of laws and regulations in integrated applications;

• further strengthening policy support in the fields of science and technology, finance, taxation, talents, pricing and IPR, etc.;

• deepening reforms to delegate power, streamline administration and optimize government services;

• eliminating industry policy barriers;

• encouraging and supporting the equal entry of multiple market players;

• fostering and expanding new technologies, industries, business forms and models related to 5G technology; and

• boosting the growth of 5G industry ecosystem.

Second, the government should actively publicize 5G achievements and improve the social awareness of 5G applications. The development of science and technology should reflect the care for people, and advanced sci-tech achievements should have higher social recognition to show their social value. The government can hold industry innovation and application competitions to pool wisdom, incubate applications, tap business opportunities and raise social awareness of 5G advanced achievements. Over the epidemic period, relevant industry associations and organizations have encouraged businesses to share with the public successful 5G applications and cases on a timely basis, and to promote the sharing of key application platforms, in a bid to maximize the application value, reduce information flow congestion and avoid resource waste. This is a laudable practice that should be further promoted across the industry.

完善供应链建设，保障粮油物资供应

——新冠肺炎疫情的启示

嘉吉公司[*]

路易达孚公司[**]

新冠肺炎病毒传染性极强，短时间即造成大量感染病例，使人猝不及防。在新冠肺炎疫情暴发期间，中国政府迅速采取有效措施，控制住了疫情传播，事实证明，这些措施极其及时、准确和高效。与此同时，我们也看到，在疫情发生初期，特别是病毒不明的情况下，中国有效控制病毒传播，全力保障医疗物资供应，但短期内疫情地区民生用品，尤其是粮油和饲料产品的供应仍带来压力。"危机"带来的是"危险"也是"机遇"，二者不可分割。英文中也有一句俗语，"Never waste a good crisis"，即"每次危机都应该带来收获"。作为粮油贸易和加工行业的从业者，我们认为政府部门和粮油行业应继续完善供应链建设，尤其是加强应急保障预案和实施机制设计，以保证灾情发生时，可以做到快速调动大量物资，通过流畅的物流组织，及时、有效地保障灾区供给，同时保障粮油生产供应链从原料生产及采购、物资生产、物流仓储、商业渠道等全链条及时启动生产，确保后续物资供应充足。

---

　*　嘉吉是一家从事生产和经营食品、农业、金融和工业产品及服务的多元化跨国企业集团，业务包括农产品供应链、动物营养、动物蛋白、食品配料及应用、运输及金属、金融服务等。由 William Wallace Cargill 先生于 1865 年创立，总部设在美国明尼苏达州。

　**　路易达孚集团由法国人列奥波德·路易达孚创建于 1851 年，是全球领先的农产品贸易和加工企业之一，每年在全球范围内种植、加工和运输约 8000 万吨农产品，为全球约 5 亿人提供食品和衣物。总部位于荷兰鹿特丹。

　特别感谢任育枝和何常君对本文的贡献。

一 新冠肺炎疫情下粮油行业基本情况

中国是世界人口第一大国，亦为世界最大的粮食生产、消费和进口国。毫无疑问，粮油行业对中国的粮食安全，对人民生活、国民经济的正常运行有着至关重要的保障作用。粮油企业不仅生产消费品，其产品更是整个食品供应链的基础。例如，养殖行业需要的饲料、食品加工行业需要的原料，均来自粮油加工行业。一旦粮油行业的运转出现问题，其传导效应将对中国甚至全球经济、社会产生巨大影响。

同所有的制造业企业一样，粮油加工企业离不开货物流动，离不开物流。无论是原料的供给，还是产品的运输，均需要通过物流加以实现。为控制成本，现代制造企业大多采用精益生产（Lean Production）、准时化生产（Just In Time）等理念，追求零库存或最小库存。没有物流的支撑，所有制造业企业都无法运转。

在整个食品供应链中，粮油属于上游，其产品供给饲料、养殖、食品甚至工业企业。但是，作为生产性企业，粮油加工企业经常也是终端用户。除原料、辅料外，其生产设备、消耗品甚至工人的防护用品等都依赖外部供应。现代供应链环环相扣，任何企业都不能脱离其供应商独立生存。

随着全球人口的激增、流动和聚集，大范围疫情的暴发和其对生命安全的潜在威胁越来越严重。在疫情等突发情况下，保障疫区及全国民生物资的稳定供应，成为帮助支援疫情救治、稳定社会情绪、凝聚社会力量、重塑社会秩序的重要基石。粮油供应链是社会的动脉。在遇到疫情或类似灾难时，如何保障粮油供应链的正常运转？我们既需要重新思考供应链的业务存续计划（Business Continuity Plan），也需要利用现代技术，提升供应链的水平，保证供应链运行通畅。

此次疫情影响了粮油供应链的正常运行。

（一）内陆物流方面

1. 道路被阻断

自新冠肺炎疫情发生以来，大量村镇采取封村封路措施（村民自发采取行动的居多），设置路障，禁止一切外来车辆通过。此类做法虽有利于防止疫情扩散，但执行中"一刀切"的方式同样封堵了生活和生产所需的车辆通行，对养殖等上下游产业造成了严重影响，导致饲料供不上、物资运不进、产品销不出、用工回不来等诸多问题。

2. 司机被隔离

防疫初期，跨省、跨市运输遇到诸多挑战，其中一项即为"有货车没人开"的窘境。因防疫限制，司机复工率偏低，加以跨地运输在目的地隔离14天，返程后有可能还要再隔离14天等要求，使物流业"雪上加霜"。在实际运行中，因恐受到隔离限制，即使能够复工，很多司机也选择不正常工作，以降低成本。

3. 物流通行受限

防疫初期，各地车辆通行证的申请要求不统一，且限量发放，导致企业很难申请到通行证，或即使拿到也满足不了正常生产需要。加之，企业的运输（比如饲料成品和原料的运输）一般外包给物流公司，但物流公司复工率不高。物流公司车辆不足，且难以找到替补车辆。同时，办理通行证时要求指定车队、指定司机、指定车号，企业基本无法满足要求。

4. 码头被封或者装卸迟缓

很多饲料原料（比如豆粕、玉米、进口饲料添加剂）的运输，要到港口、码头、粮库去装车。港口和码头封路，第三方仓库不开工，在"抗疫"初期比较常见。虽然随着秩序恢复，封锁被解除，码头仓库开工，但装卸人员到岗率较低，装卸速度迟缓。

（二）国际贸易方面

一些外国企业和消费者对疫情产生忧虑，原产自中国的动植物产品出口受阻，中国出口的货物和商品无法顺利交付。例如，巴基斯坦等国要求对原产自中国的货物出具无新型冠状病毒污染的证明并要求在卸货港加强熏蒸消毒措施；俄罗斯、韩国、土耳其等国则暂停从中国进口动植物产品。尽管世界卫生组织于2020年1月30日在宣布新型冠状病毒构成国际关注的突发公共卫生事件的声明中，不建议对中国实行旅行和贸易限制，但国际上的这些忧虑情绪并未消除。

由于出口货物目的地国家出台管制措施，叠加中国国内的物流限制，中国出口企业无法按时交付货物，被动违约。一些国内出口企业因新冠肺炎疫情影响无法履约，面临库存积压和国外客户索赔的双重打击，运营面临严重困难。值得肯定的是，中国国家贸易促进委员会和中国食品土畜进出口商会等商会、协会及时给企业纾困，据实出具不可抗力证明，助力企业渡过难关。

另外还有因票据、文件等跨境物流延迟而影响通关。码头被封、装卸迟缓也给国际贸易带来很大影响。很多货轮无法卸货；码头冷库堆满货物，迟迟无法运出，导致来华货轮只能转运他地。

以上种种问题，主要有以下原因。

（1）缺乏应急预案及统一协调机制。在灾情发生初期，如果有应急预案，可迅速行动，将灾情影响降到最低。统一协调的专项保障方案可有效地保证供应，减少各地各自为政，"牵一发而动全身"，供应链中一个环节受损导致整个链条瘫痪。

（2）供应链对人员依赖过重，自动化程度有待提高。众多物流、生产人员无法及时返工，导致企业"复工不复产"。关键岗位人员缺失，使整个工厂无法运行。

（3）供应链运行信息电子化程度不足，审批、交易依赖传统方式，既使贸易受到影响，同时也不易追溯，使有关部门难以全面掌握情况。政府大力支持企业复工复产，但在收集信息、了解情况方面仍然依靠各企业自行申报，效率不高。

二　粮油供应链应急预案设想

完善的粮油供应链应急保障预案和实施机制，可以确保灾情发生时，通过简洁的流程，紧急调动大量物资，通过流畅的物流组织和保障，及时、有效地保障灾区供给。同时保障粮油生产供应链从原料生产及采购、物资生产、物流仓储、商业渠道等全链条及时启动，确保后续物资供应充足。

从此次新冠肺炎疫情来看，未来可在中国现采用的设立政府工作组专项管理的做法上进一步完善供应链应急预案机制。在预案中根据灾情性质，确定预案触发机制，明确组成机构牵头部门、各部门职责和协动机制，实施效果动态评估和改进机制。从制度设计上需强调全产业链一体化概念，并且应该在其中：①确定重点保障物资清单，应包含粮、油、饲料等重点民生保障物资；②形成物资储备、调运和生产地图，以各地灾情发生概率、粮油物资产能、人口和养殖布局等科学布局，并充分考虑国家储备和商业储备的结合；③梳理具体行业全供应链各环节导图，包括原料、物流、仓储、设备部件、包装辅料等。以饲用原料豆粕生产为例，整个应急供应链中需协调大豆进口通关、码头装卸、工厂生产、产品物流运输和储备调运等环节，而且还应包含劳动力、设备维护、仓储等衍生因素的保障。

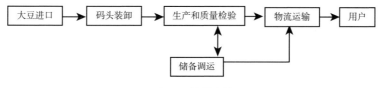

图 1　大豆压榨供应链导图

上述预案应确保一旦灾情发生，及时启动，供应链运转流畅，保障准确到位，生产恢复有序且可持续。

三　完善粮油供应链的建议

为进一步完善粮油行业供应链应急机制，结合行业的具体情况，粮油供应链可以从以下几个方面提升。

（一）生产和储备方面的建议

1. 提高粮油生产自动化、智慧化水平

目前，粮油行业自动化、智能化水平不高，难以满足应急情况下对配置弹性和高效调度能力的要求。建议，一方面，政府出台政策鼓励粮油等民生行业推进自动化建设，促进产业技术升级，大力引入 5G 视频监控、AGV 调度、数据回传、设备数据采集等技术促进行业转型升级，打造粮油智慧工厂来实现生产对大量劳动力的依赖、提质增效，未来更可以与工业互联网平台结合有效实现资源调度优化和精准决策。此外，还应鼓励推广设立一定比例的无人化工厂、产线，既可以提高生产效率，还可以避免生产被迫中断。

另一方面，也应鼓励培训技能全面的工人，以便在突发情况下，可以一人多岗应对劳动力短缺等情形，客观上也避免因劳动力短缺需要雇用临时工人造成的生产安全隐患。

2. 提高合同、生产储备在应急储备中的比例

中国供应链应急体系的粮油产品实物储备建设基本完备，此次玉米等粮食作物充足的实物储备就及时起到了满足生产需求、稳定物价的作用。但同时建议继续提高粮油产品的合同储备和生产储备的比例，推进政府储备方式多样化，充分发挥商业储备的补充作用，把饲料农资纳入应急物资保障体系，加强和完善重要农产品储备体系。

继续鼓励与龙头企业签订合同，保证在突发事件发生后能够按约定，优先租用、调用或者生产粮油产品以保障供应。同时，根据人口和养殖产业聚集程度统筹设计，对养殖优势区域的饲料和人口密集地区粮油储备进行引导和优化，与前述的分级保供企业名单相结合，建立更加完备灵活的应急粮油物资保障平台。

另外，建议指定单一政府部门在应急物资采购、存储、调拨、运输、使用等各环节的统一调度，既可以提高效率，还可以压实责任。此次医疗物资保障采用的牵头组织生产，直接将物资从企业调拨到需求单位的方法就值得借鉴和推广，大大提高了应急状态下的物资供给效率。吸取卡特里娜飓风救灾的经验教训，美国政府随后调整其应急管理政策，对联邦应急管理署（FEMA）进行了改革，其中一项重要内容就是提升后勤保障组为后勤保障委员会（LMD），整合和统一协调政府内外部应急物资。

（二）贸易和物流方面的建议

1. 利用区块链等信息技术实现物流单据电子化

区块链是分布式数据存储、加密算法等计算机技术的新型应用模式，存储于其中的数据或信息，具有"不可伪造""全程留痕""可以追溯""公开透明""集体维护"等特征。传统纸质单据等在区块链技术数字化处理后，数据的实时匹配避免了大量重复工作，令文档处理的时间缩短到了原来的1/5，完成跨境农产品贸易所需时间缩短了一半。

当前，嘉吉、路易达孚、ADM、邦吉、中粮、嘉能可六家农业大型国际化公司发起倡议，合资设立一家名为Covantis的法人实体，积极推动业界采用区块链等技术来实现国际农业运输交易标准化和数字化，并开始为交易后操作流程开发数字化解决方案。中国天津海关2019年上线的平行进口车区块链项目，充分利用了区块链技术不可篡改、可追溯等特性，解决了跨利益主体之间的互信问题，实现了流程节点可视化，提高了检验检疫通关便利化水平和效率。该技术的应用前景已经在业界和行政监管层面得到了验证，还可以推进数据共享，促进联动共治，并利用风险评估逐步构建大数据分析体系，以此提高审批效率，避免灾情下人群聚集。

建议推广区块链技术在供应链上的应用，加速推进现代化智慧供应链。实现这一目标，需要积极推动各国家间法律法规准入和电子单据互认，企业间货物提单、信用证等单据电子化，早日实现供应链单据电子化，降低成本，提高效率，降低灾情对供应链的影响。

2. 依据风险程度，分级管理水运、陆运等重要交通枢纽

分级管理机制有助于压实各级主体风险治理责任，完善供给保障的责任机制。首先，要因地制宜按照前述生产导图制定企业分级管理机制，科学地根据具体情况设立国家、省、市的分级粮油保供企业名单。其次，对名单内企业的原料进口、产品生产和物流配送分级制定全供应链运转方案，开辟涵盖水运、路运的特别绿色通道，并提前根据企业级别配发应急通行证，在突发情况下可以凭证通行，确保原料进得来、产品供得上。最后，应对码头等重要交通枢纽进行分级管理，提前梳理和优先保障产地和灾区的主要码头、公路等重要交通枢纽不间断发挥物流功能。采取工人就地隔离、机械化作业等方式，确保粮油物资可以不中断地通过这些重要节点，打破突发情况下的物流瓶颈。

3. 利用大数据等现代信息手段实现共享物流

物流业天然具有发展"共享经济"的有利条件，发展共享物流有助于消化过剩的物流产能，整合社会物流资源，降低社会物流成本，减少物流中的碳排放、资源浪费、交通拥挤、环境污染等问题，从而实现物流业集约化、绿色化、高效化转型。新冠肺炎疫情期间，邮政、顺丰等多家物流公司在司机和车辆进出疫区受限的情况下，以共享运力的方式保障了运转，其模式值得探索和推广。

我们认为，一方面，国家应继续推进车货匹配平台的建设与管理，促进物流运输与配送资源共享与合理配置。可以融合互联网、大数据、区块链等先进技术与科技，解决目前车货匹配平台存在的信息真实性、有效性

等问题。另一方面，应加快物流园区等基础设施规划布局，大力提倡智慧仓储和智慧物流管理，助力共享物流发展。未来，信息技术将加速推动物流业的进一步深度融合，大大提高对供应链应急管理的覆盖率，尤其是粮油等民生物资采购、生产、运输等环节的大数据跟踪与分析，优化物流路线，预测物资消费量与仓储量和风险防控等。

（三）加强信息公开和消费预期管理

通过此次疫情可以发现公众越来越重视灾情信息的实时披露，这不但是对公众知情权的保护，还可以帮助稳定预期，助力制造业合理安排生产计划。疫情发生后，国家及时加大了医护用品信息的公开力度，联防联控机制按照既定预案承担生产保供任务，并每天披露医护用品产能和未来增产数据，减轻了大众担忧。粮食系统也启动了粮油监测系统，针对优质企业饲料和畜禽养殖企业实施生产情况日报制度。多地推出的"菜篮子"负责制和"一日一查一报"制度，采用网络发布、手机短信等方式向民众广泛发布物价信息，稳定了民众预期。这些做法也应该推广到"米袋子""油瓶子""饲料原料"等产品中去，一来有利于生产企业合理计划，避免供应链端的生产和物流压力波动，二来有利于平抑物价和避免抢购等事件发生。

How to Improve the Supply Chain in the Grain and Oilseeds Industry to Secure Supplies for Livelihoods

By Cargill Inc. & Louis Dreyfus Company

COVID-19 became a worldwide pandemic two months after its first outbreak. The virus is highly contagious, catching people off guard and causing a large number of cases in a short time. The Chinese government has taken swift and effective measures to contain the spread of the epidemic within the country. At the early stage of the outbreak, especially when the virus is unknown and Wuhan city has been sealed off, the supply of people's livelihood, including the supply of grains & oilseeds products and feed products, met with challenges in the affected areas. As the old saying 'never waste a good crisis', the grains and oilseeds supply chain needs to be continuously improved through a joint effort from government and industry, especially to put in place emergency response plan and mechanism to ensure sustenance supply during outbreak. This will also enable grains and oilseeds production supply chain, from raw material production and purchase, production, logistics, to sales, remains functioning to ensure sufficient food supplies subsequently.

1 Basic information on the grain and oilseeds industry during the COVID-19 outbreak

China is not only the world's most populous country, but also the world's largest producer, consumer and importer of grain. There is no doubt that the grains and oilseeds industry plays a vital role in ensuring China's food safety, people's livelihoods and the normal operation of the national economy. Grains and oilseeds companies manage products, which are the basis of the entire food supply chain. For example, the feedstuff needed by the animal breeding industry and the raw materials needed by the food processing industry all come from the grains and oilseeds processing industry. If the grains and oilseeds industry was to break down, it would have a huge impact on China, the global economy and society at large.

Like all manufacturing companies, grains and oilseeds processing companies are inseparable from the flow of goods, i.e. logistics. Both the supply of raw materials and the transport of products are carried out through logistics. To control costs, most modern manufacturing companies employ the concepts of lean production and Just-In-Time production, and pursue zero or minimum inventories. The operation of all manufacturing companies is thus inseparable from logistics support.

As part of the food supply chain, grains and oilseeds are upstream, with products supplied to feed, breeding, food and even industrial enterprises. However, as producers, grains and oilseeds processing companies are often also end users. Except for raw materials and auxiliary materials, production equipment, consumables and even workers' protective articles depend on external supply. The modern supply chain is so interlinked that no company can operate without its suppliers.

As the world's population grows and people travel and gather, widespread epidemics may increasingly threaten health and human life. In the case of a sudden epidemic, ensuring the stable supply of materials for people's livelihood in affected areas and across the country is essential to support assistance during the outbreak, to maintain a cohesive social sentiment and to rebuild social order once the epidemic is over. The grains and oilseeds supply chain is the artery of society. In the event of an epidemic or a similar disaster, how can we ensure the normal operation of the grains and oilseeds supply chain? We need to ensure Business Continuity Plans for the supply chain, and to use modern technology to upgrade and ensure the smooth operation of the supply chain, even in difficult times.

During the coronavirus outbreak, we find that the following aspects affect the normal operation of the grains and oilseeds supply chain:

(1) Inland logistics

① Blocked roads. Since the outbreak of COVID-19, many villages/towns have taken measures to block the roads in or out of the villages by setting up roadblocks and forbidding external vehicles to enter the villages, most of which were taken voluntarily by villagers. Although such measures were conducive to preventing the spread of the epidemic, the "one-size-fits-all" practice blocked access for the traffic needed for livelihoods and production, with a serious impact on upstream and downstream industries. This included a short supply of feed for animals, the inability to import materials or export products, and for employees to return to work.

② Isolated drivers. During the early stages of the fight against the epidemic, inter-provincial and inter-city transportation faced many challenges, one of which was the dilemma of "trucks with no drivers". Due to anti-epidemic restrictions, fewer drivers returned to work and drivers had to be isolated for 14 days both at the destination of trans-regional transportation and after return. As a result, the logistics industry faced a worsening situation. In practice, many drivers chose not to work as normally scheduled, even if they were able to return to work, for fear of being restricted by isolation, in order to reduce costs.

③ Restricted logistic access. During the early stages of the fight against the epidemic, traffic permits for vehicles in different areas were subject to different application requirements, and limits were set to the number of permits issued, resulting in difficulties for companies to get traffic permits or the inability to meet their normal production needs, even if they did get some. Furthermore, companies usually outsource the transportation of their products (such as finished feedstuffs and raw materials) to logistics companies, who were suffering from shortages in the number of returned employees and the number of trucks, as well as difficulties to find replacement cars. Meanwhile, a traffic permit required a designated fleet, a designated driver and a designated number plate, but companies could not achieve that.

④ Closed docks or delayed loading/unloading. Many raw materials for feedstuffs (such as soybean meal, corn, imported feed additives) are handled at ports, docks or grain depots before transportation. Closed ports, docks and third-party warehouses were common during the early stages of the fight against the epidemic. Although the blockade was lifted and docks and warehouses were able to re-open, few handling staff returned to work, which resulted in delayed handling.

(2) On international trade

Some foreign companies were concerned about the outbreak and prevented exports of animal and plant products originating from China. During the worse of the COVID-19 outbreak, a lack of understanding of how the virus was transmitted, caused concern among companies and consumers in a number of countries, preventing goods and commodities exported from China from being delivered smoothly. For example, Pakistan and other countries required the issue of certificates for being free of COVID-9 contamination for goods originating from China and reinforced fumigation and disinfection measures at destination ports [1] , while Russia [2] , South Korea [3] and Turkey [4] suspended imports of

---

① Source from China Council for the Promotion of International Trade.
② Source: https://www.fsvps.ru/fsvps/laws/7073.html.
③ Source: https://cn.yna.co.kr/view/ACK20200129005200881.
④ Source: https://www.hurriyetdailynews.com/turkey-limits-chinese-imports-amid-coronavirus-outbreak-151858.

animal and plant products from China. Although the WHO did not recommend restrictions on China's travel and trade in its *Statement on the second meeting of the International Health Regulations (2005) Emergency Committee regarding the outbreak of novel coronavirus (2019-nCoV)* [①] on January 30, the concern did not go away.

Due to the introduction of control measures by destination countries of Chinese export goods, as well as China's domestic logistics restrictions, Chinese export companies failed to deliver goods on time, resulting in passive default. Some domestic export companies failed to fulfill their contracts due to the COVID-19 outbreak, and faced the double blow of inventory overstock and claims from foreign customers, as well as severe difficulties in their operations. To their credit, business associations, including the China Council for the Promotion of International Trade and the China Chamber of Commerce of Import and Export of Foodstuffs, Native Produce & Animal By-Products offered timely support to companies by issuing proof of force majeure to help them overcome difficulties.

The delay in cross-border logistics of invoices and documents also affected customs clearance. Closed docks and delayed loading/unloading had a big impact on international trade. Many cargo ships could not unload, cold storage at docks was filled with goods that could not be shipped for a long period of time, causing ships to China to be transshipped to other regions.

Reasons for the above are as follows:

① Lack of emergency plans and unified coordination mechanisms. At the early stages of a virus outbreak, an emergency plan leads to timely actions to minimize its impact. A unified and coordinated plan ensures effective supply and reduces the impact of different policies in different regions. Damage to any link

---

① Source: https://www.who.int/news-room/detail/30-01-2020-statement-on-the-second-meeting-of-the-international-health-regulations-(2005)-emergency-committee-regarding-the-outbreak-of-novel-coronavirus-(2019-ncov).

in a supply chain may cause the breakdown of the whole chain, as a slight move in one part affects the whole.

② Over-dependence of the supply chain on people and insufficient automation. As too many logistics and production personnel failed to return to work in a timely manner, companies failed to resume production even once work was supposed to have resumed. The lack of personnel in key positions meant entire plants were unable to operate.

③ Insufficient digitalization of supply chain operational information caused trade to be affected and lack of traceability, meaning the authorities did not have a full picture of the situation. Governments strongly encouraged companies to resume work and production, but they still relied on the self-declaration by companies in terms of information gathering and acknowledgment, which was inefficient.

2　Assumption on the contingency plan for the grains and oilseeds supply chain

A good contingency plan and implementation mechanism for the grains and oilseeds supply chain could ensure timely and effective supply to affected areas through simple procedures and smooth organization of logistics. This will also enable grains and oilseeds production supply chain, from raw material production and purchase, production, logistics, to sales, remains functioning to ensure sufficient food supplies subsequently.

Judging from the outbreak of COVID-19, the supply chain contingency plan mechanism may be further improved in the future, based on the special governmental managing workgroup mechanism currently adopted in China. The plan will define a trigger mechanism according to the nature of a disaster, as well as the responsibilities and coordination mechanism of leading departments and fellow departments of constituting authorities, and carry out dynamic impact evaluation and improvement. In terms of policy formulation, the plan will emphasize the concept of integration for the whole industry chain, and will:

① define the list of key guaranteed supplies, including grains, oils, feedstuff and other key guaranteed supplies for people's livelihood;

② develop maps for supply reserves, dispatching and production, so as to arrange supplies according to the probability of disasters, production capacity of grains, oils and supplies, the location of the population and breeding in different regions, and with reference to national and commercial reserves;

③ streamline the maps for every link in the supply chain of specific industries, covering raw materials, logistics, warehousing, equipment parts and auxiliary packaging materials. Taking soybean meal production as an example, the whole contingency supply chain is required to coordinate customs clearance, handling at docks, production in plants, logistics and transportation, as well as sufficient labor force, equipment maintenance, warehousing and other derivative elements.

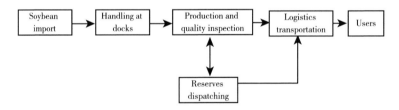

Figure 1　Map of the Supply Chain of Soybean Pressing

The above contingency plan will ensure the timely initiation of the plan, smooth operation of the supply chain, accurate and effective guarantees, and orderly and sustainable production resumption, in case of a disaster.

3　Suggestions on improving the grains and oilseeds supply chain

To further improve the grains and oilseeds supply chain contingency mechanism, the following suggestions are made according to the specific situation of the industry.

(1) Suggestions on production and reserves

① Improve the automation and intelligence of grains and oilseeds production. At present, the grains and oilseeds industry is subject to insufficient automation and intelligence, failing to satisfy the requirements for flexibility of configuration and efficient dispatching in emergency situations. It is suggested that, on the one hand, the government issues policies to encourage the automation of the grains and oilseeds industry, supporting the industrial transformation through technologies upgrade, including 5G video monitoring, AGV scheduling, data backhaul and equipment data collection technologies. These will not only enable smart grains and oilseeds plants to reduce the dependence on labor in production, but will improve product quality and production effectiveness when combining with intellectual Industry Internet in the future. Furthermore, the government should encourage the building of a certain proportion of unmanned chemical plants and production lines to improve production efficiency and avoid forced production disruption.

On the other hand, the government should encourage the training of workers with all-around skills, so that in case of emergency, one person is able to work in multiple positions to cope with labor shortage, and to avoid production safety risks caused by temporarily-hired workers due to labor shortages.

② Increase the proportion of contract reserves and production reserves in emergency reserves. China enjoys a supply chain contingency system with complete construction of physical grains and oilseeds product reserves. During this epidemic, the sufficient physical reserves of corn and other food crops played an important role in meeting production demand and stabilizing prices. However, it is still suggested to increase contract reserves and production reserves of grains and oilseeds products, to further diversify state grain reserves. It is also suggested to include feedstuffs and agricultural resources in the emergency supplies guarantee system, as part of the effort to strengthen and improve the reserve system for important agricultural products.

The government should encourage contracts with leading enterprises to ensure the prior lease, dispatch or production of grains and oilseeds products, as agreed after emergencies to secure the supply. The government should, according to population densities and the location of the breeding industry, guide and optimize the grains and oilseeds reserves close to areas where feedstuffs are needed and there are high population concentrations, building a more complete and flexible emergency grains and oilseeds supplies guarantee platform.

Furthermore, the government should assign a single government department to schedule uniformly the purchase, storage, dispatch, transportation and use of emergency supplies to improve efficiency, while defining responsibilities. During the current epidemic, the way of guaranteeing medical supplies by requiring leading companies to produce and dispatch supplies directly to client organizations is worth reference and promotion, as it greatly improved the efficiency of supply under emergency conditions. Drawing on the lessons from Hurricane Katrina, the U.S. government adjusted its emergency management policies after the disaster and reformed the Federal Emergency Management Agency (FEMA), an important part of which was to upgrade the Logistic Management Group to the Logistics Management Directorate (LMD) to integrate and coordinate uniformly the government's internal and external emergency supplies.

(2) Suggestions on trade and logistics

① Digitalize logistics documents with information technologies, such as blockchain. Blockchain is a new application pattern for distributed data storage, encryption and other computer technologies. The data or information stored in it are characterized by "unforgeable", "whole-process marked", "traceable", "open and transparent" and "collectively maintained". After the digital processing of traditional paper documents with blockchain technology, the real-time matching of data avoids heavy repetitive workloads, reducing the time for document processing by a fifth, and the time needed to complete the cross-border trade of agricultural products by half.

Currently, six large international agricultural companies, namely Louis Dreyfus Company, Cargill, ADM, Bunge, COFCO and Glencore Agriculture, have launched a joint venture called Covantis to enhance the standardization and digitization of international agricultural transportation transactions by adopting blockchain technology, and are developing a platform that will be available for post-trade operations worldwide. The blockchain program for parallel-import cars launched by Tianjin Customs, China, in 2019 made full use of the tamper-proof and traceability advantage of the technology, which addressed the problem with regard to mutual trust between different stakeholders, realized the visualization of process nodes, and made inspection and quarantine clearance more convenient and efficient. Prospects for the application of the technology has been verified in the industry.

It is suggested to further promote the application of blockchain technology in supply chains to speed up the promotion of a modern and intelligent supply chain.

② Manage water transport, land transport and other important transportation junctions hierarchically according to the degree of risk.

A hierarchical management mechanism is conducive to defining the risk management responsibilities of main bodies at all levels, and to improving the accountability mechanism of supply guarantee. First of all, a hierarchical management mechanism for companies should be developed according to the production maps mentioned earlier, with reference to local conditions. A 'white list' of grains and oilseeds companies should be put in place, based on scientific criteria and specific conditions, to ensure the companies get the support they need. Secondly, a hierarchical operation plan for the whole supply chain should be developed for the import of raw materials, production of products and logistics and delivery by companies on the list, in which special water transport and land transport channels need to open up and emergency traffic permits should be issued in advance, according to the levels of companies, to reserve access to permits in case of an emergency, so as to ensure the import of raw materials and supply of products. Thirdly, hierarchical management shall be applied to important transportation junctions such as docks, in order to streamline in advance and guarantee as a priority the continuous operation of important transportation infrastructure, including key docks and highways in production and affected areas. Workers should be isolated on the spot and operations should be mechanized to ensure that grains and oilseeds supplies are not blocked at key nodes and to break logistics bottlenecks in case of emergencies.

③ Realize shared logistics using big data and other modern information means. The logistics industry enjoys favorable conditions to develop a "shared economy", and developing shared logistics is conducive to integrating the surplus of logistics capacity in the society, lowering logistics costs, and reducing carbon emissions, waste of resources, traffic congestion and environmental pollution from logistics. This would help realize the intensive, greening and efficient transformation of the logistics industry. During the outbreak of COVID-19, some logistics companies, such as EMS and SF Express, guaranteed their operation by sharing their transportation capacity, under the condition that the access of drivers and vehicles to affected areas was restricted. Such an initiative is worth exploring and promoting.

It is suggested, on the one hand, that the country should continue to promote the building and management of a vehicle-cargo platform to enhance the sharing and reasonable allocation of logistics transportation and delivery resources. Advanced technologies, such as the Internet, big data and blockchain, may be integrated to provide solutions for problems in information authenticity and effectiveness in the current vehicle-cargo platform. On the other hand, the country should speed up the planning and layout of logistics parks and other infrastructure, and advocate vigorously for smart warehousing and smart logistics management, in order to facilitate the development of shared logistics. In the future, information technology will further enhance the in-depth integration of the logistics industry, and expand greatly the emergency management of the supply chain, especially the big data tracking and analysis of the purchase, production and transportation of grains, oils and other supplies for people's livelihood, the optimization of logistics routes, the forecasting of supply consumption and warehousing, and the prevention and control of risks.

(3) Strengthen information disclosure and consumption expectation management

During this epidemic, the public has paid more and more attention to the real-time disclosure of disaster information, which not only fulfills their right to know, but also helps the manufacturing industry to organize production plans reasonably. After the outbreak, China strengthened the timely disclosure of information on medical supplies, and allowed the joint prevention and control mechanism to undertake the task of guaranteeing production and supply by disclosing the product capacity and future production increase in medical supplies. This alleviated the public's concern. A grains and oilseeds monitoring system has also been launched in the food system to report daily on the production of high-quality feedstuff companies, and livestock and poultry breeding companies. The vegetable responsibility system and daily inspection and reporting system were introduced in many cities and regions to disclose price information to the public online, via SMS and other channels, in order to manage the public's expectations. Such practices should also be introduced for grain products, oil products and feedstuff raw materials, as they are conducive to better scheduling by production companies to avoid fluctuations, due to stress in the production and logistics parts of the supply chain, as well as helping to avoid large price fluctuations due to panic buying.

互联网医疗在疫情防控与日常医疗中的作用

辉瑞投资有限公司 [*]

2020 年突如其来的新冠肺炎疫情使整个中国社会生活和日常经济活动受到很大影响。在经历了疫情初期的严峻局面后，很快全国各地都动员起来，全力以赴投入这场疫情防控的阻击战、总体战和人民战争中。基于中国体制优势，疫情以快于很多人最初估计的速度迅速得到遏制，新发病例数在湖北尤其是湖北以外地区显著下降。中国人民在这场没有硝烟的战争中取得了阶段性的胜利。

然而，为了快速控制和阻击疫情，我们在其他很多方面都暂时付出了牺牲和代价。比如，在疫情期间，为了集中医疗资源抗疫，同时也为了避免院内交叉感染，很多医院都暂停或压缩了日常门诊，由此造成了很多其他疾病的患者无法得到及时的治疗；很多慢性疾病或需要长期服药的患者无法及时复诊、续方并配到日常服用药品，由此一些患者因无法及时复诊或服药而造成病情恶化甚至更严重的后果。我们在防止新冠肺炎的同时，也必须预防各种次生灾害的发生。

国家医疗保障局等相关部门针对这些情况，及时出台有关文件，鼓励患者在新冠肺炎疫情期间，通过网上问诊和互联网医院等线上渠道寻医问药。部分地方也出台文件将一些互联网医院纳入医保报销的范畴。世界卫生组织认为这些都是其他国家在防疫过程中值得借鉴的宝贵经验。

---

[*] 辉瑞公司是一家以研发为基础的生物制药公司，创建于 1849 年，总部位于美国纽约市。公司产品包括降胆固醇药、口服抗真菌药、抗生素等。

在中国互联网技术、电子商务、物流配送和 5G 等通信技术快速发展并在全球领先的情况下，可以以此次新冠肺炎疫情防控为契机，推动互联网诊疗的发展，使之不仅成为患者日常寻医问药的新常态，而且也可以在未来疫情发生时发挥积极的作用。对此，我们建议从以下几个方面开展积极探索。

一　通过互联网医院方便患者就医，减轻医院门诊量

中国近几年出台的相关医疗卫生体制改革的文件里都提到了将积极推进分级诊疗、互联网医疗和医生多点执业的发展。但由于各种障碍，互联网医院的发展一直比较缓慢，目前还是以网上预约挂号和轻问诊等功能为主。未来应该鼓励各级医疗机构，尤其是基层和社区医疗卫生机构开设互联网医院，处理一些日常简单的复诊和需方的工作。患者经过互联网医院实现有效分诊，导流患者至不同的医疗机构，推动分级诊疗，减轻大医院的负担，让优质医疗资源用于疑难重症的救治；对于慢性病患者，很多时候他们去医院只是为了复诊和续方配药。这点完全可以通过互联网医院实现，这样不仅能减少患者来回奔波的辛苦，也可减轻医院门诊量和医生的负担。与此同时，医生在互联网医院执业也有助于国家鼓励医生多点执业的政策落实。

更重要的是，互联网医院有助于实现患者，尤其是慢病患者的全程健康管理。与传统医院不同，医生可以通过互联网医院和患者保持长期和实时的互动交流，随时了解患者的健康情况并给予相关医学建议，真正实现患者健康的全程管理目标。

二　通过互联网医院助力疫情防控

互联网医院结合大数据系统，如短时间内发现大量患者反映有类似传染病的症状，可以有助于及早发现疫情苗头，防范潜在疫情发生，成为疫情预警机制的一部分。在疫情发生时，一方面可以通过互联网医院对其他

疾病患者进行日常问诊、复诊和续方等工作，让医院有限的医疗资源专注于疫情防控和感染患者的诊治上；另一方面也可通过互联网医院了解隔离期间感染或疑似感染患者情况，给予相关健康建议、注意事项并根据患者的情况进行分诊，避免患者和非患者蜂拥而至医院，造成医院不堪负荷，并增加交叉感染的风险。

对于一些疑似或者轻症居家隔离的患者，可以通过互联网医院随时了解患者的健康状况，并通过互联网给予患者相关的医学指导和处方。这样可以有效管理居家隔离的患者，及时掌握患者情况，一旦出现健康状况的恶化可以及时采取进一步的措施，同时也可以减少社区工作者上门的传染风险。

对于治愈出院的患者，也可以通过互联网医院定期进行复诊和随访，避免病情的复发。

三 建立高效的线下药品配送体系

互联网医院可以实现线上的问诊和处方，但药物的配送还是要线下完成。中国近年来的物流配送业发展迅速，其中包括多家专业药品配送企业的迅速发展。互联网医院可以与药品专业配送企业结合，患者在网上得到的处方可以快速传送给相关药品配送企业，患者在网上完成电子支付后可以在最短的时间里送药上门；同时也可将电子处方直接发送给患者，由患者选择零售药品等渠道自行购买。

随着各种新技术的发展和成熟，逐步探索如机器人送药和无人机送药等更加快速便捷的药品配送方式应该成为一种趋势和可能。

四 实现互联网医院的医保覆盖

目前，中国的基本医疗保险主要覆盖实体医院和部分药店。互联网医院要得到发展就必须打通医疗保险报销这条通路。此次新冠肺炎疫情期间，已有包括湖北在内的一些省市将医保报销扩展到部分互联网医院。我们建议以此为契机，逐步扩大医保覆盖的互联网医院范围，不只是实体医院开设的互联网医院，也应覆盖单纯线上的互联网医院，打通医保报销线上线下的通路。这样不仅可以减轻患者的经济负担，也有助于将更多患者分流至互联网医院。

对于互联网诊疗，防止骗保行为也很重要。这些可以通过现已成熟的人脸识别功能来实现，确保网上问诊人员和医保卡持有人一致。而相关医保部门也可以随机抽取网上处方进行审核，一旦发现骗保行为即吊销相关人员网上问诊的资质直到取消相关互联网医院的资质。

五　疫情期间通过互联网医院开展心理辅导

疫情防控期间，互联网医院还可以起到很重要的一个作用就是在线心理辅导。患者或疑似患者在长期隔离期间容易产生各种心理问题，不利于疫情的有效防控。可以通过在线的心理辅导对患者进行疏导，让患者或疑似患者积极配合居家隔离。对于病愈的患者，可能存在社会歧视和难以融入社会的问题，这方面也可以通过网上的心理辅导给予帮助。此外，互联网医院也可以在宣传疫情防控知识、个人卫生知识等方面发挥积极作用。

互联网医疗的发展需要循序渐进，不应一拥而上。相关部门应该及时出台规范互联网医疗健康有序发展的规范和配套文件，让行业发展有章可循。可以由卫生主管部门牵头，会同医保部门、市场监督管理部门、互联网管理部门一起制定相关规范性文件。在每个地区先选择几家具有一定资质和网络技术基础的医院前期开展试点，并在试点的基础上逐步扩大。积极鼓励医疗机构和相关互联网企业合作，引进先进的互联网和大数据技术及平台，搭建功能完善的互联网医院。

建议以此次新冠肺炎疫情防控为契机，积极推动互联网医疗的发展，并在疫情过后实现常态化，为进一步健全完善医疗卫生体系，并为未来更加高效地应对疫情奠定坚实的基础。

The Role of Internet Healthcare in Pandemic Control & Daily Care

By Pfizer Investment Co., Ltd.

The outbreak of novel coronavirus pneumonia epidemic in 2020 disrupted the life and normal economic activities for the entire China society. After the severe outbreak at the beginning, the nation has been quickly mobilized and fully devoted into the total war against the epidemic with the whole population engaged. Thanks to the advantages of China's political and governance systems, the epidemic is being contained at a speed much higher than initial estimated by many. The number of new cases drops significantly in Hubei province and particularly in regions out of Hubei. The Chinese people have had a periodical victory in this war without smoke.

However, we have made temporary sacrifices and paid the price in many other aspects in order to quickly control and block the epidemic. For example, for the sake of concentrating the medical resources to battling the epidemic, and avoiding in-hospital cross infection, many hospitals had suspended or even stop daily outpatient services, making many patients with other illnesses unable to receive timely treatment; a lot of patients with chronicle diseases or who need to take medication for long term could not make return visits, refill their prescriptions or have access to daily medications, which caused deterioration of conditions or even more serious consequences. We must prevent all kinds of secondary disasters while controlling the coronavirus pneumonia.

Relevant ministries such as the National Healthcare Security Administration have timely issued relevant documents targeting such cases to encourage the patients to seek consultation and medication access through online channels such as online inquiry and internet hospital during the coronavirus epidemic. Some regions also issued local documents to include some internet hospitals into medical insurance and reimbursement. WHO thinks these are valuable experiences worthy of learning by other nations for epidemic prevention.

Given the rapid growth of Internet technologies, e-commerce, logistics and 5G telecom in China that are leading in the Globe, the battle against coronavirus epidemic could be an opportunity for Internet diagnosis and treatment to develop and grow, making it a new normal for patients to seek daily consultation and medication access, while also being able to play a positive role in potential epidemic outbreaks in the future. For this, we recommend active explorations in the aspects below:

1 Make patient visit easier and reduce hospital outpatient traffic with internet hospital

The documents on healthcare system reform as issued by the central government in recent years all mentioned actively promoting the growth of tiered diagnosis and treatment, Internet healthcare and multi-sited practice by doctors. However, due to barriers of various kinds, the growth of Internet hospitals has been quite slow, right now it is mostly about online appointment-register and light inquiry. In the future, the medical institutions at all the categories especially the grass-root and community healthcare institutions shall be encouraged to set up Internet hospitals to handle some daily and simple subsequent consultations & refill of prescription. Through the effective diagnosis split by the Internet (online) hospitals, the patients are diverted to the different medical institutions, thus the tiered diagnosis and treatment are promoted to relieve the burden on major hospitals and enable the premium medical resources to be focused on treatment and cure of tough diseases. For chronicle patients, many times they visit the hospital just for subsequent consultation and refill of prescription, which can be achieved fully with online hospitals, to not only reduce the toil of travel but also alleviate the hospital outpatient traffic and the burden on doctors. At the same time, doctors practicing at online hospitals are also helpful for the implementation of national policy to encourage the multi-sited practice policy.

What's more important, online hospital helps to achieve the full-process health management for patients and especially those with chronicle conditions. Different from traditional hospitals, doctors could maintain long time and real time interactive communication with patients via the online hospital, and get to know the health conditions of patients and give relevant medical advice, thus to truly realize the full-process management for patient health.

2   The online hospitals facilitate the epidemic prevention & control

The online hospital is integrated with big data system, where if many patients complain with symptom of infectious diseases in a short period of time, it may help find the emergence of an epidemic early and prevent the potential epidemic, which becomes part of the epidemic pre-warning mechanism. In case of an epidemic happening, on the one hand the daily and normal inquiries, subsequent consultation and refill of prescription could be performed for other patients via the online hospital, thus the limited medical resources with the hospitals could be focused on prevention/control of epidemic and the diagnosis/ treatment of infected patients, on the other hand the conditions of the infected or the suspected patients could be understood via the online hospitals during the quarantine, to whom the relevant health advice could give, preventing the patients and non-patients from flocking to the hospitals to overwhelm the hospital and increase the risk of cross infection.

For some suspected patients or patients with mild symptoms in home quarantine, their health status could be accessed any time via the online hospital, so that relevant medical instruction and prescription could be given online. Thus we could effectively management the patients in home quarantine, and timely master the conditions of patients. Once their health status starts to deteriorate, we can timely take further measures while cutting the risk of infection for the community workers who drop in.

For the patients healed and discharged from the hospital, regular subsequent consultation and follow-up visit could be done via the online hospitals to prevent recurrence.

3 Set up the efficient offline medicine distribution system

Though Internet hospital could deliver online inquiry, diagnosis and prescription, the medicine distribution needs to performed offline. In China, the logistic industry has developed rapidly in recent years, including the high-speed growth of multiple professional medicine distribution enterprises. The online hospitals could be integrated with professional pharmaceutical distribution carriers, so that the prescriptions acquired by patients online can be quickly sent to relevant pharmaceutical distributors. After the patients complete the e-payment online, the medicines could be delivered to their home as soon as possible; meanwhile the electronic prescription could be directly sent to the patients who could purchase the drugs by themselves from retail drugstores.

With the growth and maturity of many new technologies, gradual exploration on robotic medicine delivery and/or drone delivery as the faster and more convenient pharmaceutical distribution model should become a trend and possibility.

4 Medical insurance coverage of online hospitals

Currently, China's basic medical insurance program mostly covers the physical hospitals and part of the drugstores. Online hospital must line up the pathway of medical insurance reimbursement in order to grow. During this coronavirus pneumonia epidemic, some provinces including Hubei have already extended the medical insurance coverage to part of the online hospitals. We recommend to take this as an opportunity and gradually expand the scope of online hospitals under medical insurance to cover not only the Internet hospital run by offline hospitals but also those that are completely online, and line up the channel or pathway of online/offline for medical insurance reimbursement. Thus we could relieve the burden on patients and help to divert more patients to the online hospitals.

For online diagnosis and treatment, it is also very important to prevent insurance fraud. It could be realized by proven face recognition function to ensure the online inquiry individual is consistent with the medical insurance cardholder. The medical insurance authority could also randomly review online prescriptions, once any insurance fraud behavior is identified, the certification of online inquiry/diagnosis for the offender(s) would be revoked, and even the certification of the offending online hospital could be canceled.

5　Psychological coaching via the online hospital in the epidemic

During the epidemic control and prevention, Internet hospitals could play an important role in online psychological counseling. Patients or suspected patients are prone to having different psychological problems during the long-term quarantine, which would cause detriment to the control and prevention of epidemic. Online psychological counseling could be leveraged to make the patients or suspected patients to actively cooperate with home quarantine. The patients healed may experience problems of social discrimination and difficulty in integrating into society, online psychological counseling could also help in these aspects. Moreover, online hospitals could also play an active role in publicizing the epidemic prevention/control knowledge and personal hygiene knowledge.

The growth of online healthcare needs to be taken as a step-by-step process and not in a rush. Relevant authorities should timely issue the codes and supporting documents to standardize the Internet healthcare for healthy and orderly growth, thus providing a guideline for the industry to follow. The public health authority may lead and join with the medical insurance, market supervision and regulatory, the Internet administration authorities to draft the normative documents together, and shortlist a couple of hospitals with certain certification and Internet technical basis in each area for early pilot, and gradually expand the scope based on the pilots. The medical institutions should also be actively encouraged to partner with Internet players to introduce advanced technology and platform of Internet and big data, and build online hospitals with elaborate functions.

It is recommended to leverage this coronavirus epidemic control and prevention as an opportunity to actively promote the growth of Internet healthcare, and make it normalized after the epidemic in order to further elaborate the medical and public health system, and lay down a solid foundation for tackling the epidemic more effectively in the future.

把握汽车行业规律，力保全球产业链

李　洁　捷豹路虎*（中国）投资有限公司　执行副总裁
苏巴鸿　大众汽车集团**（中国）　高级总监

　　新冠肺炎疫情的肆虐不仅造成数以千计生命的损失、伤害，威胁到无数人的身心健康和安全，同时给国民经济带来重创。经过举国奋战，疫情蔓延势头得到基本控制。于是，一手抓防控、一手抓复工便成为当务之急。

　　自 2020 年 2 月中旬以来，中国政府就统筹推进新冠肺炎疫情防控和经济社会发展工作做出一系列周密和详尽的部署。本文仅以汽车产业为例，沿着统筹部署路线，就产业复工和恢复正常运营的必要步骤提出一点思考与建议。

一　汽车产业在国民经济中的地位

1. 汽车工业是国民经济的重要支柱产业

　　汽车产业在推动经济增长、促进社会就业、改善民生福祉方面发挥着重要作用。汽车自诞生之始，就与人们的生活和经济活动产生了紧密的联系，并且改变了人们的生活方式和经济的发展节奏。汽车，也因此被誉为"改变世界的机器"，而汽车工业则被视为推动经济发展、社会进步的重要引擎。

---

　　*　捷豹路虎（英文简称 JLR）是一家拥有两个顶级奢华品牌的英国汽车制造商。从赛道传奇到人生旅迹，从探险利器到挑战奇迹，捷豹路虎（中国）与你一起尽享英伦风范，前瞻未来出行。

　　**　大众汽车集团是一家总部位于德国沃尔夫斯堡的汽车制造公司，于 1973 年成立。集团旗下有大众、奥迪、保时捷、宾利、斯柯达等品牌。

　　本文仅代表作者本人观点。

在21世纪"后工业化"的今天，汽车行业仍是发达国家的核心产业，美国、德国、日本、英国、法国、意大利、韩国等强大的工业国家无不拥有发达的汽车工业。而中国汽车产业，自改革开放以来迅速发展，取得了举世瞩目的成就，成为国民经济发展的支柱力量。我国国民经济统计公报显示，近年来，消费对中国GDP增长贡献超过60%，而仅汽车这一个品类就占社会消费品零售总额的10%左右。汽车工业在整个工业总产值的比重也是不容小觑的。

表1 2005~2019年中国汽车工业总产值

单位：亿元，%

年份	汽车工业总产值（A）	全国工业总产值（工业销售产值）（B）	汽车工业总产值占全国工业总产值的比重（A/B）
2005	10223.2	246946.4	4.1
2006	13937.6	310828.6	4.5
2007	17242.1	397626.7	4.3
2008	18780.6	494733.7	3.8
2009	23437.8	536134.1	4.4
2010	30248.7	684735.2	4.4
2011	33155.3	827797.0	4.0
2012	35774.4	909797.2	3.9
2013	39225.5	1019405.3	3.8
2014	42324.3	1092198.0	3.9
2015	45014.5	1104026.7	4.1
2016	39329.9	1151950.1	3.4
2017	58382.5	1292111.2	4.5
2018	52498.7	1416676.1	3.7
2019	50427.9	1472147.2	3.4

资料来源：国家信息中心。

2. 汽车产业链纵向横向延伸长

汽车从设计、生产、销售到售后服务与诸多行业有着密切的关联和深度的合作，往往带动一系列相关产业的发展。上游产业有钢铁、有色金属、橡胶、装饰织物、玻璃、线束及电子控制元件、灯具照明、塑料以及大型冲压和锻压机械制造、机械切削设备、工具制造、机器人制造甚至石化方面的油漆、机油、润滑油等，外加运输行业和生产型服务业等；在新能源车领域还有电池、电机等制造行业。下游涉及面同样很广，包括汽车维修、零部件制造、汽车信贷、汽车保险、汽车租赁、道路保养、汽车运动、汽车改装，石化方面的成品油、润滑油、冷却液和旧车回收等。发达国家的经验表明，汽车工业每增值 1 元，会给上游产业带来 0.65 元的增值，给下游产业带来 2.63 元的增值。中国的情况大致差不多，全国与汽车相关产业的就业人数，已经超过社会就业总人数的 1/6。

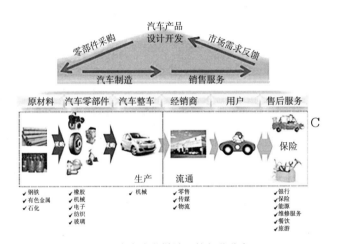

图 1　汽车产业链涉及的行业分布

3. 汽车行业是最具创新力的产业之一

在汽车的激烈竞争中，创新是提升竞争力的必由之路。因此，汽车产品变成新技术、新材料的最佳搭载平台。当今世界风起云涌，新一轮产业革命正在孕育兴起。无线通信、人工智能、新能源技术、自动化技术正在一个又一个领域推动着颠覆性的创新。而年逾百年的汽车产业，也正在吸收来自计算机、通信、新能源、新材料的技术，推动自身的"新四化"革命，成为新一轮技术革命的"主战场"。各国为了抢占这一引领创新的机遇，纷纷推出支持政策，协调产学研全速发展。2020年2月24日国家发展和改革委员会等11部委联合印发了《智能汽车创新发展战略》，将发展智能汽车定义为提升中国产业基础能力、增强新一轮科技革命和产业变革引领能力的重大战略。

4. 中国汽车产业在全球汽车产业和供应链中发挥着重要的作用

中国连续十多年来一直是全球最大的市场，也是全球最大的汽车生产国。世界上具有规模的知名汽车生产企业都在中国境内建立了合资生产企业或独资的电动车生产企业。这些企业在华耕耘数十载，使中国制造业特别是零部件供应商成为全球资源配置中一个不可或缺的生力军。根据中国海关总署统计，2019年汽车零部件出口总额超过600亿美元，较2018年增长8.9%。其中外资企业在华子公司对外出口占据了40%。这一出口规模足以说明中国汽车零部件供应商在全球产业链中的地位。

表2　外资零部件供应商在中国的分布情况

单位：家，%

地区分类	省份	企业总数	博世	电装	麦格纳国际	大陆集团	采埃孚	爱信精机	现代摩比斯	佛吉亚	法雷奥	李尔
一类	湖北	20	1	1	1	2	1	0	0	10	4	有
二类	广东	41	1	8	2	0	0	11	0	7	12	有
	浙江	18	2	1	3	2	4	4	0	2	0	有
	江苏	40	7	5	4	4	1	5	3	6	5	有
	安徽	8	2	1	0	0	1	2	0	0	1	有
	湖南	6	1	0	3	0	0	0	0	1	1	无
	河南	2	0	0	0	0	1	0	0	1	0	无
三类	其他		16	21	19	19	27	17	8	46	28	有
共计		135	30	37	33	27	35	39	11	73	51	暂无数据
重点疫区企业占中国比例			47	43	42	30	23	56	27	37	45	

资料来源：普华永道《着力眼前挑战，心怀长期发展》，2020年2月。

二 新冠肺炎疫情重创汽车产业链

中国是全球第一大汽车制造国和第一大汽车消费市场，同时又是汽车"新四化"的主要推动者，正处在推动技术革命和产品革命深入发展的关键时期，却突然遭受新冠肺炎的重袭，汽车产业顿时陷入近乎停滞的状态。突如其来的疫情给汽车行业的发展带来极大的挑战。

汽车是一件极其复杂且可靠性和安全性要求极高的产品。传统燃油汽车的零部件数量达到3万件以上，即便是结构相对简单的纯电动汽车也有将近2万件零部件。为了保证汽车产品的整体质量，整车制造商需要对重要零部件供应商进行严格的审核和验收。而庞大零部件数量的背后是不可胜数的供应商。通常整车制造商都有200家左右的供应商配套。任何一个零部件的缺失，都将迫使整个流程停摆。更为致命的是，重要零部件供应商也还需要一定数量的所谓的二级、三级乃至四级的中小企业提供零部件。其中任何供应商的停产和缺失都会影响整个供应链的正常运行，进而影响到整车制造的生产。此外，绝大部分整车制造企业也为了高效率和高效益，备货非常有限。所以，当供应链中哪怕是一个很小的环节出问题，都会带来很大的负面影响，甚至造成停工停产。

而在下游销售端，整车企业规模不一样，为其做销售服务的经销商数也不一样。大车企的经销网络拥有千家以上的经销商，小车企也有上百家（个别超豪华品牌除外）。统计数据显示，全国范围内共有3万家左右的经销商。其中大部分都是中小企业，财力及现金流有限，因而，抗险能力也相对孱弱。

值得关注的是，自2018年起，经济下行压力带来的消费信心不足，致使汽车销售连续下滑超过18个月，对整个产业形成了巨大冲击。产业链中的上游供应商和下游的经销商等服务企业大都已经感到压力重重。

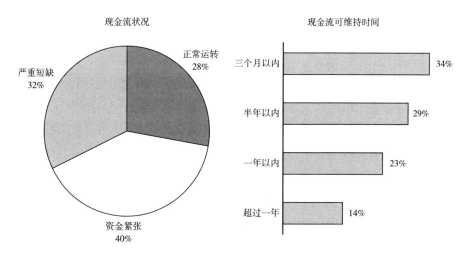

图2　2020年国内经销商经营现金流状态调查

资料来源：普华永道《着力眼前挑战，心怀长期发展》，2020年2月。

　　而这次疫情的发生，使汽车产业同许多其他产业一样处于消费和生产两端受损的状态。据乘用车市场信息联合会统计，2020年2月上半月的乘用车销售数据与上年同期相比下滑超过90%。这意味着全国绝大多数的经销商是零运营；也同时意味着所有的整车企业都在严重失血。而从供应端看，2月上半月，所有的整车车企和给其配套的供应商，原本因为春节假期而暂停生产，此后又因新冠肺炎疫情的肆虐而停工。因此，供需两端的停摆正在造成整个产业链上的企业在凛冬之后再度经受雪虐风餐般的考验，收入中断势必对现金流施予极大的压力，房租、工资、贷款利息等费用仍需支付。根据中国汽车工业协会的数据，中国目前规模以上的汽车零部件企业有1.3万余家。另外，根据中国汽车工业协会2月对212家零部件企业进行的调查，受疫情影响，零部件企业营业收入损失最高的达到20亿元，营收损失在2000万~5000万元的企业占比为16%。部分体量较小、抗风险能力较弱的中小企业将面临破产倒闭的困境。

　　汽车行业的受损肯定是支柱产业的受损，进而撼动国民经济的发展势头。这是因为，正如我们上面提到，汽车产业链上游和下游涉及面都很广，关联行业众多。更为重要的是，受创的还包括汽车产业中被定位为战略性新兴产业的新能源汽车产业。毋庸置疑，这次疫情不单单击中了汽车产业，而且击中整个国民经济的方方面面。

然而，在中国已经是深度融入全球化的大背景下，中国经济的每一个变化都在影响全球经济的脉搏。经过几十年的产业全球化发展，中国制造作为全球供应链的重要一环，已经深深嵌入全球供应链。中国供应商因疫情停工停产，就直接造成如韩国现代和日本丰田的海外工厂停产。而其他国际知名汽车制造企业在海外的工厂也将在3月面临零部件短缺、生产无以为继的局面。换句话说，如果供应商无法尽早复工恢复生产的话，中国汽车产业在全球供应链中的重要地位可能受到动摇，甚至折损。

三 实施行业统筹，抓好上下游同时施策的节奏

面对疫情对社会生产经营的冲击，中央政府及时颁布了一系列全方位的针对中小微企业复工纾困政策。各地地方政府也因地制宜地推出具体的实施细则，包括减免或降低租金、延迟或减免税款、提供金融救助以及降低或推迟缴纳社保以降低企业负担等。这些都是非常及时且必要的政策，对推动社会生产经营回归正常化有着极为重大的意义。鉴于政策的落实是在地方政府掏出真金白银扶持当地的企业而得以实现，因此，就很难避免见木不见林，缺乏产业链的视角的情况，进而找不到行业把握的切入点，难以达到行业所预期的效果。对此，我们建议如下。

1. 力保中国汽车产业在全球产业供应链中的地位

如上所述，各大汽车的生产厂家在海外的生产大都依赖在华的外资和内资的供应商，尽管依赖程度不尽相同，但因为汽车产品的特性，缺少一个零部件，其生产就无法继续，其产品就无法完成。因此，为了保证在华的供应商还会在供应链中发挥作用，就应采取精准救助的措施。

其中，第一种途径就是利用海关零部件出口数据，顺藤摸瓜列出一个

完整的出口零部件制造商名单。由工业和信息化部以及相关部门牵头，指导地方有的放矢地对名单上的企业实施扶持和支助政策。而第二种途径是让国内外的整车制造企业和零部件供应商或其在华的相关企业提供其急需零部件在国内的供应商名单，因为它们更清楚哪些零部件有库存，哪些是急需的。将两个名单进行对比，就基本可以断定哪些是时下全球产业供应链中至关重要的配套商了。工业主管部门就可以依据这样一个完整的名单来指导地方精准实施救急政策。

2. 需要指出的是，以上述途径支持相关供应商复工，并不要求地方政府提供更多额外的扶持政策，而是在现有的政策实施过程中，增加一个关注的维度，有一个更加清晰的切入点

秉持全产业链观，疏通上下游。要想让汽车产业恢复疫前正常状态，必须打通整个产业链。下游不通畅，上游复工后也会造成流通梗阻。同样，下游通畅，上游供应商没有完全复位，就会下游等水水不来，整个产业链还是无法正常运营。

日前，中央政府已经意识到下游打通的基础是首先要放松限制市场容量的政策，即要求实施限购的城市，如无法取消限购政策，至少应当放宽所限额度，扩大市场容量。这是极大的利好。另外，要提振消费者的消费信心，就要在信贷方面实施更加宽松且风险可控的政策，如降低汽车贷款的首付额度、提供相应的优惠的低息贷款、给予金融服务更多的灵活的空间。此外，鼓励汽车消费，还应一定程度采取定向明确的降税政策，例如，可以阶段性地实施减免车辆购置税，亦可取消或进一步降低 2.0L 以下小排量乘用车的消费税。另外为稳定汽车消费的长期发展，鉴于在购置环节的综合税率占比较高的问题，建议启动长期的结构性减税政策研究。还有，地方政府还可以有针对性地关注处于产业链下游的汽车经销商，根据所受冲击的严重程度，对经营有严重困难的经销商给予适当的支持补助。

3. 加快给予整车企业纾困减负，发挥其产业链的龙头作用

鉴于汽车产品的完整性特征，产业链上下游的重要性是不言而喻的。

但牵动上游和下游的是汽车整车制造商，盘活上下游的先决条件是整车企业自身运营能力无损。疫情面前，车企铁肩担道义，为纾解上下游企业困局，甚至自发组织员工参与上游零部件企业复产复工，并且自掏腰包直接补助经销商。与此同时，在目前销售几乎停滞的状态下，车企的赢利能力与现金压力也异常沉重。因此在受疫情影响的特殊时期，对于整车企业所得税进行一定程度的减免，还有确保车企的现金流，亦可成为中央和地方金融系统政策实施的切入点。

4. 应按照党中央、国务院部署，统筹推进疫情防控和经济社会发展，必须更有针对性地加大"六稳"工作力度，充分发挥中国特色社会主义的制度优势，针对疫情的短期及长期影响进行快速响应，并及时进行政策调整

（1）应在坚持促进行业长期稳定发展的大原则下，对行业管理政策进行灵活的短期调整，帮助产业度过疫情危机，以期"稳就业、稳投资、稳预期"，并保证"先生存，再发展"。疫情暴发打乱了包括研发、设计、生产、物流、销售等在内的全产业链的既有规划，进而为如期实现行业环保、节能及发展新能源汽车等方面的中短期发展目标造成困难。因此，一方面，应尽快出台包括双积分、新能源汽车发展规划等在内的前瞻性重要政策，帮助企业明确未来发展方向，稳定预期；另一方面，可以考虑适当延后或放宽部分行业政策在2020~2021年的要求，例如新能源汽车积分比例、国六排放颗粒物限值、车载 ETC 模块认证等。

（2）应继续坚持改革开放，对外资进一步开放，加快出台稳定和吸引外资的相关政策，以期"稳外贸、稳外资、稳金融"。疫情影响进一步体现了中国在全球供应链中的重要地位，但也有可能提醒一些跨国公司为了降低供应链整体风险而在其他国家寻求替代方案。因此，一方面，帮助企业有序复工复产的措施应尽快落实，以增强企业信心；另一方面，也应通过在投资及生产准入、行业管理（例如双积分中关联企业的定义）、国内外融资便利性、外汇管理等方面进一步优化外资企业的营商环境，来应对

潜在的产业转移趋势。

　　总之，中国汽车产业经历几十年耕耘后已经深度融入全球供应链中。在疫情肆虐的当下，应当首先确保中国汽车产业今天在全球供应链中举足轻重的地位稳定不变，这不仅利好中国，更能普惠全球。其次，扶持上下游企业要确保不让一家掉队，从而达到保证产业链的两端无损的目的。此外，只有让汽车制造企业顺利克服时艰，才能真正做到产业的安全和完整。最后，应将疫情的挑战作为向全世界展示中国特色社会主义制度优势的机会，做出快速且全面的响应，进一步增强国内外投资者对中国未来长期稳定发展的信心。

Grasping Automotive Industry Principle & Safeguarding the Global Industry Chain

By Jie Li, Excutive Vice President, Jaguar Land Rover (China) Investment Co., Ltd.
Bahong Su, Senior Director, Volkswagen Group China

The outbreak of COVID-19 has taken thousands of lives which not only presented a physical and mental health challenge to most people, but also crashed the economy. So far, the spread of the epidemic has been basically curbed by the whole country. Therefore, the top priority of the moment is resuming production while maintaining epidemic prevention and control.

Since mid-February 2020, the Chinese government has made a series of detailed arrangements for socioeconomic development amid epidemic prevention and control. Taking the automotive industry as an example, this article discusses some thoughts and recommendations on the essential steps for the resumption of work based on integrated strategic planning.

1 The role of the automotive industry in the national economy

(1) The automotive industry is an important pillar of the national economy

The automotive industry plays a vital role in boosting economic growth, promoting employment, and improving people's livelihood. As a critical component of people's lives and economic activities, the invention of automobile has profoundly changed people's lifestyle and economic development. Automobile is therefore known as the "The machine that changed the world", and the automotive industry is regarded as a major engine for socioeconomic development. In the "post-industrialization" era of the 21st century, the automotive industry plays a pivotal role in developed countries. The US, Germany, Japan, the UK, France, Italy, South Korea and other highly-industrialized countries have all established well-developed automotive industry. China's automotive industry has developed rapidly and achieved remarkable progress, as it has gradually grown into a pillar of the national economy since the "Reform and Opening up". According to the National Bureau of Statistics, consumption has contributed to over 60% of China's GDP growth in recent years, and the automotive category alone accounts for more than 10% of the total retail sales of consumer goods. Automotive industry also contributes a great part to the overall industrial output.

Table 1　Gross output value of China's automotive industry in 2005–2019

Unit: RMB 100 million	Gross output value of the automotive industry (A)	National industrial output value (industrial sales output value) (B)	(A/B)
2005	10,223.2	246,946.4	4.1%
2006	13,937.6	310,828.6	4.5%
2007	17,242.1	397,626.7	4.3%
2008	18,780.6	494,733.7	3.8%
2009	23,437.8	536,134.1	4.4%
2010	30,248.7	684,735.2	4.4%
2011	33,155.3	827,797.0	4.0%
2012	35,774.4	909,797.2	3.9%
2013	39,225.5	1,019,405.3	3.8%
2014	42,324.3	1,092,198.0	3.9%
2015	45,014.5	1,104,026.7	4.1%
2016	39,329.9	1,151,950.1	3.4%
2017	58,382.5	1,292,111.2	4.5%
2018	52,498.7	1,416,676.1	3.7%
2019	50,427.9	1,472,147.2	3.4%

Source: State Information Center.

(2) The automotive industry chain extends both vertically and horizontally

From design to production, sales and after-sales service, the automotive industry is structurally related with many other industries, producing upstream and downstream effects on a number of related industries. The upstream industries include steel, non-ferrous metals, rubber, decorative fabrics, glass, wiring harnesses and electronic control components, lamps and lighting, plastics; manufacturing of large stamping and forging machines, mechanical cutting equipment, tool manufacturing, robot manufacturing; paints, machine oil, lubricants, etc. in the petrochemical field; transportation industry, production service industry, etc.; manufacturing of batteries, motors in the field of new energy vehicles (NEVs). The downstream including car repair, parts manufacturing, car financing, car insurance, car rental, road maintenance, car sports, car refitting; refined oil, lubricants, coolants and used car recycling in the petrochemical field. The experience of developed countries suggests that every RMB 1 of value added to the automotive industry will bring RMB 0.65 to the upstream industries and RMB 2.63 to the downstream industries. The situation in China is almost the same. The number of people employed in the automotive-related industries nationwide has exceeded one sixth of the total employment.

(3) The automotive industry is one of the most innovative industries

In the fierce competition of automotive industry, innovation is the essential way to enhance competitiveness. Therefore, automotive products have become the best platform for new technologies and materials. The world is in the midst of the New Industrial Revolution, Wireless communications, artificial intelligence, renewable energy, and automation technologies are driving unprecedented in various fields. IT, telecom, renewable energy and other technological forces are about to ignite an outburst of innovation in the automotive arena. Considering the history of over 100 years of the automotive industry, the transformation and technology-driven trends have been revolutionizing in promoting the so called "Four Modernizations". In order to seize this opportunity to lead innovation, many countries have launched supportive policies to facilitate the development of production, education and research at full speed. **On February 24, 2020**, 11 ministries and commissions including the National Development and Reform Commission jointly issued *the Strategy for Innovation and Development of Intelligent Vehicles*, which defines the development of intelligent vehicles as a major strategy for enhancing China's leading role in the next technological revolution and industrial transformation.

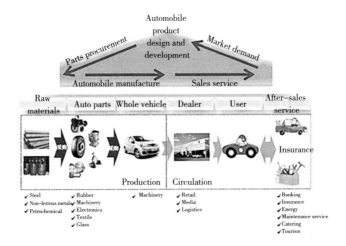

Figure 1　Industry distribution involved in automobile industry chain

(4) China's automotive industry plays a vital role in the global automotive industry and supply chain

China has been the largest automobile market and producer in the world for over ten years. Most of the world-renowned car manufacturers have established joint ventures or wholly-owned electric vehicle enterprises in China. Through decades of development in China, these enterprises have made Chinese manufacturing, especially suppliers, an indispensable force in global resource allocation. According to the General Administration of Customs of China, the total exports of auto parts in 2019 exceeded USD 60 billion, which increased positively by 8.9% year-on-year. Among them, the exports of foreign-funded enterprises' subsidiaries in China accounted for 40%. The number suggests the significance of Chinese auto parts suppliers in the global industry chain.

Table 2   Distribution of foreign parts suppliers in China

Region	Province	# of BU	Bosch	Denso	Magna	Conti-nentals	ZF	Aisin	Hyundai Mobis	Faurecia	Valeo	Lear
Tier 1	Hubei	20	1	1	1	2	1	0	0	10	4	Has
Tier 2	Guang-dong	41	1	8	2	0	0	11	0	7	12	Has
	Zhejiang	18	2	1	3	2	4	4	0	2	0	Has
	Jiangsu	40	7	5	4	4	1	5	3	6	5	Has
	Anhui	8	2	1	1	0	1	2	0	0	1	Has
	Hunan	6	1	0	3	0	0	0	0	1	1	0
	Henan	2	0	0	0	0	1	0	0	1	0	0
Tier 3	Others		16	21	19	19	27	17	8	46	28	Has
Total			30	37	33	27	35	39	11	73	51	No data
Tire 1&2 BU # Proportion of China			47%	43%	42%	30%	23%	56%	27%	37%	45%	

Source: PWC, "Facing current uncertainty and embracing the future", February 2020

2　COVID-19 epidemic hits the automotive industry chain

China is the world's largest car producer and consumer, as well as the main promoter of the "Four Modernizations" of automobiles, and it is also in a critical phase of promoting the in-depth development of technological revolution and product revolution. However, the sudden outbreak of the COVID-19 epidemic has almost stalled the industry, bringing unprecedented challenges to the development of automotive industry.

The intricacy of automobile require high standard of reliability and safety. A single traditional fuel vehicle has more than 30,000 parts, and even a pure electric vehicle with a relatively simple structure has more than 20,000 parts. In order to ensure the overall quality of automobile, OEMs need to conduct rigorous inspection and acceptance check of important parts suppliers, while countless auto parts suppliers are associated with the process. Generally, each OEM has about 200 suppliers, and the disruption of auto parts supply will result in suspended vehicle production. What's more fatal is that important parts suppliers also need a certain number of second-, third-, or fourth-tier suppliers to provide parts, and any disruption of them will affect the normal operation of the entire supply chain, and eventually impact the production of whole vehicles. In addition, most OEMs have very limited auto parts supply in inventory for cost effectiveness. Therefore, even a very small link in the supply chain goes wrong, it will generate negative effects and even disrupt the production.

At the downstream sales end, the number of dealership correlates with the size of OEMs. The distribution network of a large automobile manufacturer has more than 1,000 dealerships, and even a small automobile manufacturer has hundreds of dealerships (except for some ultra-luxury brands). Statistics show that there are about 30,000 automobile dealerships in China. Most of them are SMEs with limited financial resources and cash flow, which also have relatively poor anti-risk capacity.

It is worth noting that since mid-2018, China's car sales declined for more than 18 months in a row as the downward economic pressure took a toll on consumer confidence, which has greatly impacted the entire industry. As a result, most service enterprises such as upstream suppliers and downstream distributors in the industrial chain have already perceived the downward pressure.

Like many other industries, the outbreak has made the automotive industry suffer losses in both consumption and production. According to the statistics of China Passenger Car Association, the passenger car sales in the first half of

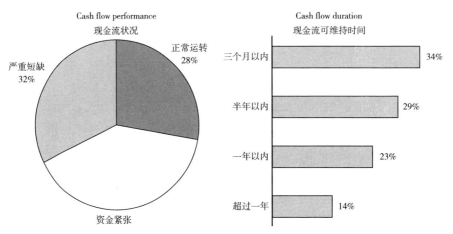

Figure 2   Survey of domestic dealers' operational cash flow in 2020
Source: PWC, "Facing current uncertainty and embracing the future", February 2020

February this year dropped by more than 90% year-on-year. This means that most of the automobile dealerships in China have nearly zero in sales, and all OEMs across the country were suffering as well. Seen from the supply side, in the first half of February, all OEMs and their suppliers suspended production due to the Spring Festival holiday, and then remained idle due to the outbreak. Therefore, the suspended supply and demand are dealing a double blow to the enterprises in the entire industry chain. The interruption of revenue will inevitably impose greater pressure on cash flow, yet expenses such as rent, salary, and interests on loans still need to be paid. According to the statistics of China Association of Automotive Manufacturers, there are more than 13,000 auto parts manufacturers above designated size in China. In addition, according to a survey conducted by China Association of Automobile Manufacturers in **February** on 212 parts manufacturers, the highest loss in operating income of parts manufacturers caused by the epidemic was RMB 2 billion, and the proportion of those with a revenue loss of RMB 20 million to 50 million was 16%. Some SMEs with small scale and low anti-risk capacity will potentially go bankrupt.

The damage to the automotive industry will inevitably affect the pillar industry, which also has ripple effect in national economy. This is because, as we mentioned above, the upstream and downstream of the automotive industry chain are related to a wide range of industries. More importantly, the NEV industry, which has been positioned as a strategic emerging industry in the automotive industry, is also suffering amid the epidemic. It is undoubtable that the outbreak has impacted not only the automotive industry, but also to every aspect of the national economy.

As China has deeply integrated into globalization, its economic prospects are intertwined with its integration into world market. After decades of industrial globalization, China's manufacturing, as an important link in the global supply chain, has been deeply embedded in the global supply chain. Chinese suppliers' suspension of production has directly caused the shutdown of overseas factories of enterprises such as Hyundai in South Korea and Toyota in Japan. And overseas factories of other world-renowned automobile manufacturers will also experience parts shortage and disruption of production in March. In other words, if suppliers are unable to resume production on schedule, the important role that China's automotive industry plays in the global supply chain may be shaken or even damaged.

3 Implementing overall industry planning and doing a good job of simultaneously implementing upstream and downstream policies

As the epidemic impact weighed on the production and operation, the central government promptly issued a series of comprehensive bailout policies for SMEs to resume operation. Local governments have also tailored implementation rules, including rent reduction and exemption, tax relief and extension, financial assistance, and flexibility in payment of social insurance to ease the burden on enterprises. These are all timely and essential measures which are of great significance to promoting the resumption of production. In the scope of providing financial assistance to local, there will inevitably be lack of the comprehensive thinking of the industrial chain, which may potentially results in inaccurate assessment of resolving the problem. The effectiveness of the measures will be difficult to achieve without big-picture thinking of industrial chain. Therefore, we put forward the following recommendations:

① Endeavor to safeguard the position of China's automotive industry in the global industrial supply chain. As mentioned above, most of the major automobile manufacturers' overseas production depends on foreign and domestic suppliers in China. Although the level of dependence varies, the characteristics of automotive products determine that finished vehicle doesn't get off the shop floor until each of those component parts are in place. Therefore, preciseness of supportive measures plays a central role when implementing supportive measures. Therefore, it is recommended to adopt the following two approaches to target suppliers that require urgent assistance:

One approach is to make a complete list of export parts manufacturers based on the customs' parts export data, the Ministry of Industry and Information Technology and other related ministries will guide local governments to implement targeted supportive measures for enterprises on the list. The second approach is to request foreign OEMs or their related enterprises in China to provide a list of domestic suppliers of their most-needed parts, because they are more familiar with parts in stock as well as urgently needed parts. By comparing the two lists, we can basically target the most important suppliers in the global industrial supply chain. Afterwards, the industry authorities can guide local governments to accurately implement urgent supportive policies based on the lists combined.

② It is noteworthy that instead of providing additional measures, the above-mentioned approaches to support production resumption are based on existing policies and measure. It simply requires a broader scope of thinking in industry chain when assessing analysis and conducting measures. Unclogging the upstream and downstream of the industry chain is essential in restoring the automotive industry back to its normalcy before the outbreak. If the downstream is not smooth, the upstream will still be blocked even after the resumption of production. Similarly, even if the downstream is smooth, the industry chain may not operate when the upstream suppliers are not in place.

Recently, the central government has recognized that the groundwork for getting through the downstream is to first loosen policies that restricting market capacity, e.g., cities with auto purchase restrictions should, if unable to revoke the purchase restriction, at least relax the quotas and expand market capacity. This is a great benefit for the industry. In addition, to boost consumer confidence, it is encouraged to implement more relaxed and risk-controllable policies on credit and loan, such as reducing the down payment of car loans, providing preferential low-interest loans, and giving more flexibility to financial services. Besides, to stimulate automotive consumption, it is encouraged to adopt targeted tax reduction policies. For example, the vehicle purchase tax shall be reduced or exempted periodically, and the consumption tax on passenger cars with displacement below 2.0L shall be revoked or further reduced. Moreover, to stabilize the long-term development of automobile consumption, we recommend launching the study on long-term structural tax reduction policies to solve the problem of relatively high comprehensive tax rate in the purchase. Furthermore, local governments shall support car dealerships in the downstream of the industry chain, and give appropriate subsidies to those with severe difficulties in operation based on the level of impact they experienced.

③ Accelerate the process of lightening the burden of OEMs, and unleash their potential in being leading roles in industry chain. In view of the integrity characteristic of automotive products, OEMs plays a significant role in linking the upstream and downstream of the industry chain. However, the condition for OEMs to revitalizing the upstream and downstream is to first ensure that the OEMs are in good shape. Faced with the epidemic, OEMs have taken the moral responsibility to relieve the predicament of upstream and downstream enterprises. They have even actively organized employees to participate in the production resumption of upstream parts manufacturers, and directly subsidized dealerships at their own expense. At the same time, under the status quo of sales stagnation, automobile manufacturers also bear extremely heavy profitability and cash flow pressure. Therefore, during the special period of epidemic, central and local fiscal policies may also consider reducing and exempting the corporate income tax of OEMs to some extent, and ensuring the cash flow liquidity of automobile manufacturers.

④ It is necessary to comply with the arrangements of the Party Central Committee and the State Council, coordinate with the measures in epidemic prevention and control and socioeconomic development, further carry out the "six stabilizations" measures in a more targeted manner, quickly respond to short- and long-term impact of the epidemic, and make timely policy adjustments by giving full play to the advantages of the socialist system with Chinese characteristics. For example:

i We should, under the principle of promoting the long-term stable development of the industry, make flexible short-term adjustments to industry management policies to help the industry weather the epidemic crisis, thus "stabilizing employment, investment, and expectations", and guaranteeing "survival and development". The outbreak has disrupted the existing planning of the entire industrial chain, including R&D, design, production, logistics, and sales, making it difficult to achieve the short- and mid-term development goals of environmental protection, energy saving and NEV development. Therefore, on the one hand, important forward-looking policies including CAFC+NEV credit rule and NEV development planning should be issued as soon as possible to help enterprises clarify the expectation on future development; on the other hand, it is suggested to consider appropriately relaying or relaxing the requirements of some industry policies in this year and the next year, such as the credit ratio of NEVs, particulate matter limits in China VI vehicle emission standards, and on-vehicle

ETC module certification.

ii It is necessary to continue to reform and open up, further attract foreign investment, and accelerate the implementation of policies related to stabilization and attraction of foreign investment, thus "stabilizing foreign trade, foreign investment, and finance". The impact of the epidemic has further shown China's important role in the global supply chain, but it may also remind some multinational enterprises to seek alternatives in other countries to reduce the overall risk of the supply chain. Therefore, on the one hand, measures for resumption of production shall be implemented as early as possible to strengthen the confidence of enterprises; on the other hand, to cope with the potential shift away of industry, it is essential to further optimize business environment of foreign-funded enterprises in terms of investment and production access, industry management (such as the definition of affiliated enterprises in CAFC+NEV credit rule), financing convenience at home and abroad, foreign exchange management, etc.

In a word, China's automotive industry has been deeply integrated into the global supply chain after decades of development. Amid the epidemic, it is necessary to maintain the critical role that China's automotive industry plays in the global supply chain, which is also beneficiary to the world. Moreover, to keep the entire industry chain safe and complete, no enterprise in the upstream and downstream should be left out in the epidemic. In addition, only by helping automobile manufacturers to get through the difficulties can truly ensure the security and integrity of the industry. Finally, we should regard the battle against the epidemic as an opportunity to show the advantages of the socialist system with Chinese characteristics, and make timely and comprehensive response to further strengthen the confidence of domestic and foreign investors in China's future prospect.

疫情对物流行业的挑战与机遇

徐俊　安博*（中国）　高级副总裁

　　庚子年初，一场新型冠状病毒肺炎疫情迅速蔓延。举国上下，众志成城，抗击疫情，共度时艰。

　　安博公司（Prologis）是全球最大的工业基础设施提供商与运营商，业务分布于全球 19 个国家，在中国多个战略区域拥有并管理现代物流仓储设施，为全球制造商、零售商、电子商务企业和第三方物流公司提供现代化、跨区域的多元化物流仓储解决方案。

　　新冠肺炎疫情期间，安博全球积极组织内部团队调动全球资源筹措相关医疗防护用品，截至 2020 年 2 月下旬已将购买的 3 万只 N95 口罩、50 万只医用一次性防护口罩、2 万只医用 N95 口罩、750 件医用防护服等物资发往武汉、鄂州、黄冈、红安等疫情较重地区。

　　全国性隔离等措施造成供应链上下游全面受阻，给供应链物流企业经营带来严重困难。作为在全球处于领先地位的供应链企业，安博公司决定除捐赠急需医疗物资产品外，积极主动发挥公司优势，无偿开放全国物流园区的仓储资源支援全国抗击疫情。

　　2 月初，安博在中国 19 个城市无偿开放 40 个物流园，用于应急周转仓储及多温区食品物流运营服务，面向各级政府及慈善机构无偿开放。同时，园区提供多温区食品的物流分装、包装、调拨、转运等运营服务，对有支援疫情防控的应急周转仓储物流需求或多温区食品的物流运营服务商

---

　　*　安博公司创立于 1983 年，是一家现代物流基础设施行业全球领袖企业，所持物业覆盖美洲、欧洲和亚洲，总面积多达 5570 万平方米，构建了覆盖全球主要物流枢纽、工业园区和城市配送中心等战略节点的高效物流网络。总部位于美国加利福尼亚州旧金山市。

提供全方位的服务。

在武汉市等部分疫情严重地区陆续采取"封城""封区""封村"举措之时，与之而来的物资供应，尤其是一线药品、医疗物资和疫区人民的食品供应成为一大问题。2020年2月3日，中共中央政治局常务委员会强调"要确保蔬菜、肉蛋奶等居民生活必需品供应……积极组织蔬菜等副食品生产，加强物资调配和市场供应"，保障人民生活必需品的正常供给[①]。

一　物资及时供应除受当地分配方式与效率影响外，运输环节亦是影响时效的关键因素

影响供应链企业物流运输成本的因素很多，控制措施既涉及运输环节本身，也涉及供应链的整个物流流程。要想降低物流运输成本，就必须调整运输系统的观点和方法，并进行综合分析，发现问题，解决问题，使物流运输活动更加优化、物流成本更加合理化。受疫情影响，作为民生保障基础的物流运输行业，面临不同程度的经营压力，也因此迎来了非常规性的发展机会。物流数字化和智能化成为未来创新发展的方向。安博在大数据、智能分拣、机器人等方面早有布局。疫情过后，中小型企业所积压的运输需求将集中爆发，这为企业外包物流服务提供了机会，安博将凭借仓储、物流规模优势，提供弹性运力解决方案[②]。

新冠肺炎疫情对供应链企业的影响到底有多大？企业经营风险到底有哪些？有哪些可以对应？

我们对新冠肺炎疫情的影响阶段进行分析。

---

① 《中共中央政治局常务委员会召开会议研究加强新型冠状病毒感染的肺炎疫情防控工作》，中华人民共和国中央人民政府网站，2020年2月3日，http://www.gov.cn/xinwen/2020-02/03/content_5474309.htm。

② https://www.prologis.com/logistics-industry-research/prologis-research-special-report-COVID-19-and-implications-logistics.

（一）新冠肺炎疫情对供应链企业经营影响的三个阶段 [1]

第一阶段，"暴发阶段"。全国经济持续停摆，员工复工困难，业务持续萎缩。员工染病风险大，销售收入同比大幅度下滑。

第二阶段，"动荡阶段"。企业的客户经营、市场需求、经营资源、社会经济都处于一个较大幅度的动荡中，整个经济社会不安定性较大，客户的市场、供应链的关系、社会上的供需关系都会出现变化甚至出现全面调整，各种管理、运营、服务、市场、人员、资金等各种问题和风险会层出不穷，企业经营管理重点不得不放在应对各种应急状态上，努力维系企业稳定生存和经营的平衡。

第三阶段，"恢复阶段"。疫情结束后，经济社会逐步恢复正常，企业经营开始消化第二阶段造成的成本及资金风险，逐步恢复到正常的经营发展轨道。

（二）新冠肺炎疫情给供应链企业带来的经营风险 [2]

根据经营判断，我们重点分析新冠肺炎疫情对供应链服务企业可能带来的重大经营风险（仅分析受疫情影响的供应链企业，不包括在疫情中业务量饱和的其他企业）。

1. 资金风险

①资金风险是最大的风险。

②固定成本、防控及人员成本等持续支出带来的流动资金严重不足。

③由于供应链企业市场充分竞争的特点，企业将会面临重大突发性经营困境，给企业带来重大的经营风险。

---

[1] 《新冠肺炎疫情对全球供应链体系的冲击与应对》，江苏智库，2020年3月20日，http://www.jsthinktank.com/zhikuyanjiu/202003/t20200320_6568436.shtml。

[2] 《新冠肺炎疫情背景下中国企业面临的新风险及其应对措施》，人民网 强国论坛，2020年2月21日，http://bbs1.people.com.cn/post/1/1/2/174908068.html。

2. 员工风险

①由于全国性封锁，外地员工无法按期回企业复工，企业员工不足。

②在休假期间员工被感染，短期内丧失工作能力。

③员工在紧急业务期间被感染，构成工伤，对企业造成重大经营风险。

④员工出现心理性障碍，影响业务的正常开展与团队的稳定性。

⑤多种因素叠加造成人力资源不足，影响企业正常运营。

3. 成本风险

①由于整体经济停滞，收入大幅度下降，低于盈亏平衡点。

②用于疫情防范所需的设备与设施的购置与使用造成成本大幅度上升。

③经营必需品、消费品成本大幅上升，造成经营成本的上升。

④由于全国运输通道不畅，资源紧缺，很多业务被隔离造成无法按时返回，业务及外包的成本大幅度上升。

4. 法律风险

①由于延长假期，各地复工时间不一，政策解释不一，复工后因加班与工资计算方法造成的劳动关系法律风险增加。

②由于疫情期间部分业务无法履行造成的合同履约法律风险增加。

5. 市场风险

①复工后宏观经济恢复需要时间，客户业务量出现较大下降，业务收入阶段性大幅度下滑。

②客户业务调整及供应链调整加快，造成企业现有合约业务量变化下滑。

③各地由于疫情控制及市场需求的情况变化，客户的供应链及业务出现较大的不确定性造成原有市场波动。

6. 运营风险

①由于人员到岗不足，各种应急措施不到位，运营流程变形，管控变形，运营服务能力下降。

②供应商困难重重，业务能力大幅度下降，全国运营服务出现严重困难。

③各地不同的管控措施造成运营服务受阻，服务时间拖延，成本大幅

度上升，客户投诉增加。

7. 疫情风险

①企业复工中一旦出现员工染病造成员工传染，将可能造成企业集体性感染事件，企业有被封闭的可能，形成巨大经营风险。

②企业出现员工染病现象，造成员工健康风险继而带来企业经营风险。

（三）建立系统性企业战略——供应链企业应对疫情危机时的管理 [①]

面对突发的全国性疫情，供应链企业决策者最关键的是需要正确的认识，将此次疫情作为"对企业经营发展的一次严峻的考验与倒逼"，面对严峻的市场与经营风险，抓住经营的关键要素，实现经营管理上的突破与经营服务上的创新是战略对策的关键。

疫情将造成市场剧烈波动，在给企业带来风险的同时，也带来了新的机会。因此供应链企业特别需要系统性的思维，重视经营发展战略的及时调整，对应快速动荡的市场，重点关注市场变动带来的机会，利用企业的决策优势，采用系统化战略思维，科学制定企业的发展战略。

1. 做好对经营困境的常态化经营战略准备

疫情下供应链企业除了保障疫区的体系，其他复工复产很慢，原材料供给不足，从而导致无法顺利开展生产运输，物流企业面临极大压力。推动供应链企业物流节点的多功能性和多业务兼容能力提升，加强运力部署的弹性，构建整体连接、局部可调整的柔性网络。

2. 塑造共识力，强化团队建设

自身层面，看清自身短板，提升内部专业管理能力；客户层面，与客户在持续沟通下互相理解，保证业务正常运转；应急管理层面，重视应急措施，随时应对突发情况。

---

① 《疫情趋于平稳，企业该如何调整战略赢得市场》，KNX 肯耐珂萨，2020 年 2 月 28 日，http://www.knx.com.cn/news/detail/202002281042.html。

3. 经营思维的转变

由于疫情的长期影响，市场需求与经营环境将出现重大的变化，企业经营团队需要以自我批判的高度研判企业的经营思维，在新的市场中找机会，在企业的现有经营思维中找问题，重点在现有经营业务中找到新的发展商机的同时，重点拓展新的服务市场，创新服务模式，抓住变革时期探索供应链技术平台的建立，根据当地的实际情况与变化，创新经营思维，创造新的服务和体系。

4. 坚持抓住供应链企业经营战略三要素

需要紧紧抓住企业经营发展的"效益 + 高管 + 战略"三要素，高级管理层要站在战略的角度考虑问题、经营企业，提升经营管理能力与水平，加强各种形式的管理层培训，保持企业的团队健康发展，所有工作的重点向"创效益"集中，一切工作以效益为目标，带领企业尽快安全走出疫情影响期。

5. 建立供应链企业共生共赢的生态观

企业的发展需要突破自我发展模式，更多的创新应该向资源重新整合与服务创新模式发展。因此，供应链企业经营团队需要注重建立共生共赢的生态观念，不仅对外部资源，在企业内部与企业的团队中也需要推进建立企业共赢生态体系。

二 抗击疫情期间，面对经济下行压力，供应链企业应该如何采取有效措施渡过难关、稳健发展？

疫情期间，整体供应链企业监控和响应计划缺少较低层的透明性，这源于供应链的数字化程度并不高。在整个供应链中，数字化平台的应用还并不普遍，这对在应急供应链中的及时响应与调度带来困难。对于需要员工较少、便于疫情管控的智能化工厂与智能化供应链中心成为一大亮点。相反，对劳动力依赖程度较高的产业或企业受到较大影响。

每经历一次社会重大事件，都会对相应的产业提出新的要求，在疫情蔓延下，众多不确定性会持续发生，我们不仅需要有直面它的勇气，更需要有认知它的能力，与它共处。在本次新冠肺炎疫情中，供应链企业虽然发挥了较为及时与稳定的作用，但是效率与质量上还需要进一步提高。经过本次疫情，线上线下业务齐头发展的业务模式将成为标配，基于线上线下全生态业务的供应链建设将成为常态。

1. 完善供应链数字化信息平台

疫情常态化下，越来越多的企业将运用供应链数字化管理平台，与此同时，整个社会要求通过数字化平台快速了解变化，保证供应链状态的及时性、透明性、可控性。供应链数字化的信息平台将成为企业信息化建设的必备内容，基于软件平台建设的迭代性特点，整个技术平台都会按照应急供应链的高要求来设计与部署。

2. 提高供应链智能化

疫情期间，对劳动力依赖程度较高的企业都受到较大影响。从发展趋势来看，基于无人化、少人化的供应链场景将会有较大的发展，对与其相匹配的智能供应链技术的需求也会增多，因此供应链企业更要加深智能供应链技术的应用。

3. 增强供应链多功能性

基于疫情对供应链响应的高要求，供应链设施的共用性与通用性成为关注焦点，这也要求在今后的供应链系统建设中，基础设施应具备多功能性、对多种业务的兼容性、对紧急业务的包容性；其次还体现在增设部署的便利性，实现在较短的时间内完成供应链产能的补充或扩大，这对规划、软件与智能硬件的融合都提出了更高的要求。

4. 挑战极限式地降低物流成本

2019年，很多企业已经有了自我调整发展的模式，有了转型业务及增长方式的新探索，但遇到疫情，还需要有更强的危机意识，更坚定地自我救赎，缩减费用和剥离不良业务，杜绝亏损及没有质量的增长，确保现金流，同时要确保较强竞争力。要做到这一点的关键是，一定要挑战极限式地降低物流成本，根本目的就是保住现金流。具有良好现金流的企业，建议重构自己的成本能力，因为应对不确定性是一种常态能力。

三　对应新冠肺炎疫情重大风险的抗风险经营对策 [①]

面对突发疫情，供应链企业除做好持久战准备外，还应根据各地情况与企业经营的实际，制定抗风险经营对策，主要包括以下几点。

1. 员工与企业安全是第一位

员工安全，企业才安全。一旦企业内部出现新冠肺炎疫情，企业将可能面临集中传染和隔离停业的重大风险，经营将受到严重的影响。因此，企业应把确保员工健康放在首位，制定详尽的应急预案，明确各级管理层职责，提高全员安全防范意识。

2. 资金挑战

供应链企业普遍存在收款账期，且规模普遍较小，财务风险承受能力较弱。同时，供应链企业以个体司机为主，其财务风险承受能力更弱，会直接造成广大的微小车队或个体户的生存难以维系，亦可能引发潜在的社会风险。

3. 关注市场变化主动出击，抓住创新机遇

疫情期间，客户需求是否改变，消费者习惯是否改变，线上线下业务占比变化，数字化时代如何跟客户黏在一起，分享更多价值等，及时捕捉这些变化，对开拓创新发展机遇至关重要。

4. 加强培训，练内功，储备经营实力

自身层面，明确自身短板，提升内部专业管理能力；客户层面，加强与客户在持续沟通下的互相理解，保证业务正常运转；应急管理层面，重视应急措施，随时应对突发情况。

---

① 《CWM50 报告：新冠肺炎疫情对经济的影响及对策建议》，新华网，2020 年 2 月 18 日，http://www.xinhuanet.com/money/2020-02/18/c_1125590528.htm。

5.降低成本

应对企业现金流危机及企业在疫情中生存关键措施之一，就是降低成本，主要包括以下几点。

①降低人力成本重点应该放在提高劳动生产率、提高员工工作效率、降低人员成本方面。

②降低运营成本包括仓储、设备租赁等固定成本及运营业务的变动成本。

③降低管理成本尽量减少与经营收入无关的管理成本支持。

6.降低法律风险

在疫情情况下，法律风险将会相对集中。因此，针对劳动风险可能集中出现的情况进行预判，企业人力资源部门需要加强人力资源疏导，使企业劳动风险提前得到控制和合理化解。

7.加强运营管理

供应链企业竞争力的核心永远是运营能力。疫情期间，企业的车辆、员工随时可能被隔离或者被封在某个区域外，对运营业务的组织带来重大挑战。因此，特别需要加强运营组织管控来保证疫情期的业务稳定和完成。与此同时，利用现有业务量不大的情况，梳理与修订供应链业务流程与服务流程，努力强化服务流程与服务项目，提升服务水平，为快速恢复运营做好准备，配合好未来市场开发与业务拓展。对供应链物流服务企业，同时需要加强对供应商的支持管理，加强与供应商的共同沟通与支持。

8.做好疫情防范策略

供应链企业是劳动密集型企业，在新冠肺炎疫情结束前，特别需要做好疫情防范的口罩、消毒液、红外测温仪等防范物资准备，加强全员防范培训与全覆盖干部责任制，建立应急汇报与送医隔离制度，一旦出现发热、乏力等症状立即按各地政府的规定到指定医院就诊，积极治疗，保证员工安全与企业安全 ①。

---

① 《关于依法科学精准做好新冠肺炎疫情防控工作的通知》，中华人民共和国中央人民政府网站，2020 年 2 月 25 日，http://www.gov.cn/xinwen/2020-02/25/content_5483024.htm。

四 一些思考：供应链将引领"新零售时代"

对于供应链企业来说，这次疫情可能成为一个分水岭。

一些中小企业在交通阻断的情况下，供应链遭遇重创，导致末端销售、客服等其他方面出现价格、服务、响应机制等失控极端情形，以及面对投诉以及处罚。不难预见的是行业集中度将由此提升、马太效应不可避免，客户流量将越来越集中到类似于大型、连锁等高端大型企业。

（一）强者恒强

大型、连锁行业坐拥渠道和高端定位优势，在经营的同时通过供应商获得了性价比高的优势。这将意味着供应商、企业、消费者三者之间形成一种正平衡，这种平衡对于消费者和供应商来说都能产生向心力，构成永续高品质经营的基础。

从这个意义上看，"新零售时代"的大型连锁等行业，或许正在经历一个供应链企业竞争的新阶段，尤其是在叠加大数据、云平台等先进技术情况下，供应链开始变得更加"智能"，从而可以精准匹配消费者更加多元化的需求，持续提供高品质的差异化供应链服务。

（二）物流在地产资本市场环境变化中处于有利位置

尽管长期供应链企业仓储租赁可以抵抗波动，但由于金融市场波动以及随之而来的分母效应，资本流动可能会放缓。尤其是物流基础设施领域，一直存在投资者分配不足的情况。利率已经开始下降，并且很可能维持在较低水平。从基本面来看，考虑到仓储管理和电子商务对长期需求的潜在推动作用，总体而言，物流行业的处境要优于其他行业。此外，资本可能更偏爱那些在表现强劲地区的优质核心资产，因此会流向这些地区进行避险[1]。

"十三五"规划中强调了工业和物流在国民经济体系中的支柱作用[2]，其作用将会对中国推进"一带一路"建设产生重要的影响。各地各级政府应继续出台相应的支持和鼓励的政策和措施，推动该产业的发展，进而为整个国民经济的健康协调发展提供保障和支持，确保"一带一路"倡议的成功推进。

（三）中国物流基础设施发展趋势良好，但供应链企业在获取相关项目土地方面仍存在问题，希望相关部门予以关注

支撑供应链企业的物流基础设施产业项目有其相对的独特性和专属性，就物流基础设施项目土地的获取对于商业企业还是必须设置相应的准入条件，以保证地尽其用，让真正有实力有信誉的企业得到发展。

我们认为，物流基础设施产业作为与国民经济和社会民生紧密相关的基础性产业，还具有一定的公益性，需要政府从土地、税收、资金、人力资源成本等多方扶持。如果将供应链企业的物流与其他产业不加区别地等同对待，势必造成供应链企业在投入上的却步，给行业和企业发展造成冲击。

当前，中国正处于经济转型与高质量发展的进程中，越是逆境，越要发展。对于供应链行业而言，疫情期间考验的是企业资源调度能力，应急组织能力；疫情过后考验的是企业自救速度、持续运营能力，大家都在同时间赛跑。中国的供应链企业是最具战斗力也是最具激情的企业，供应链企业是复工复产的先行官，这既是信任重托，更是使命责任。风雨过后见彩虹，寒冬消散是春天，2020 年是全面建成小康社会和"十三五"规划

---

① Gerald Eve、世邦魏理仕研究部、高纬环球、仲量联行、高力国际、世邦魏理仕计量经济顾问、安博研究部，https://www.prologis.com/logistics-industry-research/prologis-research-special-report-COVID-19-and-implications-logistics。

② 《中华人民共和国国民经济和社会发展第十三个五年（2016 - 2020 年）规划纲要》，中国共产党员网，2016，http://www.12371.cn/special/sswgh/wen/#7。

的收官之年。习近平总书记明确强调，坚决打赢疫情防控的人民战争、总体战、阻击战，努力实现 2020 年经济社会发展目标任务①。我们供应链企业作为国民经济发展的基础性、战略性、先导性产业，是社会经济实现目标任务的坚强保证。

广大供应链企业和千百万供应链从业者，做好一手抓防控、一手抓发展工作，全面打通供应链生命线，实现疫情防控阻击战和经济社会发展目标双胜利是我们的重要任务。

---

① 《坚决打赢疫情防控的人民战争总体战阻击战——习近平总书记在北京调研指导新冠肺炎疫情防控工作时的重要讲话》，《人民日报》2020 年 2 月 12 日，http://www.12371.cn/2020/02/12/ARTI1581462495242410.shtml。

Challenges & Opportunities of the Epidemic to the Logistics Industry

By John Xu, Senior Vice President of Prologis（China）

At the beginning of 2020, the coronavirus epidemic spread rapidly. The whole country works together to fight against the epidemic and pass the hard times.

Prologis is the world's largest industrial infrastructure supplier and operator with business in 19 countries. It owns and manages modern logistics and warehousing facilities in multiple strategic regions in China. It provides modern, cross-regional and diversified logistics and warehousing solutions for global manufacturers, retailers, e-commerce companies and third-party logistics companies.

During the coronavirus epidemic, Prologis actively organized internal teams to mobilize global resources to raise related medical protective supplies. As of late February, 30,000 N95 masks, 500,000 medical disposable protective masks, 20,000 N95 medical masks, 750 pieces of medical protective clothing and other materials were sent to Wuhan, Ezhou, Huanggang, Hongan and other severely affected regions.

Due to national isolation and other measures, the upstream and downstream of the supply chain have been blocked, which has brought serious difficulties to the operation of supply chain logistics enterprises. As a leading supply chain company in the world, in addition to donating urgently needed medical supplies and products, Prologis has decided to actively take advantage of the company's superiority, and freely open the warehouse resources of the national logistics park to support the nation's fight against the epidemic.

From the beginning of February, Prologis has opened 40 logistics parks in 19 cities in China for free to governments and charities at all levels, which are used for emergency turnover storage and multi-temperature food logistics operation services. At the same time, the park provides operational services such as logistics sub-packaging, packing, allocation, transfer of multi-temperature food and provides comprehensive services to those who need emergency turnaround warehousing and logistics to support epidemic prevention and control.

When the lockdown measures of city, district and village were successively adopted in some severely affected areas such as Wuhan, the supply of materials, especially the front-line medicines and medical supplies, and the food of the people becomes a big problem. On February 3, The Standing Committee of the Political Bureau of the Communist Party of China (CPC) Central Committee stressed that "ensure the supply of necessities for residents, such as vegetables, meat, eggs, and milk...Actively organize the production of non-staple food such as vegetables, strengthen the allocation of materials and market supply" to ensure the normal supply of people's daily necessities [1].

1　First of all, in addition to the local distribution methods and efficiency, transportation links also affects the timeliness of materials supply

There are many factors that affect the logistics and transportation costs of supply chain enterprises. Control measures involve both the transportation link itself and the entire logistics process of the supply chain. If you want to

---

[1]　The Standing Committee of the Political Bureau of the Communist Party of China (CPC) Central Committee held a Meeting on the Prevention and Control of Pneumonia Epidemic Caused by the Novel Coronavirus, 2020-02-03 20:10 Source: Website of the Central People's Government of the People's Republic of China. http://www.gov.cn/xinwen/2020-02/03/content_5474309.htm.

reduce the logistics cost, you must adjust the perspectives and methods of the transportation system, and carry out a comprehensive analysis to find and solve problems, making logistics activities more optimized, and logistics costs more rational. Affected by the epidemic, the logistics and transportation industry, which is the basis for the guarantee of people's livelihoods, faces varying degrees of operating pressure, but also encounters unconventional development opportunities. Digitization and intelligence of logistics have become the direction of future innovation and development. Prologis has long been involved in big data, intelligent sorting, and robotics. After the epidemic, the backlogged transportation needs of small and medium-sized enterprises will break out intensively, which provides opportunities for outsourcing logistics services. Prologis will provide flexible capacity solutions relying on the advantages of warehousing and logistics scale [1] .

What is the impact of COVID-19 on supply chain companies? What exactly are business risks? Which can be dealt with?

We analyzed the impact stages of COVID-19:

(1) Three stages of the impact of COVID-19 on the operation of supply chain enterprises [2]

The first stage, "outbreak". The national economy has continued to stagnate; employees have difficulty returning to work; business has continued to shrink; employees are at risk of illness; and sales revenue has fallen sharply year-on-year.

The second phase, "turbulent". The enterprise's customer operation, market demand, operating resources, and social economic situation are all in a large

---

[1] Gerald Eve, CBRE Research, Cushman and Wakefield, JLL, Colliers, CBRE-EA, Prologis Research; https://www.prologis.com/logistics-industry-research/prologis-research-special-report-COVID-19-and-implications-logistics.

[2] The Impact and Response of COVID-19 to the Global Supply Chain System, 2020-03-20 14:39:00, Source: Jiangsu Think Tank. http://www.jsthinktank.com/zhikuyanjiu/202003/t20200320_6568436.shtml.

turbulence. The overall economic society is unstable. The customer's market, supply chain relationship, and social supply-demand relationship will change or even appear full adjustments, various problems and risks such as management, operations, services, markets, personnel, and funds will emerge endlessly. The focus of business management must be on responding to various emergencies and striving to maintain a balance between stable survive and operation.

The third stage, "recovery". After the epidemic, the economy and society gradually return to normal, and companies begin to digest the cost and capital risks caused by the second stage and gradually return to the normal operation development track.

(2) Operational risks brought by COVID-19 to supply chain companies [1]

Based on operational judgments, we focus on analyzing the major business risks that COVID-19 may cause to supply chain service companies (only analyze the supply chain companies affected by the epidemic, excluding other companies with saturated business in the epidemic).

Funding risk:

① Funding risk is the biggest risk;

② The serious shortage of liquidity caused by continuous expenditures such as fixed costs, prevention and control costs, and personnel costs;

③ Due to the characteristics of full competition in the supply chain enterprise market, the enterprise will enter a major sudden operating dilemma, which will bring significant operational risks to the enterprise;

Employee risk:

① Due to the national blockade, out-of-town employees cannot return to the company to work on schedule, so that the company has staff shortage;

---

① New Risks Faced by Chinese Enterprises in the COVID-19 Epidemic and Countermeasures, 2020-02-21 20:33:14 Source: People's Daily Online BBS. http://bbs1.people.com.cn/post/1/1/2/174908068.html.

② Employees became infected during vacation and lost their ability to work in a short time;

③ Employees are infected during the emergency business period, which constitutes work injury and causes significant business risks to the enterprise;

④ Employees have psychological obstacles that affect the normal business development and team stability;

⑤ Various factors cause the human resources shortage which affects the normal operation of the enterprise;

Cost risk:

① Due to the stagnation of the overall economy, income has fallen sharply and is below the breakeven point;

② The purchase and use of equipment and facilities required for epidemic prevention causes a significant increase in costs;

③ The substantial increase in the cost of business necessities and consumer goods causes the increase in operating costs;

④ Due to poor transportation channels and scarce resources in the country, many businesses are isolated and cannot be returned on time, and the cost of business and outsourcing has increased significantly;

Legal risk:

① Due to prolonged holidays, the time of work resumption varies from place to place, and the interpretation of policies is different. The legal risk of labor relations due to overtime and wage calculation methods after resumption of work is increased;

② Increased legal risks of contract performance due to the inability to perform certain businesses during the epidemic;

Market risk:

① It will take time for the macroeconomic recovery after the work resumption, the customer's business volume will decline significantly, and thus the business income will decline sharply in stages;

② Acceleration of customer business adjustment and supply chain adjustment, causes decline of the company's existing contract business volume;

③ Due to epidemic control and changes in market demand in various places, the customer's supply chain and business are subject to greater uncertainty, causing original market fluctuations;

Operational risk:

① Due to insufficient staffing, various emergency measures are not in place, resulting in deformation of operational processes, management and control, and reduction of operational service capabilities;

② Suppliers have many difficulties. Their business capabilities have fallen sharply, and there have been serious difficulties in operating services across the country;

③ Different management and control measures in various places have caused obstruction of operation services and delayed service time, which causes a significant increase in costs and customer complaints;

Epidemic risk:

① Once an employee becomes infected and causes employee contagion during work resumption, it may cause a collective infection of the enterprise, and the enterprise may be closed, posing a huge operational risk;

② The contagion between employees in enterprises causes employees' health risks, which will in turn lead to business risks;

(3) Establish a systematic corporate strategy-management of supply chain companies in response to epidemic crisis [①]

Facing the sudden national epidemic situation, the most important thing for decision makers in supply chain companies is to correctly understand

---

① The epidemic has stabilized, how should companies adjust their strategies to win the market, 2020-02-28 Source: KNX. http://www.knx.com.cn/news/detail/202002281042.html.

the epidemic situation as a "serious test and inverse force of the business development of enterprises". In the face of severe market and operating risks, grasping the key elements of operation, achieving breakthroughs in management and innovation in operating services are the keys to strategic countermeasures.

The epidemic will cause violent market fluctuations. While bringing risks to enterprises, it will also bring new opportunities. Therefore, supply chain companies particularly need systematic thinking, pay attention to the timely adjustment of business development strategies, respond to the rapidly turbulent market, focus on the opportunities brought by market changes, accelerate the decision-making advantages of enterprises, adopt systematic strategic thinking, and scientifically formulate corporate development strategy.

Establish preparations for normalized operating strategies for operating dilemma. In the epidemic, except the system that guarantee the affected area, other systems of supply chain companies resumed the work and production slowly and the supply of raw materials is insufficient. As a result, production and transportation cannot be carried out smoothly, and logistics companies are facing great pressure. It is necessary to promote the versatility and multi-service compatibility of logistics nodes in supply chain enterprises, strengthen the flexibility of capacity plan, and build a flexible network that is overall connected and partially adjustable.

Build consensus and strengthen team building. At its own level, see its own shortcomings and improve its internal professional management capabilities; at the customer level, understand each other through continuous communication with customers to ensure the normal operation of the business; at the emergency management level, attach importance to emergency measures and respond to emergencies at any time.

Change business thinking. Due to the long-term impact of the epidemic, there will be major changes in market demand and business environment. Enterprise management teams need to judge the business thinking of the company with a high degree of self-criticism, find opportunities in new markets, and find problems in the existing business thinking of the company. While focusing on finding new development opportunities in existing business, also need to focus on expanding new service markets, innovating new service models, seizing the period of change, exploring the establishment of supply chain technology platforms, and innovating operating thinking and creating new services and systems according to local actual conditions and changes.

Persist in grasping the three elements of the supply chain's business strategy. It is necessary to tightly grasp the three elements of "benefit + executive + strategy" for business development. The senior management should consider issues and operate enterprises and departments from a strategic perspective, improve business management capabilities and levels, and strengthen various forms of training management to maintain the healthy development of the company's team. The focus of all work should concentrate on "creation of benefits", which means all work is aimed at benefit to lead the company out of the period of impact of the epidemic situation.

Establish an ecological concept of symbiosis and win-win for supply chain enterprises. The development of the enterprises needs to break through the self-development model, and the re-integration of resources and the service model should be innovated. Therefore, the management team in the supply chain enterprises needs to pay more attention to establishing an ecological concept of symbiosis and win-win. It is necessary to promote the establishment of a win-win ecosystem for the enterprise not only for external resources, but also within the company and the team.

2　During the fight against the epidemic, in the face of economic downward pressure, how should supply chain companies take effective measures to overcome difficulties and develop steadily?

During the epidemic, the overall supply chain enterprise monitoring and response plan lacked lower-level transparency because of the low degree of digitization of the supply chain. In the entire supply chain, the application of digital platforms is not universal, which makes it difficult to respond and deploy timely in the emergency supply chain. Those intelligent factories and intelligent supply chain centers that require fewer employees and are easy to control the epidemic have become a highlight. Conversely, industries or enterprises that are more dependent on labor are more affected.

Every time when a major social event occurs, new requirements are imposed on the corresponding industry. As the epidemic spreads, many uncertainties will continue to occur. We need not only the courage to face it, but also the ability to recognize it and live with it. In this COVID-19 epidemic, although the supply chain companies have played a relatively timely and stable role, the efficiency and quality still need to be further improved. After this epidemic, the model of common development of online and offline business will become standard, and the supply chain construction based on full ecological business of online and offline will become the norm.

(1) Improve the supply chain digital information platform

Under the regular epiclemic prevention and control measures, more and more enterprises will use digital management platforms of supply chain. At the same time, the entire society requires rapid understanding of changes through digital platforms to ensure the timeliness, transparency, and control of the supply chain status. The digital information platform of supply chain will become an indispensable content for enterprise information construction. Based on the iterative characteristics of software platform construction, the entire technology platform will be designed and deployed in accordance with the high requirements of the emergency supply chain.

(2) Improve supply chain intelligence

During the epidemic, companies that have a high degree of labor dependency are greatly affected. From the perspective of development trends, unmanned and less-populated supply chain scenarios will have greater development, and the demand for matching intelligent supply chain technologies will also increase. Therefore, supply chain companies need to deepen the application of intelligent supply chain technology.

(3) Enhance supply chain versatility

Based on the high requirement of the epidemic for the supply chain response, the commonality of supply chain facilities has become the focus of attention, which also requires that in the future supply chain system construction, the infrastructure should be multifunctional, compatible with multiple businesses and applicable to emergency services; Secondly, it is also reflected in the convenience of additional deployment to achieve the completion or expansion of the supply chain capacity in a short period of time, which proposes a higher requirement of planning, integration of software and intelligent hardware.

(4) Challenge the limit of logistics costs reduction

In 2019, many companies already have self-adjusting development models and new explorations of transforming business and growth methods, but in the event of an epidemic, they also need to have a stronger sense of crisis and save themselves more resolutely by reducing costs, quitting bad business, eliminating losses and growth without quality, ensuring cash flow, and meanwhile ensuring strong competitiveness. The key to achieve this is to challenge the limit of logistics costs reduction with the purpose of maintaining cash flow. For companies with good cash flow, it is recommended to rebuild their own cost capabilities, because dealing with uncertainty is a normal capability.

3 Anti-risk operational countermeasures against major risks of COVID-19 epidemic [①]

In the face of sudden outbreaks, in addition to preparing for protracted battle, supply chain companies should also formulate anti-risk operational countermeasures based on local conditions and the actual situation of business, which mainly includes:

(1) Safety of employees and enterprises comes first

When the employees are safe, the company is safe. Once the COVID-19 occurs within the enterprise, the enterprise may face major risks of centralized infection and quarantine, which will affect severely its operations. Therefore, enterprises should give priority to ensuring the health of their employees, formulate detailed emergency plans with specific responsibilities of management at all levels, and distribute them to management and ordinary employees to improve their safety and prevention awareness.

(2) Funding challenges

Supply chain companies generally have collection periods, their scale is generally small, and their financial risk tolerance is weak. At the same time, supply chain companies are dominated by individual drivers whose financial risk tolerance is weaker, which will directly make it difficult for the survival of small fleets or self-employed individuals, and may also cause potential social risks.

---

① CWM50 Report: Impact of COVID-19 on the Economy and Countermeasures, 2020-02-18 11:45:29 Source: Xinhuanet. http://www.xinhuanet.com/money/2020-02/18/c_1125590528.htm.

(3) Pay attention to market changes and take the initiative to seize opportunities for innovation

During the epidemic, it is vital to capture timely those things whether customer needs have changed, consumer habits have changed, how online and offline business share analysis is, how to stick with customers and share more value in the digital age for exploring opportunities for innovation and development.

(4) Strengthen training, practice internal skills and reserve operating capability

At its own level, clarify its shortcomings and improve internal professional management capabilities; at the customer level, strengthen mutual understanding with customers through continuous communication to ensure normal business; at the emergency management level, attach importance to emergency measures and respond to emergencies at any time.

(5) Reduce costs

One of the key measures to deal with corporate cash flow crisis and survive in the epidemic is to reduce costs, mainly including:

① The focus of reducing labor costs should be on improving labor productivity, staff efficiency, and reducing staff costs;

② Reduce operating costs includes fixed costs such as warehousing and equipment leasing and variable costs of operation;

③ Reduce management cost support that is not related to operating income;

(6) Reduce legal risk

In the epidemic, legal risks will be relatively concentrated. Therefore, the human resources department of the enterprise need prejudge the possible occurrence of labor risks and strengthen human resource counseling so that the enterprise's labor risks can be controlled and resolved in advance.

(7) Strengthen operation management

The core of supply chain enterprise competitiveness is always operational capabilities. During the epidemic, the vehicles and employees of the enterprise may be isolated or sealed out in a certain area at any time, posing a major challenge to the operating organization. Therefore, it is particularly necessary to strengthen the management and control of the operating organization to ensure the stability and completion of the business during the epidemic. At the same time, taking advantage of the current situation of small business volume, sort out and revise the supply chain business processes and service processes, strive to strengthen service processes and items, improve service levels, prepare for the rapid resumption of operations, and support future market and business development. For supply chain logistics service companies, it is also necessary to strengthen the support and management of suppliers and the communication with suppliers.

(8) Prepare strategies for epidemic prevention

Supply chain enterprises are labor-intensive enterprises. Therefore, before the end of the COVID-19 epidemic, those companies in particular need prepare precautionary materials of epidemic such as masks, disinfectants, infrared thermometers, and strengthen preventive training for all staff and responsibility systems of full coverage. And the emergency reporting and medical isolation system also should be established. Once symptoms such as fever and fatigue appear, immediately go to the designated hospital according to the regulations of local governments, and get active treatment to ensure the safety of employees and the company[1].

---

① Notice on Scientific and Accurate Prevention and Control of COVID-19, 2020-02-25 13:53 Source: Website of the Central People's Government of the People's Republic of China. http://www.gov.cn/xinwen/2020-02/25/content_5483024.htm.

4 Some thoughts: supply chain determines "post-epidemic era"

For supply chain companies, the epidemic could become a divide.

In the case of traffic disruption, some small companies suffered severe damage to the supply chain, resulting in extreme situations such as out-of-control of prices, services, and response mechanisms in terminal sales, customer service, and other aspects, complaints and punishment. It is not difficult to foresee that the industry concentration will be increased, the Matthew effect will be inevitable, and customers will be increasingly concentrated in large-scale enterprises and chain enterprises.

(1) The stronger is always strong

Large-scale and chain industries have channel and high-end positioning advantages, and have obtained cost-effective advantages through suppliers while operating, which will mean that a positive balance is formed between suppliers, enterprises and consumers. This balance can generate centripetal force for consumers and suppliers, and form the basis for sustainable high-quality operations.

In this sense, large-scale chains and other industries in the "post-epidemic era" may be experiencing a new stage of competition among supply chain companies. Especially in the context of advanced technologies such as big data and cloud platforms, the supply chain becomes smarter, which can precisely match the more diverse needs of consumers and continue to provide high-quality differentiated supply chain services.

(2) The logistics is in a favorable position in the change of real estate capital market environment

Although long-term warehousing leasing of supply chain enterprise can resist fluctuations, capital flows may slow down due to financial market fluctuations and the denominator effect that follows. Especially in the field of logistics infrastructure, there has been a shortage of investor allocation. Interest rates have begun to fall and are likely to remain low. From a fundamental point of view, considering the potential driving role of warehousing management and e-commerce on long-term demand, the logistics industry is generally better than other industries. In addition, capital may prefer high-quality core assets in regions with strong performance and therefore flow to these regions for hedging [1] .

The 13th Five-Year Plan emphasized the pillar role of industry and logistics in the national economic system [2] , which will have an important impact on promoting the "the Belt and Road" strategy. Local governments at all levels should continue to issue corresponding support and encouragement policies and measures to promote the development of the industry, and then provide guarantee and support for the healthy and coordinated development of the entire national economy, and ensure the successful promotion of the "the Belt and Road" strategy.

(3) The development trend of Chinese logistics infrastructure is good, but supply chain companies still have problems in acquiring land for related projects. I hope relevant departments will pay attention to it

The logistics infrastructure industry projects that support supply chain enterprises have their relative uniqueness and specificity. Must set up appropriate access conditions on the acquisition of land for logistics infrastructure projects for commercial enterprises to ensure that they can make the best use of the land and let the truly powerful and reputable enterprises develop.

We believe that the logistics infrastructure industry, as a basic industry

---

[1] Gerald Eve, CBRE Research, Cushman and Wakefield, JLL, Colliers, CBRE-EA, Prologis Research;https://www.prologis.com/logistics-industry-research/prologis-research-special-report-COVID-19-and-implications-logistics.

[2] The Outline of the 13th Five-Year Plan (2016-2020) of the National Economic and Social Development of the People's Republic of China, 2016 Source: Chinese Communist Party Member Network. http://www.12371.cn/special/sswgh/wen/#7.

closely related to the national economy and the people's livelihood, which has a certain degree of public welfare, requires the government to support it from various aspects including land, taxation, capital, and human resource costs. If the logistics of supply chain companies is treated in the same way as other industries, it will inevitably cause the supply chain companies to deter investment, which will impact the industry and corporate development.

At present, China is in the process of economic transformation and high-quality development. The more adversity, the more development. For the supply chain industry, what is tested during the epidemic is the ability of enterprise resource allocation and emergency organization; what is tested after the epidemic is the speed of self-rescue and the ability of continuous operations. Everyone is racing against time. Chinese supply chain companies are the most aggressive and passionate companies. They are the forerunners of resumption of work and production, because of the trust and the mission. Rainbow comes after the storm, and spring comes when the winter ends. This year is the year to complete the construction of a well-off society and the 13th Five-Year Plan. General Secretary Xi Jinping clearly emphasized that must be determined to fight and win the battle against the epidemic, block the spread of the virus and strive to achieve this year's economic and social development goals and tasks [1]. As a basic, strategic and pioneering industry for the development of the national economy, supply chain enterprises are a strong guarantee for achieving the goals and tasks of society and economy.

All supply chain enterprises and millions of supply chain practitioners should prevent the epidemic and develop at the same time, fully opening up the lifeline of the supply chain. It's our important task to achieve the both goals of epidemic prevention and control and economic and social development.

---

[1] Be Determined to Fight and Win the Battle against the Epidemic – An Important Speech by General Secretary Xi Jinping during the Investigation and Guidance of Prevention and Control of the COVID-19 in Beijing, 2020-02-12 07:11 Source: People's Daily. http://www.12371.cn/2020/02/12/ARTI1581462495242410.shtml.

国际突发公共卫生事件对航空业的影响及对策建议

刁志辉　太古集团*（中国）董事

　　2020 年突发的新冠肺炎疫情直接冲击包括交通运输业和旅游业在内的服务行业，航空运输业（以下简称"航空业"）受到空前打击。

　　太古集团旗下的国泰航空有限公司（以下简称"国泰"），包括国泰航空、国泰港龙航空、香港华民航空以及香港快运四家航空公司，拥有 236 架次的机队规模，以中国香港为基地连接中国内地及全球 200 多个城市。新冠肺炎疫情与 2003 年的非典疫情具有高度的相似性，在经历了非典疫情后，航空业积累了应对突发公共卫生事件的经验，各类应急机制也不断完善。本文希望通过回顾整理 2003 年非典疫情期间航空业的经验和措施，探讨此次国际突发公共卫生事件对航空业的影响及国家在疫情期间及过后如何扶持航空业的恢复和发展。

一　新冠肺炎疫情对全球航空业的影响

　　受疫情影响，全球各国加强入境限制导致航空需求疲弱。根据国泰分析航空数据公司 OAG 的统计，疫情中的 2020 年 2 月对比疫情前的 2019 年 12 月，中国内地的国内及国际航线客运可用座位公里分别减少 52% 和 59%，货运可用吨位公里则分别减少 50% 和 41%。

---

　　*　太古集团是一家涉及地产、航空、零售、饮料及食物链、海洋服务和贸易等业务的高度多元化的环球集团，成立于 1816 年，总部位于英国伦敦。

2003 年非典疫情的暴发让全球航空业损失近 100 亿美元，疫情之后整个航空业花了 9 个月的时间才恢复到正常水平。中国香港作为受非典疫情影响的主要地区之一，国泰 2003 年的客运收入同比下降 16.6%，货运收入则同比增长 5.6%。

此次新冠肺炎疫情相比 17 年前的非典疫情，对中国航空业的影响将更大。根据中国民航局的数据，2019 年全国民航旅客运输量达到 6.6 亿人次，国际航线数 849 条（2018 年），而 2003 年全国民航旅客运输量仅为 8759 万人次，国际航线数 194 条。同时，近年来中国出入境人数也不断增长。国家移民管理局公布的数据显示，内地居民出入境人数从 2003 年的 3973 万人次增加到 2019 年的 3.5 亿人次，17 年间增长了近 8 倍；外国人出入境人数从 2003 年的 2269 万人次增加到 2019 年的 9767 万人次 [①]。国际航空运输协会（IATA）最新发布的新冠肺炎疫情对全球航空业的财务影响数据显示，根据疫情的传播范围，2020 年全球客运业务的收入将损失 630 亿~1130 亿美元。

二 新冠肺炎疫情为航空业带来的挑战及应对措施

1. 疫情发展速度及规模带来的应变能力的挑战

航空公司面临的最主要挑战来自新冠肺炎疫情的发展速度。由于疫情的发展速度和规模不断变化，全球各机场口岸的政策和限制措施也在不断调整，航空公司因此需要及时准确应对。比如，在机组排班时，需考虑本次航班的机组是否此前 14 天内执飞过目的地国家禁止入境的口岸；机场值机人员需要熟悉每个目的地的入境限制，以及在全球各个机场关闭自助值机设备和暂停网上值机后，确保不符合规定的旅客不准登机。考虑到疫情于春运期间扩散的风险，中国民航局 1 月 23 日果断公布关于民航免收机票

---

① 数据来源于国家移民管理局。

退票费的政策，而文化旅游部于 1 月 24 日宣布即日起暂停所有团队旅游及"机票 + 酒店"旅游产品。在有效协助控制疫情的同时，航空公司必须面对数以十万计的改签以及退票处理的挑战。2 月 1 日，越南宣布禁止往来中国的航班，越捷航空当天下午一架从越南富国岛前往中国香港的航班在途中不得已只能返航岘港。这些挑战需要航空公司安排更多的资源应对。

航空公司在应对突发公共卫生事件时，首先需要与政府的卫生部门建立直接沟通机制。准确的信息对航空公司制定应对措施很关键，包括加强航空器消毒、对旅客体温检测及协助旅客健康申报等。以国泰为例，公司迅速成立了由行政总裁直接领导的应变小组，公司作为一个整体在疫情不断变化的情况下快速做出响应，同时与香港特区政府相关部门保持紧密沟通。

另外，航空公司可以通过官方网站、手机程序和社交媒体即时发布准确的消息，保持与公众、旅客、旅行中介、货运代理、政府部门及机场等外界沟通时的信息一致性，减少公众的疑虑。

2. 保障旅客及员工健康与安全的挑战

航空公司有责任去保护旅客和员工的健康与安全。同时，需要采取措施应对病毒可能通过航空器传播的风险。中国民航局从 1 月底开始发布关于航空公司以及机场疫情防控技术指南，并随着防控工作的进展加以修订。

以降低人与人接触的次数为目标，国泰迅速调整并简化航班上的各项服务包括商务舱餐饮改为头盘、主菜及甜品均以单一餐盘奉上，暂停餐前饮料及餐车服务；对员工而言，相关措施把正常的 7 道服务工序缩减成 2 道，降低前线员工的顾虑，体现了公司对员工的关怀。同时，国泰每日于航班之间进行的消毒已经达到并超过业界标准，目前使用的消毒剂是一款医院级消毒剂，通过了针对如冠状病毒等亲脂性病毒的欧盟 EN 测试。另外，国泰还加强了对旅客有关疫情的相关教育。在客机上通知旅客入境口岸的要求，并提醒乘机过程中需要注意的卫生事项，帮助旅客在旅行途中更好地保护好自己及他人。

为了与员工及时沟通，国泰在新引进的内部网站建立特定防疫页面，让全球 90 多个城市的 2 万多名员工同步收到公司及不同政府的各项政策措施，并举行相关说明会，确保员工在执勤时遵守这些规定。

3. 各机场口岸不同检疫政策的挑战

各级地方政府在疫情暴发的短期内迅速采取措施，包括进出港限制、健康申报等。这些措施对于疫情的防控是及时而有效的，但航空公司在实际执行的过程中却面临着诸多挑战，特别是各地方政策的不一致性。对于在中国不同城市都有航线网点的国际航空公司而言，海外机场值机人员办理登机手续时需要分清这些要求并有可能需要向乘客逐一解释入境政策。政策的不一致性还体现在应对飞机落地后发热乘客的处理措施，登机口旅客的体温检测等方面，航空公司需要及时了解各机场口岸的最新政策并及时应对。

4. 航班营运网络规划的挑战

由于需求骤减，航空公司必须考虑部分航线的成本效益，以保持现金流为目标。调整运营网络和班次可考虑以下因素。首先，保证主要城市之间的基本运力。以中国内地为例，国泰继续运营北京、上海、成都及厦门四座门户城市，以保证华北、华东以及西南地区与中国香港的联通。其次，航点和班次调整的先后顺序需要考虑到受困旅客。由于航班取消，很多旅客被困海外，取消航班计划公布前，需充分考虑旅客有备选的航班改签。另外，如阿联酋航空、新加坡航空和国泰航空等枢纽航空公司有很多中转旅客通过枢纽机场前往全球各地，航路的调整难度更大。例如，当意大利对往返中国的航班发布禁令后，国泰在取消意大利的航班后，温州到中国香港的航班也很难继续运营，因为大部分温州旅客都是搭乘这班机经中国香港前往意大利的。中国民航局于 2020 年 1 月 23 日宣布因疫情防控工作调减的航班将不计入航班执行率、正常率、投诉率等各类考核，能给予航空公司更大的弹性，灵活处理航班规划。

5. 现金流的挑战

应对航空需求减弱，航空公司需要削减航班班次，这有助于降低包括燃油费、起降服务费、停机费等变动成本。但航空公司依然面临着飞机租赁费、固定资产折旧及员工薪酬开支等高额的固定成本。由于出行需求骤减，数以十万计的退票，对航空公司的现金流带来另一重挑战。航空公司可以推出暂停招聘非关键岗位、全员无薪假期、非重要项目延期及与供应商协商延迟应付款项等措施。随着疫情在全世界多个国家扩散，荷兰皇家航空、汉莎航空、阿联酋航空、韩亚航空和越南航空等都陆续推出了无薪假期的措施来维持稳定的现金流。另外，3月4日财政部及中国民航局出台了关于疫情防控期间资金支持政策，缓解航空公司现金流方面的压力。

6. 应对健康申报工作的挑战

在疫情期间，航空公司需要协助完成外国旅客进入中国前的健康申报工作。除了中国海关要求填报的健康申报表外，大多数省市的卫生健康委员会要求入境旅客在线填报健康及旅行信息。但在线申报表格通常只有中文，为不懂中文的外国旅客填报带来了困难。另外，部分在线申报表格需要微信扫描二维码，很多外国旅客并不使用需要实名认证的微信。健康申报工作让外国旅客在疫情期间入境中国更加复杂，也给航空公司员工增添了额外的工作压力。

7. 航空货运的角色变得更加重要

对比客运，在疫情期间，航空货运的需求有所增加，当中包括海外为国内捐赠的口罩、防护服等紧缺的医疗物资。因此，在突发公共卫生事件期间保持航空货运通道的畅通很重要，也能体现航空公司的企业社会责任。另外，航空货运收入也在一定程度上缓解了客运航班缩减所带来的现金流压力。此次疫情期间，国泰的全球货机网络包括北京、上海、郑州、重庆、成都和厦门均正常运行，只有部分到内地的货班在航线和时刻上做出调整，使机组人员可以当天往返中国香港。各地航空公司利用货运网络积极支持防疫物资的运输工作，除了完成日常机场到机场的运输外，还可以帮助捐赠方协调地面的物流公司并协助防疫物资在海关的清关工作。另外，面对客运航班减少、防疫物资又猛增的情况，也可以考虑安排部分客机以"只载货"模式营运，以充分利用客机的腹舱运力。

三 疫情后的政策建议

面对未来可能发生的国际突发公共卫生事件，航空公司需要加强自身的应对机制，包括危机应变的组织架构及产品的替代方案等。中央及各省市地方政府面对新冠肺炎疫情已经做出非常迅速的决策安排和方案指导，在此基础上，为帮助业界提升处理未来突发公共卫生事件的能力，可以参考以下建议。

1.疫情管理的政策统一

新冠肺炎疫情暴发后，中国各地方的卫生健康委员会也参与到机场的卫生检疫工作中。而有别于国际航班的惯例由海关统一对入境旅客检疫，新冠肺炎疫情期间各省市机场口岸的入境标准并不统一。有的机场禁止过去14天内有湖北省旅行史的旅客入境，其他机场则禁止持有湖北省签发护照的旅客入境。还有个别城市的检疫单位要求航空公司员工，陪同来自疫情高发地区的旅客，前往特定的隔离点或小区进行居家隔离。不同城市机场疫情管理的要求存在差异，以致在实际操作层面给旅客和航空公司带来很大困扰。

在机组人员安排方面，中国民航局统一规定外籍机组人员可以返回基地隔离，但个别地方卫生部门在执行时却有不同的要求。由于隔离措施的不可预见性，国际航空公司在人员的安排上受到很大影响。综上可见，在面对突发公共卫生事件时，统一各省市的疫情管理政策可大幅降低公众的疑虑以及航空公司在执行方面的难度，并提高落实相关措施的效率。

从技术层面看，可以拓展现有的 iAPI 系统，即出入境航空器载运人员信息预报预检系统。目前该系统会收集旅客的航班信息和护照信息，在疫情暴发期间可以增加旅客的座位信息及当地联系方式以备日后使用。以上措施的有效实施都要建立在各机场口岸政策统一的基础上。

2. 建立多语种的统一数据信息平台

旅客在网上进行健康申报并填写联络信息增加了信息收集的有效性和准确性。为确保入境外国旅客了解并遵守中国的防疫措施，根据此次应对新冠肺炎疫情的经验，建议建立统一的数据平台，通过海内外通用的手机程式收集相关信息，并提供多语种的服务。同时，由于外国旅客对于个人信息的收集比较敏感，统一平台也可降低外国旅客对信息被泄露的担忧。

3. 保障主要货运航线的畅通

突发公共卫生事件暴发后，航空公司保障货运航线的畅通对于支持疫情的防控以及减少疫情对国家经济的长期影响非常重要。如前所述，抗疫物资的运输由于需求的紧迫性而高度依赖空运。而在突发公共卫生事件期间，客运航班的运力下降，保障货运航班凸显重要。在这样一个充满挑战的时期，民航监管机构的工作效率和灵活性将发挥关键作用。例如，在批准航班时刻、包机业务、改变航路和升级货机类型等方面民航监管机构都可以发挥积极作用进行引导和支持。事实上，中国民航局在新冠肺炎疫情暴发期间已经采取了类似的做法。如果这类政策能有一个明确的指导方针，就可以帮助航空公司和货运公司更好地提前进行规划。

4. 疫情后的市场重建

中国政府采取的控制疫情及促进经济增长的措施，有助于减轻疫情对中国乃至世界经济的中长期影响，全球包括中国在内的航空业长期增长的趋势未变。随着疫情得到有效控制，以旅游及商务为代表的航空出行需求将很快得到恢复。疫情之后为促使航空业能够快速恢复，各地政府可以考虑如下建议。

航空业复苏的第一个迹象是对旅行限制的解除，根据疫情控制情况，世界卫生组织可以及时协调各国政府，宣布疫情的结束。鼓励公民出游是刺激旅游业和航空旅行恢复的有效途径。疫情过后，建议各国政府的旅游推广部门通过举办大型市场活动增加访客人数并通过游客消费来刺激经济的增长。

简化入境程序是促进游客增长的另一个关键因素。建议各国政府可以考虑免除游客签证等政策来鼓励国际旅客旅游。同时，各地机场可以采用新技术，简化通关和安检程序提升旅客的体验，例如，使用手机登机牌，使用通关程序中的一码通关，使用常旅客的快速通关等举措。建议各地政府还可以考虑通过减税、减免社保以及其他公共费用的方式来减轻此次疫情对居民的影响，这些措施也可以在一定程度上增加居民的可支配收入并刺激其在国内外旅游等方面的支出。

航空业的恢复预计将是相当漫长的过程。为了使航班尽快恢复到正常规模，通过减免机场相关费用包括飞机起降、停机、导航和旅客服务费等政策以鼓励航空公司尽快复飞航班。2020 年 3 月 9 日，中国民航局发布了关于积极应对新冠肺炎疫情有关支持政策的通知，通过实施积极财政政策和推进降费减免等方面促进航空业稳定发展。

四 结语

2020 年 2 月 14 日，习近平总书记在中央全面深化改革委员会第十二次会议上提出，"抗击新冠肺炎疫情是对国家治理体系和治理能力的一次大考，要研究和加强疫情防控工作，从体制机制上创新和完善重大疫情防控举措，健全国家公共卫生应急管理体系，提高应对突发重大公共卫生事件的能力水平"。航空业是受传染病疫情影响较大的行业，也是健全国家应对突发公共卫生事件防控体系的重要环节。

国泰作为中国航空业重要的一员，理应肩负起肩上的重任，共同为健全国家公共卫生应急管理体系做出贡献。太古集团和国泰相信，疫情的影响是短期和阶段性的，无论是管理层还是员工，均对中国政府对疫情的管控以及航空市场未来的恢复充满信心。国泰依旧会将乘客的安全放在第一位，并根据各级政府的要求配合做好防疫工作，保证不断航的同时拿出运力支持国家防疫物资的运输工作。只有在配合这场抗击防疫的战争中站好岗，才能保证旅客的信任和支持，使疫情后的复工有序进行。国泰相信在中央政府的有序领导下，中国最终将赢得抗击疫情的胜利，迎来新的市场增长。

参考文献

《2020 年全国民航工作会议召开》，中国民航网，2020 年 1 月 6 日。

《国家移民管理局：2019 年出入境人员达 6.7 亿人次》，新华社，2020 年 1 月 5 日。

IATA:《国际航协升级新冠肺炎疫情的行业损失预测》，中国民航网，2020 年 3 月 6 日。

《暂停旅游企业经营活动的紧急通知》，中华人民共和国文化和旅游部，2020 年 1 月 26 日。

Impacts of International Public Health Emergency and Recommendation of Countermeasures on Aviation Industry from the Epidemic

By Titus DIU, Director of John Swire & Sons (China) Ltd.

The outbreak of the COVID-19 epidemic in early 2020 has exerted a direct impact on service industries including the transportation and tourism industries. The global aviation industry in particular has been impacted on unprecedented levels.

The Cathay Pacific Group (hereinafter referred to as "Cathay Pacific") operates four airlines. These are Cathay Pacific, Cathay Dragon, Air Hong Kong, and Hong Kong Express. With a fleet size spanning 236 aircraft, Cathay Pacific is based out of its home hub in Hong Kong Special Administrative Region (HKSAR) and connects Mainland Chinese cities with more than 200 cities worldwide. COVID-19 shares significant resemblance to SARS in 2003. After experiencing the SARS epidemic, the aviation industry has accumulated an understanding of the importance of an effective response to public health emergencies and has been prepared with various emergency mechanisms. This paper will review the experience and measures taken by the aviation industry during the SARS epidemic in 2003, discuss the impacts of the current impact of COVID-19 on the industry and explore how governments can support the recovery and rebound of the industry during and after the epidemic.

1 Impacts of the COVID-19 epidemic on the global aviation industry

Affected by the epidemic, the strengthening of entry restrictions by countries around the world has resulted in weak global travel demand. Cathay Pacific's analysis of flight information data provider OAG's statistics showed that in February 2020 during the epidemic, compared with December 2019 before the epidemic, the passenger ASK(Available Seat Kilometers) on domestic and international routes in Mainland China declined by 52% and 59% respectively, and cargo ATK (Available Tonne Kilometers) declined by 50% and 41% respectively.

The SARS outbreak in 2003 cost the global aviation industry a loss of nearly USD10 billion. It took nine months for the entire aviation industry to return to normal levels after the epidemic. As one of the main regions affected by the SARS epidemic, HKSAR saw Cathay Pacific's passenger revenue in 2003 decreased by 16.6% year-over-year while cargo revenue increased by 5.6% year-over-year.

The COVID-19 epidemic will have a greater impact on China's aviation industry than the SARS epidemic 17 years ago. According to the data of the Civil Aviation Administration of China (CAAC), the number of passenger trips nationwide reached 660 million in 2019 (CAAC, 2020) across 849 international routes (2018). Comparatively in 2003, the number of passenger trips nationwide was only 87.59 million spanning 194 international routes. At the same time, the number of entry and exit trips to and from China has grown significantly in recent years. According to data released by the National Immigration Administration (NIA), the number of mainland residents entering and exiting increased from 39.73 million in 2003 to 350 million in 2019, a nearly 10-fold of increase in 17 years; the number of foreigners entering and exiting increased from 22.69

million in 2003 to 97.67 million in 2019 (NIA, 2020). The latest data of financial impact of the COVID-19 epidemic on the global air transport industry released by the International Air Transport Association (IATA) demonstrates depending on the scope of the epidemic spread, 2020 global revenue losses for the passenger business may range from USD63 billion to USD113 billion (IATA, 2020).

2 Challenges and countermeasures stemming from the COVID-19 epidemic

(1) The challenge of responding effectively to the speed and scale of the epidemic

The main challenge for airlines stems from the speed at which the COVID-19 epidemic has developed. As the speed and scale of the epidemic continues to transform, policies and restrictions at airports around the world are constantly under adjustment and as a result, airlines need to respond in a timely and accurate manner. For example, when crew management teams are scheduling crew rostering patterns, it is necessary to consider whether the crew of this flight have flown within the previous 14 days to a port from where it is forbidden to enter the destination country. Additionally, airport check-in personnel need to be familiar with the evolving entry restrictions of each destination. Many airlines have taken to suspending self-service check-in systems at various airports around the world while simultaneously suspending online check-in to thoroughly ensure that passengers adhere to the specific-country regulation requirements. Given the risk of the epidemic spreading during the Spring Festival travel peak, CAAC announced decisively on January 23 the implementation of a policy that would exempt any fees applicable to passengers applying for refunds on their air tickets, while the Ministry of Culture and Tourism (MCT) announced on January 24 to suspend all group travel and "air tickets and hotel accommodation" tourism products (MCT, 2020). Airlines now face the challenges of handling vast numbers of rebooking and refund applications. On February 1, Vietnam announced a ban on flights to and from China. On the afternoon of the same day, VietJet Air had a flight scheduled from Phu Quoc in Vietnam to HKSAR and ultimately had to turn back to Da Nang. These challenges demonstrate the necessity for airlines to mobilize significant resources to respond.

When airlines respond to public health emergencies, they must first establish a direct communication mechanism with the government's health authorities. Accurate information is critical for airlines to formulate response measures, including strengthening aircraft disinfection procedures, detecting passenger temperatures and assisting in passenger health declarations. Taking Cathay Pacific as an example, the company quickly set up a taskforce directly under the leadership of the CEO. The company then responded unilaterally to the rapid changing external environment while maintaining close communication with HKSAR's health authorities.

In addition, airlines have been pressed to release accurate and timely information through official websites, mobile applications and social media to maintain a consistent flows of information in order to communicate with the public, passengers, travel agents, freight forwarders, government agencies, and airports, among other external parties in order to ease stakeholder anxiety.

(2) The challenge of protecting the health and safety of passengers and employees

Airlines have a responsibility to protect the health and safety of both passengers and employees. At the same time, measures need to be taken to address the risk that the virus spread through in-flight. CAAC released technical guidelines on epidemic prevention and control for airlines and airports at the end of January, and revisions have been made with the development of the epidemic.

With the goal of reducing the frequency of person-to-person contact, Cathay Pacific quickly adjusted and simplified various services in-flight, including meal-service in business class to be served on a single plate while suspending pre-takeoff drinks and cart services. For crew, relevant measures have reduced the normal seven meal service procedures to two, alleviating concerns of frontline employees and embodying the company's care for employees. At the same time, Cathay Pacific's daily disinfection procedures between flights has exceeded industry standards. The disinfectant currently in use is a hospital-grade disinfectant that has passed EU EN testing for lipophilic viruses such as coronavirus. In addition, Cathay Pacific has also demonstrated passenger service quality by notifying passengers of the requirements of the final destination port of entry while reminding them of simple personal hygiene measures that can be taken during the flight to better protect themselves and others during the journey.

In order to communicate with employees in a timely manner, Cathay Pacific has also established a specific epidemic prevention page on the newly introduced internal website, allowing over 20,000 employees in more than 90 cities around the world to receive the company's and various governments' policies and measures in the same pace, while holding relevant briefings to ensure employees abide by these rules while on duty.

(3) The challenge of different quarantine policies at airport ports

Local governments at all levels have quickly adopted measures in a short period after the outbreak, including restrictions on entry and exit and health declaration, etc. These measures are timely and effective for the prevention and control of the epidemic, but airlines face many challenges in the actual implementation process, especially due to inconsistencies across various local policies. For international airlines that have flights in different cities within China, check-in personnel at overseas airports need to distinguish between these requirements when processing check-in and may need to explain the entry policy to passengers individually. The inconsistency in policies is also reflected in the passenger landing process and the temperature monitoring procedures at departure gates, etc. Airlines need to keep themselves updated with the latest policies at different airports and respond timely.

(4) The challenge in flight operation network planning

As demand has plummeted, airlines must consider the cost-effectiveness of some routes with the goal of maintaining cash flows. The adjustment of frequency and network plans is based on the following factors: firstly, to ensure basic capacity between major cities. Taking Mainland China as an example, Cathay Pacific continues to operate in the four gateway cities of Beijing, Shanghai, Chengdu and Xiamen to ensure the connectivity between North China, East China and the Southwest and HKSAR. Secondly, the sequence of port and frequency adjustments requires considering the stranded passengers. Due to flight cancellations, many passengers are stranded overseas. Before announcing flight cancellation decisions, full consideration must be given to allow alternative flights for rebooking passengers. In addition, airlines such as Emirates, Singapore Airlines, and Cathay Pacific have many transit passengers who travel through their city-hubs to various parts of the world, making network adjustments even more difficult. For example, when Italy issued a ban on flights to and from China, and after Cathay Pacific cancelled its flights to and from Italy, it became commercially unviable to operate the Wenzhou to HKSAR route, given that a vast number of passengers on this route are often transit passengers between Wenzhou and Italy. CAAC announced on January 23 that flights affected due to epidemic prevention and control measures would not be counted in various performance metrics such as flight execution rate, on-time performance rate, complaint rate, etc., allowing airlines greater flexibility for flight planning.

(5) The challenge of cash flows

In response to the weakening of travel demand, airlines have need to reduce flight frequencies, which have helped reduce variable costs including fuel costs, take-off and landing service charges, and parking charges. But airlines still face high fixed costs such as aircraft leasing fees, depreciation of fixed assets, and employee compensation expenses. As travel demand has plummeted, hundreds of thousands of refunds have come into play, posing another challenge to airlines' cash flows. Airlines have sought to further maintain healthy cash flows through introducing measures to suspend the recruitment of non-critical positions, offer unpaid leave to employees, postpone non-critical projects, and negotiate with vendors on payment terms and potential reductions. As the epidemic spread in many countries around the world, KLM, Lufthansa, Emirates, Asiana Airlines and Vietnam Airlines have successively introduced unpaid leave schemes to maintain stable cash flows. In addition, the Ministry of Finance and CAAC issued a policy on funding support during the epidemic prevention and control on March 4 to ease the pressure on airlines' cash flows.

(6) Response to the challenge of health declaration

During the epidemic, airlines need to assist in completing health declarations for foreign passengers before they enter China. In addition to standard health declaration forms required by customs, most provinces' and municipalities' health commissions have required inbound passengers to submit a health and travel history declaration form online. However, online declaration forms are usually only available in Chinese, which makes it difficult for foreign passengers who may possess limited Chinese-language proficiency to complete the forms. In addition, some online declaration forms require WeChat to scan the QR code, but many foreign passengers do not use WeChat that requires real-name authentication. The health declaration process has made the process for inbound foreign passengers entering China during the epidemic outbreak more complicated, and has also put extra pressure on airline employees.

(7) The role of air cargo becomes more important

Compared with the sharp decline in passenger traffic during the epidemic, the global demand for air freight has increased, with transportation of medical supplies such as masks and protective clothing in high-demand and being donated from overseas. Therefore, the maintenance of freighter lanes during public health emergencies is crucial, and also allows airlines the capability to make their contribution to corporate social responsibility. In addition, air cargo revenue has helped to alleviate cash flow pressures caused by the reduction of passenger flights. During the epidemic, Cathay Pacific's global freighter network including Beijing, Shanghai, Zhengzhou, Chongqing, Chengdu and Xiamen have been operating under normal conditions, and only some adjustments have been made to routes and schedules for cargo flights to and from the Mainland, including benefiting from the enablement of crew members to travel to and from HKSAR on the same day. Airlines around the world have been harnessing their freighter networks to actively support the transportation of medical supplies. In addition, they can also help donors coordinate with ground logistics companies and assist in the clearance of epidemic prevention materials at customs. In the face of a reduction in passenger flights and a surge in epidemic prevention supplies, it has also been possible to consider flying passenger aircraft to operate "cargo-only" flights, in order to make full use of the belly-hold capacity of passenger aircrafts.

3　Policy recommendations after the epidemic

In face of potential international public health emergencies in the future, airlines need to strengthen their own response mechanisms, including organizational structures and product alternatives for crisis response. The central government and local governments of various provinces and municipalities have made rapid arrangements in the face of the COVID-19 epidemic. Based on this and in order to help the industry strengthen its ability to handle future potential public health emergencies, the following suggestions can be referred to.

(1) Unification of epidemic management policies

After the outbreak of COVID-19, health commissions in various provinces and municipalities have also participated in health quarantine work at airports. In contrast to the general practice of international flights, where customs uniformly quarantine inbound passengers, the entry criteria of the provincial and municipal airport ports during the COVID-19 epidemic are not unilateral. Some airports have banned the entry of passengers who have traveled to Hubei Province within the previous 14 days, while other airports have prohibited the entry of passengers who hold a passport issued by Hubei Province. There are also health authorities in some particular cities that require airline employees to accompany passengers from regions with high infection rates to specific isolation facilities or communities for home quarantine. Different cities have different requirements for the management of the epidemic which has caused great confusion to passengers and airlines at the operating level.

In terms of crew arrangements, CAAC has uniformly stipulated that foreign crew members can return to their bases for isolation, but some particular local health authorities have different requirements, meaning that the unpredictability of quarantine measures has greatly affected airlines' staffing arrangements. In summary, when facing public health emergencies in future, unifying the epidemic management policies in various provinces and municipalities can greatly reduce the public's doubts and the difficulties airlines face when implementing them.

From a technical point of view, the existing iAPI (interactive advanced passenger information) system can be expanded. At present, the system will collect passengers' flight information and passport information. During the epidemic, passenger seat information and local contact information can be added. The effective implementation of the above measures must be based on unified policies at airports.

(2) Establish a multilingual unified data platform

Passengers making health declarations online and filling in contact information have increased the effectiveness and accuracy of information collection. In order to ensure that inbound foreign passengers understand and comply with China's epidemic prevention measures, it is recommended to establish a unified data platform to collect relevant information through popular mobile application and provide multilingual services, based on the experience learnt from the COVID-19 outbreak. At the same time, as foreign passengers may be more sensitive to the collection of personal information, a unified platform would also serve to address their concerns about potential information leakage.

(3) Ensure the smooth flow of major freighter routes

After the outbreak of a public health emergency, it is important for airlines to ensure the smooth operation of freighter lanes to support the prevention and control of the epidemic and mitigate the long-term impact of the epidemic on the national economy. As mentioned earlier, the transportation of medical supplies is highly dependent on air transportation due to the urgency of demand. During public health emergencies, the capacity of passenger flights will ultimately decline and therefore the security of cargo flights become increasingly important. In these times, the efficiency and flexibility of civil aviation regulators will play a key role. For example, civil aviation regulators can play an active role in providing guidance and support in approving freighter schedules, charter flights, changes in routes and upgrading freighter types. In fact, CAAC has already taken a similar approach during the outbreak of COVID-19. If such policies possess clear guidelines, they can help airlines and freighter operators plan more effectively.

(4) Market reconstruction after the epidemic

Measures taken by the Chinese government to control the epidemic and promote economic growth will help mitigate the mid- and long-term impacts of the epidemic on the Chinese and the world economy. The long-term growth trend of the global aviation industry, including that of China, has remained unchanged. With the effective control of the epidemic, the demand for air travel represented by tourism and business will soon recover. To facilitate the rapid recovery of the aviation industry after the epidemic, local governments can consider the following suggestions.

The first sign of recovery within the aviation industry will be the lifting of travel restrictions, stemming from the World Health Organization coordinating with governments in a timely manner to declare the end of the epidemic. Encouraging citizens to travel is an effective way to stimulate the recovery of tourism and air travel. After the epidemic, it is suggested that tourism promotion agencies of various governments organize large-scale marketing events to stimulate travel demand.

Simplifying entry procedures is another key factor in promoting tourist growth. It is suggested that governments consider policies such as exempting tourist visas to encourage international tourists to travel. At the same time, airports can adopt new technologies to simplify customs and security procedures and improve passengers' experiences. For example, the use of mobile boarding passes, one-code clearance in customs and safety check procedures, fast track channel for frequent travelers and other measures. It is suggested that local governments also consider reducing income tax and reducing or exempting social security contributions and other public service fees to lower the impact of the epidemic on residents. These measures will serve to increase public disposable incomes which in turn may facilitate an increase in tourism expenditure levels at home and abroad.

The recovery of the aviation industry is expected to be a long-term process. In order to return to operating levels experienced pre-outbreak, policies related to the reduction or exemption of airport fees including aircraft take-off and landing, parking, navigation, and passenger service fees can be considered to motivate speedier flight resumption plans. On March 9, CAAC issued a notice on the relevant support policies for actively responding to the COVID-19 epidemic in order to promote the stable development of the aviation industry through the implementation of proactive financial policies and promotion of fee reductions and exemptions, etc.

4 Conclusion

On February 14, 2020, General Secretary Xi Jinping put forward, at the 12th Meeting of the Central Commission of Comprehensively Deepening Reform, that "the current fight against the novel coronavirus pneumonia epidemic is a major test of China's system and capacity for governance. We must study and strengthen the efforts of prevention and control of the epidemic, innovate and improve the systems and institutions in place that act to contain the spread, improve the national public health emergency management system and improve capabilities to respond to major public health emergencies. The aviation industry has been significantly affected by epidemics of infectious diseases, and serves as a case in point of the importance of building a robust system of prevention and control in response to a potential future public health emergency.

Cathay Pacific, as an important member of China's aviation industry, shoulders the heavy responsibilities of the industry and will continue to contribute to the improvement of the national public health emergency management system. Swire Group and Cathay Pacific believe that the impact of the epidemic is short-term. Both management and employees are fully confident in the Chinese government's control of the epidemic and the future recovery of the aviation industry. Cathay Pacific will continue to put the safety of passengers first, and cooperate with the government at all levels to combat the epidemic by ensuring the provision of cargo flights to support the transportation of medical supplies while maintaining a small number of passenger flights for essential travel necessities. Our duties to combat the epidemic will guarantee the trust and support of our passengers, duties that will facilitate the eventual resumption of work after the epidemic. Cathay Pacific believes that under the trusted leadership of the central government, China will eventually win the fight against the epidemic and usher in new market growth.

Bibliography

CAAC. (2020, Jan 6). CAAC 2020 Work Conference. Retrieved from CAAC: http://www.caac.gov.cn/ZTZL/RDZT/2020QGMHGZHY/2020TPXW/202001/t20200107_200213.html

NIA. (2020, Jan 6). Entry and Exit Trips Reached 670 Million in 2019. Retrieved from NIA: https://www.nia.gov.cn/n741440/n741567/c1199336/content.html

IATA. (2020). IATA Updates COVID-19 Financial Impacts -Relief Measures Needed. Singapore: IATA.

MCT. (2020, Jan 26). Notice on Suspending All Group Travel. Retrieved from MCT: https://www.mct.gov.cn/whzx/ggtz/202001/t20200126_850571.htm

2020 年大变局之文化影视行业新思考

甄超凡　环球 * 影业中国区　执行副总裁兼董事总经理

黄志湘　环球影业中国区　副总裁

2020 年初暴发的 COVID-19 肆虐中国及全球，打破了世界一切原有的正常运营秩序和模式。在这场百年罕见的全球危机中，中国经过两个多月的抗疫，终于有效控制住疫情并逐步开始复工复产。中国医护人员和社会各界的艰苦牺牲、中国人民上下一心的力量又一次让世界惊叹。抗疫的初步成功让中国成为许多其他国家学习的对象。

这场世纪大疫不仅是一场全球公共卫生危机，而且对全球经济也造成了重大冲击，它不可避免地给全球各个行业带来前所未见的严峻挑战。以文化影视行业为例，由于电影院线运营模式的特殊性，电影行业成为受疫情严重冲击的行业之一，电影产业损失惨重。疫情对整个电影行业的冲击是全方位的，影院、制片公司、宣发公司等都面临着生死存亡的压力。

一　疫情严重影响全球电影业

1. 新冠肺炎疫情导致中国电影市场损失巨大

这场疫情造成的影响是全球性的，电影行业遭受的重创更是前所未有的。中国市场从 2020 年春节前夕开始就出现影片撤档、影院集体关门。《每日经济新闻》3 月初报道：2019 年内地春节档票房为 59.1 亿元。如

---

　　* 环球是全球领先的媒体、娱乐公司，面向全球观众制作、发行、营销娱乐、新闻和资讯等节目。拥有新闻娱乐电视网络、知名电影公司、电视节目制作公司、主题公园以及基于互联网的数字业务等，是美国康卡斯特旗下的子公司，总部位于美国洛杉矶。

果没有疫情，多位业内人士曾预测，2020年春节档票房有望突破70亿元大关。

不但观众看不到电影，各大剧组也面临停工。为抗击疫情，保证人员安全，各大影视基地以及已经开机的剧组纷纷发布停拍公告。影视停拍、延拍无疑对片方经济实力进行了一次大考。

尽管现阶段疫情已有所好转，人们因为担心疫情会卷土重来，对于人流密集性场所依然十分谨慎。像影院这种人员密度高的封闭空间，人们的信心恢复起来肯定需要一些时间。人们与影院之间的信任关系将在复工后面临考验，需要花费一段时间重新建立。

2. 新冠肺炎疫情令全球电影业进入停摆期

据《好莱坞报道者》预测，由于票房收入的下滑及对制作进度的影响，新冠肺炎疫情已对全球电影业带来至少70亿美元损失；如果持续到5月，损失将增加100亿美元；5月后损失将难以估计。

根据韩国电影协会数据，韩国首尔的票房成绩跌至16年来的最低水平；作为全球影业第三大票仓，日本目前虽没有让影院集体停业，但影院营业状况大受影响。欧洲市场也深受疫情冲击，法国、西班牙、意大利、荷兰和爱尔兰等32个国家的大多数影院都已关门歇业。同样，北美电影市场也深受重创，《007：无暇赴死》《寂静之地2》《速度与激情9》《花木兰》《黑寡妇》等纷纷延期或撤档；《蝙蝠侠》《神奇动物3》《黑客帝国4》《灰姑娘》《小美人鱼》《尚气》等好莱坞重头电影宣布停拍。

二 院线电影转向网络播放

随着此次疫情的暴发，大部分企业和单位都不得不停工停产，传统行业和经济遭受了重创。但另外，应对疫情的需求和人们工作生活方式的改变，意外地加速催生了各种线上业务的快速兴起和成长：远程医疗、远程办公、视频会议、线上教育、网络视听、在线游戏等，成为新的产业发展亮点和未来方向。同时，数字技术的发展也为线上业务的实现提供了技术上的可能性，线下向线上转移的时刻正在来临。疫情在某种程度上意外加速催生了全球电影产业新一轮的变革。

国内《囧妈》《大赢家》在头条系免费网播之后，好莱坞也开始尝试对新上映的影片开通付费点播业务，随着 NBCUniversal 环球影业宣布将通过康卡斯特和 SKY 提供《狩猎》《隐形人》《艾玛》三部影片的点播服务，《魔发精灵2》亦被其所属公司提早可在线上点播，至此好莱坞各大公司相继缩短美国院线传统"窗口期"，同时，各公司也将和苹果公司的 iTunes、亚马逊等科技巨头合作推行点播业务。

好莱坞巨头"院网同步"或者"网络首发"的尝试对于全球电影行业来说无疑为一次新的尝试和突破。电影产业在这一特殊时期的格局性变化引发了业内人士的热议和思考。

其实，电影的院线与网络之争在这次疫情之前就早已开始。线上点播的灵活性、技术优势及个性化推荐模式，导致它与传统院线发生不可调和的冲突，根本上是观影需求模式的市场争夺。《电影发展研究报告》显示，近几年院线电影在视频平台上线比例稳定在 80% 左右，且影院上映到视频平台上线之间的窗口期缩短，2019 年窗口期为 47 天，较 2016 年缩短一半。互联网时代，网络平台已成为院线电影发行的"第二战场"。美国电影协会公布的《2019 主题报告》显示，2019 年全球电影票房为 422 亿美元，较 2018 年上升了 1%。而全球家庭娱乐市场（包括流媒体、电视、DVD）的规模达到 588 亿美元，较 2018 年增长了 14%。全球的数字影视内容市场规模达到 487 亿美元（这个数字不包括付费电视），较 2018 年增长了 25%。其中北美市场增长了 18%，海外市场增长了 29%。落实到更具体的流媒体市场，其规模为 448 亿美元，超过电影院线。2019 年上海网络视听产业周上发布的消息称，截至 2019 年 6 月，中国网络视频用户规模达 7.59 亿人，较 2018 年底增长 3391 万人，占网民整体的 88.8%，网络剧、网络电影、网络纪录片等节目样态呈现井喷式发展，节目数量呈爆发式增长。

互联网时代，所有行业的游戏规则都会或主动或被动地发生改变。我们认为，这次疫情给消费者生活模式带来的前所未有的变化，也是大家为观众提供影院和家庭观影双重选择的重要原因。各公司这次的决定除了有实际需要外，也有一定试水的成分，这不代表 2020 年的其他影片也会以同样模式发行，各公司将根据这次实验的成效和各方的反应进行评估，亦要通过与各合作方包括院线充分协商和沟通才会进行下一步的改革，确定每个市场的最佳发行策略。

其实这几部影片的转网并不意味着线上模式会完全取代传统院线模式：一是在短期内线上模式是难以取代影院观影效果的，尤其是特效大制作影片；二是对头部影片而言，窗口期院线发行更符合片方及产业链各方利益。目前院线渠道仍是头部内容的首选渠道，而线上影院实际上是为部分差异化竞争以及中长尾电影作品提供了增量的分发渠道和变现方式。

可以明确看到的是，随着疫情在全球的暴发，作为并非绝对刚需的电影产业的确受到极为严重的冲击，疫情促进了线上消费模式的加速发展。此外，"90 后"逐渐成为主流观影人群，他们更愿意在互联网上付费以获取个性化的服务。但是疫情对院线的影响应该是暂时的，等疫情彻底结束后，积压的很多优质产品都会找到更好的机会放映，大众也需要娱乐活动，重新回到正常生活，这时候院线将会迎来显著的市场回暖。同时，院网之争同时也会倒逼传统院线进行思考和创新，进一步提升其硬环境和软环境，为观众提供更好的观影环境和观影体验，以期将观众从小屏幕吸引回大银幕。

因此，无论行业将来如何发展，线上观影并不会彻底取缔线下模式或者对院线电影市场造成毁灭性打击，可以预计要经过很长一段时期，院线和视频点播才会达成最合乎各方需求和利益的平衡。全球数字化是一个大趋势，院线无法完全排斥流媒体，流媒体也暂时无法完全取代院线，双方将在一段时间内并存、相互适应、相互改变、有机融合。目前网络平台与传统电影产业的融合尚处于相互试探的阶段，两者其实可以互相借力。例如，两者通过进行广泛深入的版权合作可以有效降低内容采购成本；平台自制电影的宣发依靠传统发行放映业进行内容产品分销，同时为传统电影作品提供新的放映渠道以及宣传渠道；资金方面，流媒体平台也可以给优质电影内容版权需求提供新的融资渠道。相互借力之后，流媒体平台和传统电影企业将在新的电影产业链上形成合力，这股合力的核心是优秀内容创制。优秀的内容创制离不开人才和技术，这两个层面互联网平台与传统电影各具优势。①

三 对电影产业未来的期待

无可否认这场疫情引发了一些另类产业模式的试探，虽然没有人能在变革中准确预测电影产业的未来，但可以看到互联网将对传统院线业务形成挑战且两者之间将有旷日持久的跨界市场竞争。事实上，美国影业更早些时间就面临了类似的问题，只不过它们的对手是流媒体或家庭视频点播服务，而中国院线业务的对手则是在线视频平台。

流媒体全球化的趋势已经形成，互联网内容的地域性不断减弱，而优质内容更是在全球范围内得到广泛传播。中国作为互联网人口大国，应该充分了解全球优质流媒体平台和内容，在与全球流媒体不断交流与接触中，逐渐建立适合自己的操作和经营模式。这不但满足了人们对优质内容的需求，还可以为行业的发展方向提供参考，为中国互联网影视产业技术和理念迭代升级时刻做好准备。

鉴于此，中国电影在互联网时代渠道变革的进程中，可以考虑以更开放包容的态度拥抱互联网，更广泛深入地开展国际合作，引进国外先进的创制技术和运营管理经验，实现电影产业外资规制的效益最大化。

---

① 章霖轩：《迭代、破窗与共融：流媒体平台撬动电影产业的当下与未来》，《电影文学》2019/17，P12-P13

1. 有利于优化电影产业资源配置

猫眼专业版数据显示，2019年上半年分账票房和观影人次同比都出现下降，为2011年来首次，表明电影行业规模驱动的发展模式已经接近尾声。中国电影行业正处于从规模到质量的历史节点。

同时，随着中国网络视频用户的规模不断增加，中国网络用户对高质量内容的渴求也是日益凸显。视频影视产业也已经告别高增长阶段，转向高质量发展时期。但中国电影市场的"互联网化"是两个体系，一个是院线电影市场的高度互联网化，另一个是以用户流量为基础的视频平台，二者短时期内很难实现融合。

而好莱坞则具备积淀几十年的内容制作体系，同时又有流媒体平台的分发渠道，在维护自有版权体系的基础上成功构建起"流量闭环"或者说"渠道闭环"。允许有成熟模式及运营经验的外资进入中国电影产业，有利于打破目前国内发展困局，加速产业资源优化配置。

2. 有利于接轨和开拓国际市场

尽管中国电影票房快速增长、电影市场不断扩张，但国产电影通过有限的海外发行资源开发国际市场的成效不甚明显，本土电影在海外市场的份额较低。而美国电影不仅是美国市场的电影，还是面向全球市场的电影，很多美国电影海外票房要远远高于本土收入。

扩大和深化发展"中外合拍"的制片模式，使更多本土制作公司可以借鉴外方投资制作理念、借用外方的全球发行资源，深度融合中西方文化。更多海外的资本进入，同时简化对外资进入的限制也将使中国电影在海外发行销售更为容易，并能够在国外的主流院线公映进而提升中国电影的国际竞争力和影响力，有利于中国电影拓展海外市场。

3. 有利于形成完整电影产业价值链

长期以来，以好莱坞为代表的美国电影产业已经形成了以电影票房为核心，通过整合其他媒体资源、文化旅游资源，并通过研发IP衍生产品来满足消费者的各类需求，形成了完整的电影产业价值链。比如

NBC 环球影业公司，它不仅拥有环球影片、照明娱乐、梦工场等顶级电影片厂，还有多个电视频道包括 NBC、CNBC 等，美国和海外的主题公园，新媒体网站包括售票平台 Fandango 和电影电视评分权威网站 ROTTEN TOMATOS（烂番茄），以及授权产品包括消费品和手游电游业务，等等，这些业务已经覆盖全球。而环球的母公司康卡斯特（纳斯达克：CMCSA）是全球领先的媒体和技术公司，主要业务包括康卡斯特有线电视、NBC 环球以及欧洲的天空集团。康卡斯特有线电视以 Xfinity 为品牌提供服务，是美国最大的家用及商用视频、高速互联网和电话供应商之一，并同时提供商用服务。康卡斯特还通过 xfinity 提供家用无线网络、安全服务及自动化服务。NBC 环球经营新闻、娱乐和体育有线电视网络、NBC 和 Telemundo 广播电视网络、电视制作公司、电视台、环球影业，以及环球主题公园及度假区集团。天空集团是欧洲媒体及娱乐业领军企业之一，通过付费电视服务为观众提供丰富的视频内容，包括家用高速互联网、电话及无线等多项服务。天空集团旗下有天空新闻、体育和娱乐网络，制作原创内容并享有独家内容权益。

放宽引入外资的限制将进一步推动中国电影产业结构调整，完善中国电影产业价值链。

4. 有利于电影产业法制化发展与完善

好莱坞由于建立了强大的内在的商业法则和产业化影响力，并渗透在制片、发行、放映等各个环节和方面，不断驱动了整体产业的建立和良性发展。

逐步放开外资对电影市场的经营资格准入、产品准入、资本准入和技术标准准入制度，降低准入门槛，鼓励一切有条件的民营和外资文化企业进入电影制片、发行、放映领域，为企业营造公开、公平、公正的市场经营环境，将促进贯穿电影产业的各个链条协调发展，有利于中国电影行业建立依法行政、科学调控的政策法规体系和政府监管体系，形成完整的包含行业投资主体、多元化经营、多样化生产、多渠道发行、多层次开发的一整套格局清晰的电影产业化计划，从而提升中国电影在国际影坛的地位，弘扬中华文化影响力，促进电影产业的繁荣发展。

四　结语

2020 年，全球面临着百年不遇的疫情和经济危机。影视行业也同其他行业一样，面临一场世纪大考。但危中总有机，面对挑战，我们更需要珍惜所有的机会。疫情之后，整个行业如何积极反思，与国际接轨，创新求变，重塑行业活力，迎来更健康持续的发展，成为重中之重。

当今正值数字革命的重要契机，前几次技术革命都成就了世界格局的重构和新兴产业的兴起，数字技术将引发更全面、更深刻的重大变革，产业格局和国际关系都有可能重新洗牌。这次疫情，又进一步加速促进线下向线上的转移，将带来文化影视产业转型升级的新考量。

中国影视行业进一步开放发展，将有力地增进中国与世界的沟通交流。中国本土文化市场的开放，会促进中国与世界的良性互动，增强中国软实力以及经济实力，提升中国国家品牌形象。

自 2014 年环球影业正式落户中国以来，环球影业在中国市场的业务稳步发展，包括协助国内合作单位在院线、传统电视和网络视频点播平台上发行其电影和电视内容、电影电视合拍项目等业务，以及电游手游和消费产品的开发和授权等。目前，环球影业正在与中国合作方在北京倾力打造全球最大的环球影城主题公园，2021 年将在北京盛大开业；作为奥运会的主要转播机构，环球影业在 2008 年成功转播北京奥运会后，并将与冬奥组委会再度合作，向世界转播 2022 年冬奥会。

中国是环球影业的重要市场和合作伙伴。我们期待着在应对疫情冲击及未来发展的同时，与中国媒体娱乐行业加强合作，共同迎接全球大变局带来的挑战和机遇。

Film and Television Industry in the Disruptive Changes of 2020

By Jo YAN, Excutive Vice President and Managing Director &
Shauna HUANG, Vice President of Universal China

During early 2020, the COVID-19 virus outbreak impacted China and other countries all over the world, causing disruption to all normal operations worldwide. China has thus far effectively managed the pandemic and is gradually resuming work and production after more than two months of anti-epidemic efforts during this once-in-a-century global crisis. The selfless dedication of Chinese medical staff, various sectors of society and the concerted efforts of all Chinese people have garnered global admiration. The initial success of the fight against the pandemic has made China a model for many other countries.

This pandemic has not only created a global public health crisis, but also taken a heavy toll on the global economy. It has brought unavoidable and unprecedented severe challenges to various industries around the world, including the film and television culture industry. Due to the nature of cinema operations, the theatrical business in particular has been severely hit by the pandemic, causing heavy losses to the film industry. All segments of the film industry have been affected by this pandemic. Cinemas, studios and publicity companies are all under pressure to survive.

1 The pandemic and its impact on the global film industry

(1) China's film market has suffered huge losses due to the pandemic

The pandemic has had a global impact, and the film industry is suffering unprecedented losses. In the China market, films have been withdrawn and all cinemas have been closed since the eve of the Spring Festival in 2020. It was reported in National Business Daily in early March that the mainland box office during the Spring Festival of 2019 was RMB 5.91 billion. It was predicted by several insiders that the box office during the Spring Festival of 2020 would have exceeded RMB 7 billion had the pandemic not taken place.

Not only has the audience had no access to movies, but the major production teams also faced shutdown. In order to fight against the pandemic and ensure the safety of personnel, all major film and television bases and the production teams that had already started shooting issued suspension announcements. There is no doubt that the suspension and postponement of the film and television brings a huge financial challenge to film producers.

Although the pandemic is now more under control, the public are still very cautious about occupying crowded locations for fear that the situation may worsen again. It will definitely take some time for general confidence to recover enough to see a return to enclosed spaces with a high density of people, such as cinemas. The trust between filmgoers and cinemas will be tested during this recovery period and will take some time to be re-established.

(2) The global film industry entered a shutdown period during to the pandemic

According to the Hollywood Reporter, the pandemic has caused a loss of at least USD 7 billion to the global film industry due to the decline in box office revenue and its impact on production progress. If COVID-19 continues until May, the loss will increase by USD 10 billion, and further loss will be harder to predict should COVID-19 continue beyond May.

According to data from the Korean Film Association, the box office revenue in Seoul, South Korea, has fallen to its lowest level in 16 years. Japan, which represents the world's third largest box office market, has also experienced significant impact on its theatrical business despite not implementing an entire industry shutdown. The European market has also been hit hard by the pandemic. Most cinemas in 32 countries, including France, Spain, Italy, the Netherlands and Ireland, have been closed. Similarly, the North American film market has also been greatly affected. 007: No Time to Die, A Quiet Place, Fast & Furious 9, Mulan, Black Widow and other films have been postponed or withdrawn. The Batman, Fantastic Beasts 3, The Matrix 4, Cinderella, The Little Mermaid and Shang-Chi and other Hollywood blockbuster movies have also been suspended in production.

2   Transition from cinema to online viewing

With the outbreak of the pandemic, most corporations and related business units have suspended operations, so traditional industries as well as the wider economy have suffered heavy losses. Conversely, this has given rise to pandemic-driven business changes and changes in people's work and lifestyle behavior, unexpectedly accelerating the rapid rise and growth of various online services such as telemedicine, telecommuting, video conferencing, online education, online audio-visual and online games, which have become new bright spots and future opportunities for industry development. At the same time, the development of digital technology also provides technical possibilities for the realization of online services, bringing closer the era of transfer from offline to online. To some extent, the pandemic has unexpectedly accelerated and given rise to a new round of disruptions in the global film industry.

After Lost in Russia and Winner Takes All were broadcast free of charge on Douyin in China, Hollywood also launched a paid video-on-demand service for newly released films. Following the announcement made by NBCUniversal on providing an on-demand service on Comcast and SKY of the three films, "The Hunt", "The Invisible Man" and "Emma", "Trolls World Tour " was also made available for streaming online by its affiliated company in advance of a theatrical release. As of now, major Hollywood companies have begun shortening the traditional theatrical release window. At the same time, major studios are also planning to work with Apple's iTunes, Amazon and other technology giants to implement on-demand services.

The attempt by Hollywood majors to implement a "day-and-date" release or "first release on the internet" is undoubtedly an experiment and a breakthrough for the global movie industry. The change in the traditional film industry process during these exceptional times has provoked much debate and reflection in the industry.

In fact, competition between cinemas and the internet for movies began long before the pandemic. The flexibility, technical advantages and user-recommendation capabilities of online on-demand presents irrefutable differences between the online on-demand and traditional cinema-going experience, highlighting the competition for the movie-watching business. According to the Film Development Research Report, the proportion of cinema movies released on video platforms in recent years has stabilized at around 80%, and the window between cinema release and video platform release has been shortened to 47 days in 2019, half of what it was in 2016. Internet has become the "second battlefield" for cinema movie distribution. According to the 2019 Theme Report released by the American Film Association, the global box office in 2019 was USD 42.2 billion, a YOY increase of 1%. The global home entertainment market (including streaming media, TV and DVD) reached USD 58.8 billion, an increase of 14% since 2018. The global market for digital film and television content reached USD 48.7 billion (excluding pay TV), a 25% increase since 2018, whereas the North American market increased by 18% and the overseas market increased by 29%. Specifically, the streaming media market reached USD 44.8 billion, surpassing the theatrical market.

According to the news released during the 2019 Shanghai Network Audio-Visual Industry Week, as of June 2019, the number of online video users in China had reached 759 million, an increase of 33.91 million since the end of 2018, accounting for 88.8% of the total number of netizens. Online dramas, online movies, online documentaries and other programs showed a growth spurt, with a dramatic increase in available programming.

In the age of the internet, all industries will go through game-changers, actively or passively. We believe that the unprecedented changes brought about by the pandemic to consumers' lifestyles are also an important reason why companies decide to provide audiences with the dual choice of cinema and home theater. This decision was not only made out of practical necessity but also as a chance to test the water; it does not mean that other films will be distributed in the same way in 2020. Companies will need to evaluate the impact of this trial run and assess reactions from all parties affected. Only through full consultation and communication with all partners, including cinema chains, will the next stage be considered to determine the best distribution strategy for each market.

In fact, the move towards online distribution for these films does not mean this will in future replace watching films in traditional cinemas. Firstly, it is difficult at least in the short term, for online viewing to achieve the full cinematic experience, especially for large-scale production films with special effects. Secondly, for top movies, maintaining initial theatrical distribution windows is in the interests of film producers and all players throughout the industry supply chain. At present, theatrical channels are still preferred for major productions, while online distribution can provide incremental distribution channels and monetization methods for a broader range of content and medium- and long-tail movies.

It is obvious, however, that the film industry, regarded as a non-essential lifestyle purchase, has been severely impacted by the global outbreak of the pandemic and this in turn has accelerated the development of online content consumption. Additionally, the post-90s generation has over time become the mainstream audience, and they are more willing to pay for personalized services online. However, the impact of the pandemic on cinema chains should be temporary. Once the pandemic is completely under control, the backlog of high-quality products will find more theatrical distribution opportunities, and the public will return to normal life with a need of entertainment activities, bringing a significant market recovery to cinema chains. At the same time, the competition between cinemas and online viewing will also force traditional cinema chains to rethink and innovate to further improve the quality of their facilities and services in order to provide a better environment and viewing experience for the audience, thus luring audiences from the small screen back to the big screen.

Therefore, no matter how the industry evolves in the future, online movie viewing will not completely replace offline, nor cause a devastating blow to the theatrical movie market. It can be expected that it will take a long period of time before cinema and video-on-demand are balanced to best meet the needs and interests of all parties. Despite the trend of global digitization, cinema will not completely overcome online streaming, and online streaming will not completely replace cinemas. Both will coexist, adapt, and change to be organically integrated with each other over a period of time. Presently, network platforms and the traditional movie industry are tentatively figuring out the best way to co-exist, and the two may ultimately actually help each other. For example, the two can work in tandem to effectively reduce the cost of content procurement through extensive and in-depth copyright cooperation; the marketing and promotion of "online" movies can be supported by traditional distribution and cinematic screenings, while online platforms can provide new pre-screening and publicity channels for traditional theatrical releases. In terms of funding, streaming media platforms can also provide new financing channels for copyrighted demand of high-quality movie content. Through mutual cooperation, streaming media platforms and traditional movie businesses will form a joint force in the new movie industry chain, with excellent content creation at the core. Excellent content creation relies on talents and technology, for which internet platforms and traditional movie distribution methods have their respective advantages.

3　Expectations for the future of the film industry

There is no denying that the pandemic has triggered the exploration of some alternative business models. Although no one can accurately predict the future of the movie industry while undergoing the process of change, it's apparent that the internet will pose certain challenges to the traditional business of cinema chains and there will be, for the foreseeable future, intense market competition between the two. In fact, the American film industry faced similar problems earlier; their competitors are streaming media or home video-on-demand services, while the rivals of China's cinema chains are online video platforms.

The trend towards the globalization of streaming media is taking shape, and it is less about regionalized internet content and more about high-quality content being distributed globally. As a country with a large number of internet users, China will be well-versed in high-quality streaming media platforms and their content, and continually align communication and interface between them to gradually establish new operating and business models. This will not only meet people's demand for high-quality content, but also provide direction for industry development, preparing China's internet film and television industry well for the iterative upgrades in technology and concepts.

In view of this, while distribution channels adapt to the internet era, the Chinese movie industry can consider embracing the internet with a more open and inclusive attitude, carrying out more extensive and in-depth international cooperation, to import advanced production technology and operational management experience, thereby maximizing the benefits of foreign investment in the film industry.

(1)　Supporting resource optimization in the film industry

According to data from Maoyan Pro, for the first half of 2019, both box office revenue split and cinema admissions declined year-on-year for the first time since 2011, suggesting that the movie industry's scale-driven development model is coming to an end. China's film industry is at an historical turning point as it transforms from a scale-driven to a quality-driven model.

At the same time, with the increasing number of China's online video users, China's online users' demand for high-quality content is also becoming increasingly prominent. The streaming platforms are also bidding farewell to the era of high growth and entering the era of high-quality development. However, the "Internet-based" development of China's film market is divided into two systems, one is the highly internet-based ticketing market of movie theatres, and the other is the video platform based on user traffic. It is difficult to merge the two in a short period of time.

Hollywood has decades of experience in content production, and well-established distribution channels for streaming media. It has successfully built a "closed traffic loop" or "closed channel loop" on the basis of maintaining its own copyright system. Giving access to foreign investment from countries with mature sector experience would allow China's film industry to break the current content development difficulties and accelerate the optimal allocation of industry resources.

(2) Supporting international market integration and development

Despite the rapid growth of local box office for Chinese films and the continuous expansion of the Chinese film market, Chinese films have not gained success internationally, and due to limited overseas distribution resources, Chinese films have taken a relatively low international market share. Conversely, American movies are not only distributed in the US, but globally. Many American movies achieve much higher overseas box office revenue than domestic.

We should try to expand and deepen the development of the "Sino-foreign co-production", so that more Chinese production companies can learn from foreign investors and producers, and leverage their global distribution resources, to more properly integrate Chinese and Western cultures. Increased overseas investment and the relaxation of foreign capital entry restrictions will also facilitate the international distribution and sale of Chinese films. This will enable Chinese films to be released in foreign mainstream cinemas, and ultimately enhance the international competitiveness and influence of Chinese films, leading to the expansion of overseas markets for Chinese films.

(3) Supporting the formation of a complete film industry value chain

For a long time, the U.S. Film industry, represented by Hollywood, has formed a complete value chain through the film industry, commencing with box office as the central pillar, and expanding through integration with other media channels, cultural tourism channels and the development of extended franchise products to meet the various needs of consumers. Take NBC Universal as an example, in addition to several top film studios, such as Universal Pictures, Illumination, DreamWorks Animation, etc., Universal also has multiple television channels, including NBC, and CNBC, theme parks located in the U.S. and overseas, new media website (including the ticketing platform *Fandango*) and the ranking authority for movie and TV, *ROTTEN TOMATOES*, as well as post-movie products such as consumer products, mobile games and computer games, the business for which has already expanded globally. Meanwhile, Comcast Corporation (Nasdaq: CMCSA), the parent company of NBC Universal, is a global media and technology company with three primary businesses: Comcast Cable, NBC Universal, and Sky. Comcast Cable is one of the United States' largest video, high-speed internet, and phone providers to residential customers under the Xfinity brand, and also provides these services to businesses. It also provides wireless and security and automation services to residential customers under the Xfinity brand. NBC Universal is global and operates news, entertainment and sports cable networks, the NBC and Telemundo broadcast networks, television production operations, television station groups, Universal Pictures, and Universal Parks and Resorts. Sky is one of Europe's leading media and entertainment companies, connecting customers to a broad range of video content through its pay television services. It also provides communications services, including residential high-speed internet, phone, and wireless services. Sky operates the Sky News broadcast network and sports and entertainment networks, produces original content, and has exclusive content rights.

Relaxing the restrictions on the introduction of foreign capital will further promote the restructuring of China's film industry and improve the value chain of China's film industry.

(4) Supporting the legal development and improvement of the film industry

Hollywood has established strict commercial laws and industry influence which permeate all aspects of production, distribution and screening, continuously driving the establishment and stable development of the overall film industry.

We should gradually open up the Chinese film market for foreign investment, relax access measures based on business qualifications, products, capital and technical standards, and lower the entry threshold to encourage all qualified private and foreign-funded cultural enterprises to enter the fields of film production, distribution and screening, thereby creating an open, fair and just market environment for enterprises and smoothing the way for industry-wide development. Such measures will support Chinese movie industry to have a government regulated system that includes legal oversight and clear policies, proper data-based measures and controls, and a clearly structured plan comprising industry investment, diversified management, and the diversification of production, distribution and development of films. This will enable Chinese films to establish a competitive presence in the international marketplace, support the growth of Chinese cultural influence at an international level and enable the Chinese film industry to thrive and prosper.

4 Conclusion

In 2020, the world is facing the worst pandemic and economic crisis in a century. The film and television industry, like other industries, is facing a great challenge. However, there are always opportunities arising from crises, and in the face of the challenges we need to make good use of all the opportunities we get. After the pandemic, it will become a top priority for China to reflect on the whole industry, integrate globally, and revolutionize, innovate and restore the vitality of the industry to achieve more healthy and sustainable development.

An important opportunity for digital revolution is taking place right now. Previous technological revolutions have all resulted in the reconstruction of the world order and given rise to emerging industries. Digital technology will lead to more comprehensive and profound changes, disrupting current industry patterns and cross border relations. The pandemic has accelerated the shift from offline to online, launching new considerations for the transformation and upgrading of the cultural film and television industry.

The further opening-up and development of China's film and television industry will greatly enhance communication between China and the world. The opening of China's local cultural market will promote positive interaction between China and the world, enhance China's soft as well as economic power, and improve China's national image.

Since officially starting its operations in China in 2014, Universal Pictures has steadily grown its collection of businesses which includes assisting local partners in the theatrical distribution and marketing of its movies and TV content in cinemas, on television and internet video-on-demand platforms, co-production of movies and TV content, as well as the development and licensing of PC and Mobile games and Consumer Products based on its rich portfolio of IP. Currently, Universal is building the world's largest Universal Theme Park in Beijing with its

Chinese partners, set to open in 2021. As the major broadcasting partner of the Olympic Games, after successfully broadcasting the Beijing Olympic Games in 2008, NBCUniversal will cooperate again with the Winter Olympic Committee to broadcast the Winter Olympic Games in 2022 to the world.

China has always been an important market and valuable partner for Universal. We look forward to strengthening our cooperation with the Chinese entertainment industry as we take on the impact brought by COVID-19 and rebuild our business for the future. Together we shall embrace the challenges and opportunities resulting from this global phenomenon.

第二部分
抗击疫情在行动
Part II
Actions for Fighting COVID-19

齐心必胜！赛诺菲通过中国红十字基金会捐赠 100 万元人民币

赛诺菲中国

【2020-01-24】

微信号： SanofiChina

公司介绍： 赛诺菲是一家全球领先的医药健康企业，以患者需求为本，研究、开发并推广创新的治疗方案。主要业务涵盖三个领域：制药、人用疫苗和动物保健。于 1982 年成立，总部位于法国巴黎。

新型冠状病毒肺炎疫情近日牵动了全国人民的心，全社会积极动员抗击疫情。作为一家在华 38 年的跨国药企，赛诺菲责无旁贷、即刻行动，在除夕夜宣布向中国红十字基金会捐赠 100 万元，用于购买相关防护物资以支援湖北和武汉一线医护人员抗击疫情，包括护目镜、防护服、口罩、手套和消杀设备等。

赛诺菲集团坚定支持中国政府和人民抗击疫情，并将竭尽所能贡献力量。我们将持续关注此次疫情的发展，并随时准备继续做出贡献。在政府的指导下，我们有信心与社会各界齐心协力，最终战胜此次疫情！

Sanofi Announced the Donation of RMB 1 Million to Chinese Red Cross Foundation

The outbreak of new coronavirus drew great attention across China. The whole society has been mobilized to fight against the coronavirus. As a responsible corporate citizen, Sanofi took prompt actions and announced the donation of 1 million RMB to Chinese Red Cross Foundation on the Lunar New Year's Eve. The donation will be used to purchase goggles, protective suits, masks, gloves and disinfection equipment etc. to support Wuhan and Hubei based hospitals to fight against the epidemic.

We are strongly committed to supporting the Chinese government and population in combating the epidemic and will contribute our effort whenever possible. We are also confident that with joint efforts from the government and the whole society, we will win the war against the coronavirus!

共抗疫情，嘉吉捐赠 350 万元现金及防护物资

嘉吉集团

【2020-01-26】

微信号： CargillChina1

公司介绍： 嘉吉是一家从事生产和经营食品，农业、金融和工业产品及服务的多元化跨国企业集团，业务包括农产品供应链、动物营养、动物蛋白、食品配料及应用、运输及金属、金融服务等。由 William Wallace Cargill 先生于 1865 年创立，总部设在美国明尼苏达州。

近日，嘉吉向中国红十字基金会捐赠 200 万元现金用于支持武汉蔡甸火神山医院建设。此外，嘉吉还将同步捐赠价值 100 万元的防护物资，支持疫情防控。同时，嘉吉还向韩红爱心慈善基金捐赠 50 万元，驰援武汉。

这个春节，在武汉，一场没有硝烟的战争正在进行。奋战在一线的医护工作人员、"闭关"在家里的武汉人民，牵动着亿万中国人的心。

随着疫情的发展，政府部门上下联动，医护人员紧急驰援，社会群众也积极响应加强防护。作为全球粮食和食品配料的供给者，嘉吉情牵疫区群众，希望在这场没有硝烟的战争中发挥企业力量，通过此次捐款捐物，以实际行动与各方共渡难关。

此刻，保护好自己和家人是首要任务。我们也呼吁，所有的员工、客户、合作伙伴，始终将安全置于首位，做好健康检查和疫情防护工作。

关爱无界，大爱无疆！攻坚时刻，嘉吉与你心手相连。相信，通过社会各界的支援和聚力合作，疫情一定会被早日击退，还大家一个平安、健康的 2020！

Cargill Donates RMB 3.5 Million to Help Fight the New Coronavirus Pneumonia

On Jan 26 of 2020, Cargill announced a donation of 2 million Yuan to the Chinese Red Cross Foundation, to support construction of the second makeshift hospital (named Huoshenshan Hospital) in Wuhan. In the meantime, medical supplies worth of 1 million Yuan will be donated by Cargill to help prevent the new coronavirus-related pneumonia. In addition, another 500000 Yuan will be donated to Han Hong Foundation in support of Wuhan.

As a responsible global supplier of ag products and food ingredients, Cargill wants to make possible contributions to help people affected by this unexpected incident. At this special moment, we truly hope that everyone works for and with Cargill stays in a healthy status by following protection guidance issued by central and local governments. We believe that, with joint efforts of all walks of life, the China society will be recovered from the epidemic, and everyone will enjoy a brighter and healthier year of 2020.

雅诗兰黛集团累计捐赠现金及物资 1500 万元人民币驰援新冠肺炎疫情

雅诗兰黛集团

【2020-01-26】

微信号： EL_China

公司介绍： 雅诗兰黛集团是全球最大的护肤、化妆品和香水公司之一。公司由雅诗·兰黛夫人在 1946 年创立，公司的名字也是用自己的名字命名。公司总部位于美国纽约市。

雅诗兰黛集团于 2020 年 3 月 8 日宣布再次启动驰援新冠肺炎疫情防控工作，捐赠价值 1000 万元的护肤用品，希望通过此次捐赠帮助一线医护人员更好地呵护肌肤。这些护肤用品来自雅诗兰黛集团旗下所有护肤品牌，涵盖精华水、眼霜、乳液和面膜。此前，雅诗兰黛集团累计捐赠人民币 500 万元用于抗击新冠肺炎疫情。截至目前，雅诗兰黛集团已累计捐赠现金及物资 1500 万元。

雅诗兰黛集团中国区总裁樊嘉煜女士表示，"我们心系坚守在一线的医护人员，他们始终为全面战胜疫情而持续艰苦努力，这其中更有很大一部分女性医护人员。我们希望可以通过自身的绵薄之力，在节日来临之际为她们送上祝福"。除此之外，雅诗兰黛集团正在进一步积极协调，推进后续的各项援助举措。

进入中国市场 27 年，集团始终伴随中国市场共同成长。樊嘉煜女士强调，"我们希望能和这片土地产生更紧密的命运联系，更好地为中国消费者和社会服务。我们同时坚信，在政府的领导下，疫情终将过去。着眼于未来，我们对中国市场充满信心。我们刚刚也宣布了在中国投建世界级研发中心的计划，为进一步协助深化中国美妆行业在全球科研领域的领导地位"。

Estée Lauder Companies has Donated Cash and Supplies in the Cumulative Amount of RMB15 Million to Support the Fight against the Novel Coronavirus-infected Pneumonia

On 8 March 2020, Estée Lauder Companies announced another support for the female frontline medical workers in Hubei who fight the novel coronavirus pneumonia with donation of RMB 10 million-worth of skincare products. Estée Lauder Companies' donation is intended to help frontline medical workers take care of their skins. The skincare products donated include all brands under the group including toners, eye creams, lotions and facial masks. Prior to the in kind donation, the Estee Lauder Companies has accumulatively donated RMB 5 million to support the fight against the novel coronavirus-infected pneumonia. By now, Estée Lauder Companies has donated cash and supplies in the cumulative amount of RMB15 million.

"We show great concern for the frontline medical workers, many of whom are females, who spare no efforts to fight the outbreak. We would like to do our mite and send them blessings on this special day," said Ms. Joy FAN, China President for Estée Lauder Companies. Besides, the group is further coordinating proactively for more supports to follow.

Since making its debut in China 27 years ago, the Estée Lauder Companies has always enjoys co-development with the Chinese market. "We want a still closer tie with the fate of this nation, and better serve the Chinese consumers and society. We also firmly believe that the epidemic will diminish eventually through leadership of the Chinese government. Looking into the future, we have full confidence in the Chinese market. We have just announced our investment plan to set up a world-class research and development center in China to further help China's cosmetics industry gain leading status in the global R&D field," Ms. FAN emphasizes.

太古集团宣布捐赠人民币 1000 万元用于支援抗击新型冠状病毒感染的肺炎疫情

太古集团

【 2020-01-27 】

微信号： SwireinChina150

公司简介： 太古集团是一家涉及地产、航空、零售、饮料及食物链、海洋服务和贸易等业务的高度多元化的环球集团，成立于 1816 年，总部位于英国伦敦。

2020 年 1 月 27 日——太古集团今天宣布，面对新型冠状病毒感染肺炎疫情严峻态势，决定向中国红十字会总会紧急捐款人民币 1000 万元，专项用于抗击新型冠状病毒感染的肺炎疫情。通过中国红十字会总会，该笔捐款将根据疫情防控和一线医务人员需求，购买紧缺医疗物资和设备，全力支持抗击新型冠状病毒感染肺炎疫情防控工作。

同时，太古可口可乐旗下湖北太古可口可乐饮料有限公司向武汉经济技术开发区（汉南区）政府捐赠人民币 150 万元，用于购买医疗设备及用品，并通过武汉市慈善总会向一线救援（医护）人员捐赠"纯悦"瓶装水和"怡泉 +C"瓶装饮料共 50 万瓶。此前，湖北太古可口可乐饮料有限公司于 1 月 25 日，与可口可乐中国、壹基金和云豹救援队的专业人士合作，捐赠 20400 瓶"冰露"纯净水，用于武汉当地医院医护人员饮用。1 月 26 日，通过武汉市慈善总会捐赠 24000 瓶"纯悦"瓶装水，为奋战在火神山医院建设工地的工作人员提供安全饮用水。

心系中国，太古将持续密切关注疫情发展，根据疫情防控工作需要，采取后续相关行动，积极支持抗击疫情工作。太古深信，在政府的领导下，全国人民定能众志成城，攻克难关，取得这场阻击战的最终胜利。

Swire Group Announcement of Donation of RMB 10 Million for Providing Aid in Combating the Novel Coronavirus Pneumonia Epidemic

Beijing, Jan. 27,2020—Swire Group has announced today about the decision to donate 10 million RMB to The Red Cross Society of China. The donation will be dedicated to fight against the outbreak of pneumonia caused by the novel coronavirus. Through the Red Cross Society of China, the donated amount will be used to purchase medical supplies and equipment in need for medical workers and provide full supports to the control and prevention from the novel coronavirus pneumonia epidemic.

Meanwhile, Swire Coca-Cola Beverages Hubei Limited, under the Swire Coca-Cola has made a donation of 1.5 million RMB to the government of Wuhan Economic and Technological Development Zone (Hannan District) for purchasing medical equipment and supplies and has donated 500,000 bottles of "CHUNYUE" bottled water and "Schweppes+C" bottled beverages through the Wuhan Charity Federation to the rescue team of medical staff on the front line. Earlier on Jan. 25th the Swire Coca-Cola Beverages Hubei Limited cooperated with Coca Cola China, One Foundation and YB Rescue Team and donated 20,400 bottles of "Ice Dew" purified water for the medical staff in hospitals in Wuhan. On Jan. 26th, through the Wuhan Charity Federation, they donated 24,000 bottles of "CHUNYUE" bottled water to working personnel fighting day and night on the construction site of Huoshenshan Hospital.

Swire's heart goes with China and will keep closely watching the development of the epidemic. Swire is ready to take subsequent actions to support the work of control and prevention of the epidemic. Swire has a firm belief that under the leadership of the government, the whole nation will unite as one and overcome difficulties to win this battle.

抗击疫情，路易达孚在行动

路易达孚集团

【2020-01-27】

公司介绍： 路易达孚集团由法国人列奥波德·路易达孚创建于 1851 年，是全球领先的农产品贸易和加工企业之一，每年在全球范围内种植、加工和运输约 8000 万吨农产品，为全球约 5 亿人提供食品和衣物。总部位于荷兰鹿特丹。

新冠肺炎疫情暴发以来，路易达孚集团一直密切关注新型冠状病毒肺炎疫情及其给大众带来的影响，积极采取相应措施，全力保障员工的健康和安全。我们于 2020 年 1 月 27 日通过中国红十字基金会向湖北捐赠 100 万元，此笔款项已被用于黄冈市疫情防控临时医院的建设项目，来帮助紧急收治罹患 COVID-19 的患者。此后，我们又通过天津市滨海新区红十字会向当地定点医院捐赠了价值 40 万元的"金掌门"食用油等物资，向奋战在抗疫一线的医务工作者送去慰问。

尽管面临劳动力短缺和物流受限的挑战，路易达孚在中国的油籽油料加工厂均已于 2020 年 2 月上旬恢复生产。路易达孚也积极参加到由国家市场监督管理总局指导、中国食品工业协会主办的"三保"行动倡议中，保价格、保质量、保供应，将食用油和饲料原料等民生相关重要物资运送到最需要的地方去。疫情期间，路易达孚克服重重困难，不计成本向湖北省紧急调运豆粕近 3 万吨，供应当地养殖企业的生产需要；针对深受疫情冲击的餐饮行业，路易达孚与美团、美菜等电商合作伙伴联手，对 16 万箱食用油产品提供补贴，支持餐饮企业渡过难关。

作为一家在中国扎根逾 40 年的企业，我们将全力以赴支持中国渡过难关，共迎春天!

LDC in Action: Fighting COVID-19

Louis Dreyfus Company (LDC) is very concerned about the COVID-19 outbreak and the many people it has affected. We have taken steps to help ensure the health and safety of our employees, our partners and our customers. We have donated RMB 1 million in cash to the Red Cross Society of China to support frontline efforts to combat the virus. The donation has been used for the renovation project of a Huanggang anti-epidemic hospital for the emergency treatment of patients with COVID-19. Later, we also donated 400000 RMB worth of 'Mastergold' cooking oils to the local designated hospital through the Red Cross Society of Binhai District, Tianjin, to support the medical workers fighting the epidemic.

Despite of labor shortage and logistic challenges, all our oilseeds crushing plants in China resumed work in early Feb 2020. LDC also took part in the local initiatives to ensure food and feed supply for people's livelihood. In addition, since the outbreak of the epidemic, we have overcome difficulties and coordinated resources to transport close to 30,000 tons of soybean meal to Hubei Province, supplying the production needs of local feed industry, to ensure people's needs for high-quality proteins. We also worked jointly with E-commerce partners, including Meituan and Meicai, to provide subsidies for 160,000 boxes of packaged oil products, supporting catering enterprises to tide over the difficulties.

As a company rooted in China for over 40 years, LDC stand together with China in fighting COVID-19 and overcome the difficulties!

高通捐款 700 万元人民币，支持抗击新冠肺炎疫情

Qualcomm 中国

【2020-01-29】

微信号： Qualcomm_China

公司介绍： 高通（Qualcomm）是一家无线电通信技术和芯片研发公司，于 1985 年 7 月，由美国加州大学圣地亚哥分校教授厄文·马克·雅各布和安德鲁·维特比创建，总部位于美国加利福尼亚圣迭戈市。

Qualcomm 将向中国相关组织捐款 700 万元，支持新型冠状病毒感染肺炎疫情的防控工作。我们向所有受到疫情影响的人们表示衷心的慰问，向所有奋战在疫情防控一线的工作人员致以崇高的敬意！

Qualcomm Donates RMB 7 Million in Support of Efforts to Combat the Coronavirus

Qualcomm donates RMB 7 million to relief agencies in China in support of efforts to combat the impact of the Coronavirus. Our Thoughts go out to all those affected.

IBM 捐款 200 万元支持中国抗击新型冠状病毒肺炎疫情

IBM 中国

【2020-01-30】

微信号： IBM

公司介绍： IBM（国际商用机器公司）是一家集信息技术、咨询服务和业务解决方案于一体的外资公司，由托马斯·沃森于 1911 年创立，总部位于美国纽约州阿蒙克市。

IBM 宣布将通过中国相关组织捐款 200 万元，支持新冠肺炎疫情的防控工作。

IBM 十分关注疫情的发展，在做好公司内部的疫情防控、确保员工自身防护与健康的前提下，将积极响应客户和社区的需求，做出应有的贡献——与全国人民一起，共克时艰！

向所有奋战在一线的医务人员致敬！

武汉加油，中国加油！

IBM Donated RMB 2 Million to Support China's Fight against Novel Coronavirus

IBM announced that it would donate 2 million RMB through relevant organizations in China to support the prevention and control work of novel coronavirus.

IBM pays close attention to the development of the epidemic. Under the premise of preventing and controlling the epidemic within the company and ensuring the health of employees, we will actively respond to the needs of customers and the community, make due contributions to overcome the difficulties together!

To all who are in the front line

Salute to all the medical workers!

Go Wuhan, Go China!

霍尼韦尔捐赠价值 100 万美元物资助力武汉抗击新型冠状病毒肺炎疫情

霍尼韦尔中国

【2020-01-31】

微信号: honeywell_china

公司介绍: 霍尼韦尔是一家多元化高科技制造企业,于 1885 年在美国新泽西成立。企业业务涵盖航空产品和服务、家庭和工业控制技术、汽车产品等领域。

霍尼韦尔今日宣布捐赠价值 100 万美元的物资,全力支持武汉医院抗击新型冠状病毒。捐赠物资包括空净和水净产品、ICU 空气管理系统,针对医院管理的扫描、打印设备,以及赠予武汉学校的霍尼韦尔儿童萌宠口罩。

自暴发新冠肺炎疫情以来,霍尼韦尔始终高度关注疫情发展,并采取紧急行动。春节前以及春节期间,霍尼韦尔及时组织相关合作伙伴调配库存和物流,以最大限度保证防护物资的供应。霍尼韦尔是全球领先的个人安全防护用品制造商,为消防、电气安全、通用工业以及建筑行业的工人提供从头到脚的保护。

通过积极协调各方资源,霍尼韦尔全力以赴为市场总计供应了超过2000 万只口罩,并以公司全部产能积极配合政府保障疫情严重地区一线工作人员防护用品的供应。

与此同时,霍尼韦尔和授权经销商密切合作维持价格稳定,并提供公开渠道鼓励消费者在非常时期举报经销商私自上涨价格的行为;公司也和电商平台积极配合进行限购，坚决抵制倒买倒卖等不良行为，最大限度地保护消费者的权益。

霍尼韦尔中国总裁张宇峰说："我们全体员工心系疫情发展地区，并立刻展开行动，全力保障防护物资供应给最需要的人员。为了支持武汉医院更好地抗击新型冠状病毒，公司已经决定捐赠霍尼韦尔的相关技术和产品协助进一步武装好武汉地区的医院。接下来，霍尼韦尔将继续持续配合中国政府抗击新型冠状病毒肺炎。"

张宇峰说："霍尼韦尔一直以来秉承'东方服务于东方'的发展战略支持中国市场。霍尼韦尔向抗击新型冠状病毒第一线的医务人员勇士、第一响应者、媒体以及其他乐于奉献的专业人士和志愿者等致以最崇高的敬意。"

Honeywell Donates US $1 Million in Equipment to Support Fight against Coronavirus in Wuhan

Honeywell today announced that it will donate US $1 million worth of equipment to support hospitals in Wuhan in their fight against the coronavirus outbreak. The donation includes technologies such as air and water purification systems, ICU air management solutions; and scanning and mobile printing equipment. Honeywell will also provide children's masks to Wuhan schools as part of the donation.

Since the coronavirus outbreak, Honeywell has paid close attention to the situation and taken immediate actions. Honeywell has been working with partners to manage our protective products' inventory allocation to ensure supply before and during the Spring Festival. Honeywell is the world's leading personal protection equipment (PPE) producer with head-to-toe solutions for workers in the fire service, electrical safety, and general industrial and construction environments.

Honeywell has also actively coordinated resources and supplied 20 million masks to the market, and we have committed all our available manufacturing capacity to the government to help ensure supply to the front-line operators in the most affected areas.

In addition, Honeywell has worked diligently with dealers to maintain price stability, offering an open channel for end users to report dealer price increases in the wake of the sharp increases in demand. Honeywell has actively cooperated with e-commerce platforms to limit purchases and firmly resist hoarding to protect consumers' rights and interests to the greatest possible extent.

Honeywell China President Scott Zhang said, "All our employees extend their hearts to the people in the affected areas, and we are making every effort to ensure the supply of protective equipment to those who need it most. To show our fullest support, we have decided to donate relevant products and technologies to better equip hospitals in Wuhan, which are at the forefront of the fight against novel coronavirus. Going forward, Honeywell will continue to support the Chinese government in addressing this outbreak."

Zhang added: "Honeywell has long maintained its 'East for East' commitment to support China and its markets. Honeywell would like to pay its highest respect to those who have been fighting against coronavirus at the front lines, including the courageous health professionals, first responders, media, and many other dedicated professionals and volunteers."

凯雷及员工捐助 300 万元善款物资驰援湖北疫区一线

凯雷

【2020-01-31】

公司介绍： 凯雷投资集团是一家全球性资产管理公司，于 1987 年在美国华盛顿特区创立，已发展成为世界上最大且最成功的投资公司之一。

新冠肺炎疫情在全球不断蔓延，对世界各地都造成巨大冲击。在这一艰巨时刻，凯雷投资集团依靠其遍布全球的网络和渠道，积极动员全球的资源，为中国疫区一线采购抗疫急需的医疗产品。凯雷集团及其员工一共捐助价值 300 万元的医疗物资及现金，支持中国抗击此次疫情，其中定向捐赠 5 万只 N95 口罩和 1 万件防护面罩给受影响最严重的疫区。此外还通过湖北省慈善总会捐赠 200 万元，支援湖北省抗击疫情。

同时，凯雷极力帮助中国的被投企业在全球范围内购买医疗防护用品，以保护员工和客户的安全。

凯雷投资中国 20 多年，有扎根中国的团队和庞大的被投企业大家庭。凯雷旗下众多被投企业也各自积极发挥资源优势，为支援疫情防控贡献力量，截至 2020 年 1 月 31 日，旗下被投企业共捐赠了 1800 万元，调集运输超过 100 万件医疗用品。

凯雷将持续深挖全球网络资源，与员工、投资者和被投企业一道共同应对疫情蔓延的挑战。

Carlyle and Its Employees Donate RMB 3 Million in Cash and Medical Supplies to Support Frontline Medical and Support Staff in China's Most Affected Areas

The continuing spread of the coronavirus has become a great cause of global concern. In this extraordinary time, Carlyle has mobilized its global network and resources to source medical supplies for front-line medical and support staff in China, with the firm and its employees donating RMB 3 million in cash and medical supplies to fight against the COVID-19 crisis. As part of this, Carlyle has donated 50000 N95 protective masks and 10000 faceshields to the most affected communities in China. The firm has also donated RMB 2 million to the Hubei Charity Federation to help Hubei Province contain the outbreak.

Furthermore, Carlyle has been helping its Chinese portfolio companies to source protection gear to protect the safety of their own employees and customers.

With a presence in China spanning more than 20 years, Carlyle has a strong local team and an extensive portfolio of companies. These companies have also drawn on their own resources and strengths to help those affected by the coronavirus. As of January 31, 2020, they had donated RMB 18 million and delivered more than 1 million medical supplies to those in need.

Through mobilizing its global resources and network, Carlyle continually looks for ways to support its employees, investors and portfolio companies as we work through this challenging period.

安博与武汉同在，与湖北同在，与中国同在

安博

【2020-02-02】

微信号：Prologis

公司介绍：安博公司创立于 1983 年，是一家现代物流基础设施行业全球领袖企业，所持物业覆盖美洲、欧洲和亚洲，总面积多达 5570 万平方米，构建了覆盖全球主要物流枢纽、工业园区和城市配送中心等战略节点的高效物流网络。总部位于美国加利福尼亚州旧金山市。

岁末年初，一场突如其来的新冠肺炎疫情肆虐神州大地，严重威胁人民群众生命健康安全。安博全球董事会主席兼首席执行官何慕德先生（Mr. Hamid R. Moghadam）第一时间在全球员工视频会议上说："非常时期我们需要采取非常措施，携手同行，共抗疫情。当今社会，各方高度交融，牵一发而动全身。消灭疫情不是哪一个部门、哪一个群体的事，需要全社会、全要素密切配合、共同参与。公司将调动一切有力资源全力保障，各方面恪尽职守、各尽其责，形成支持战胜疫情的强大合力。"

自疫情发生以来，安博中国克服种种困难，积极有效地联系防疫物资供货渠道，为湖北和武汉等疫情严重地区采购最急需的抗疫物资，及时关注全国疫情重灾区，为举国抗疫之战贡献力量。截至目前，安博采购的所有物资均已捐赠交付给武汉相关部门。

安博的捐赠物品包括 50 万只普通医疗口罩、2 万只 N95 医疗口罩、3 万只 N95 普通口罩、750 套医疗防护衣。此次抗疫捐赠行动体现了安博

团结合作的实干与高效，全员全力支持全国范围内的新冠肺炎疫情防控工作。"青山矗立，不堕凌云之志。"疫情面前，你我不分彼此。安博仍将坚持践行"引领未来"的企业理念，坚定地与全中国人民站在一起，齐心协力共同面对这场疫情防控的阻击战。疫情挡不住春天的脚步，更割舍不断安博全员对疫区人民的牵挂。我们相信，万众一心，我们必将赢得这场战疫，安博与中国同在，与湖北同在，与武汉同在，抗疫之战必胜！

PROLOGIS with Wuhan, with Hubei & with China

At the beginning of the year, the outbreak of coronavirus raged on the land of China, seriously threatening the health, safety and lives of the people. Mr. Hamid R. Moghadam, chairman and CEO of Prologis, said at the first time in a global employee video conference, "In extraordinary times, we need to take extraordinary measures and work together to fight the epidemic. In today's society, all parties are highly intertwined, which means even a tiny change can affect the whole. Eliminating the epidemic is not a matter of a certain department or group. It requires close cooperation and joint participation of the whole society and all elements. The company will mobilize all powerful resources and urge all parties to fulfill its due diligence and responsibilities to form a strong joint force to support the fight against the epidemic."

Since the outbreak of the epidemic, Prologis China has overcome all kinds of difficulties, actively and effectively contacted the supply channels of epidemic prevention materials, purchased the most urgently needed anti-epidemic materials for severe epidemic areas such as Hubei, paid attention to the severely affected areas in the country in time, and contributed to the national anti-epidemic fight. So far, all materials purchased by Prologis have been donated to relevant departments in Wuhan.

Prologis donated 500000 ordinary medical masks, 20000 N95 medical masks, 30000 N95 ordinary masks, and 750 sets of medical protective clothing, which shows the solid work and efficiency of Prologis's cooperation and full support to the nationwide prevention and control of the coronavirus. In the face of

| 责任与担当——抗击新冠肺炎疫情中的跨国公司（中英双语版）

the epidemic, we are same. Prologis will still adhere to the corporate philosophy of "Ahead of What's Next", stand firmly with the entire Chinese people, and work together to fight against the epidemic. The epidemic can't stop the pace of spring, and it can't stop all members of Prologis care about the people in the affected area either. We believe that when we fight together, we will win this war against epidemic. Prologis is with China, with Hubei, and with Wuhan. The battle against epidemic will prevail!

大众汽车集团（中国）携旗下大众、奥迪、保时捷、宾利和斯柯达等品牌，与合资企业一道，共同捐资 1.2 亿元人民币抗击疫情

大众中国

【2020-02-03】

微信号： gh_0a0889848a37

公司简介： 大众汽车集团是一家总部位于德国沃尔夫斯堡的汽车制造公司，于 1973 年成立。集团旗下有大众、奥迪、保时捷、宾利、斯柯达等品牌。

大众汽车集团（中国）携手合资企业，共同捐资 1.2 亿元，用于支持新型冠状病毒肺炎疫情的相关防治工作。捐款将主要用于湖北及其他疫情严重的省市地区购置防护用品、医疗器械、医药等物资，并支持相关疫情防控及抗击工作。该款项由大众汽车集团（中国）与旗下大众汽车品牌和奥迪、斯柯达、保时捷和宾利等众多品牌，及合资企业一汽－大众、上汽大众共同捐赠。

"我们高度关注疫情的发展态势，并向英勇奋战在疫情抗击前线各个岗位上的工作人员致以崇高的敬意。大众汽车集团（中国）与全国人民并肩作战，全力以赴抗击疫情"，大众汽车集团（中国）CEO 冯思翰博士表示，"对于大众汽车集团而言，中国是我们的第二故乡，面对疫情的突袭，我们与中国民众万众一心，共克时艰"。

捐赠款项还将在国家相关部门统一部署下，用于全力驰援中国境内其

他有迫切需求的地区，为其提供医疗物资及医护救治等疫情防护方面的支持。

大众汽车集团（中国）CEO 冯思翰博士就疫情在个人领英平台上发出的呼吁："请世界睁开眼睛，以开放的心态听中国、看中国。我们要对抗的是病毒，而不是受害者！在中国的十余年里，我结识了许多善良、友好的中国人。疫情当前，去指责一个国家更是有失公正的。无论时值顺境抑或当下这般艰难时刻，我们都是人民的、大众的汽车企业，是中国社会以及中国汽车发展 40 年历程中的一分子，为此我们深感自豪。此时此刻，我们与中国客户和我们的同事以及全体中国人民站在一起！"

Volkswagen Group China and Its Joint Ventures to Collectively Donate RMB 120 Million to Combat Coronavirus Outbreak

Volkswagen Group China and two of its joint ventures are putting on a united effort to collectively donate RMB 120 million in support of novel coronavirus (COVID-19) relief work. The donation will go towards securing medical supplies and providing urgently needed aid, such as protective equipment, medical equipment, medicine, and other materials, to hospitals across Hubei Province and other Chinese provinces facing a serious situation. The donation will be made by Volkswagen Group China and its brands, such as Volkswagen, Audi, ŠKODA, Porsche and Bentley, together with its Chinese joint ventures, FAW-Volkswagen and SAIC VOLKSWAGEN.

"The current situation concerns us, and we would like to express our deepest gratitude to the hardworking and determined people on the front line of disaster relief. They have our full commitment and support," said Dr. Stephan Wöllenstein, CEO of Volkswagen Group China. "For us at Volkswagen Group, China is our second home. In times like these, we must stay together as one and take all necessary measures to assist the Chinese people wherever needed."

The overall donation will be used to combat the virus throughout mainland China, wherever relevant government authorities deem the need is greatest.

During this challenging period, Dr. Stephan Wöllenstein also made appeal on his social platforms:"Please open your eyes, ears and minds for China. Fight the virus, not the victims! During my 10 years in China, I got to know its kind people. It is simply wrong to blame an entire nation. Whether in good times or difficult ones like now, we are the People's car company, part of this society and its people's lives for 40 years. And we are proud of it. Therefore we stand firm alongside our Chinese customers, colleagues and all citizens!"

亚马逊筹措全球逾百万件医疗物资驰援疫情严重省份，中国加油！

亚马逊全球

【2020-02-03】

微信号： cn_amazon

公司介绍： 亚马逊（Amazon）创立于 1995 年，是一家全球领先的互联网高科技公司，服务于全球超过 3 亿消费者，业务范围涵盖网上零售、云计算、人工智能技术及硬件设备、物流运输、医疗保健等领域。总部位于美国华盛顿州西雅图市。

    面对中国多个省市和地区发生的新型冠状病毒肺炎疫情，亚马逊将向包括武汉在内的疫情严重省份和城市捐赠逾百万件医疗防护防疫用品。

    亚马逊通过全球物流和运营网络，积极筹措了逾百万件包括医用防护口罩、医疗防护服、医疗手套等在内的医疗防护防疫用品，将捐赠给奋战在包括武汉在内的疫情严重省份和城市的一线医疗人员，以支持抗击新冠肺炎疫情的救援工作。

    此外，亚马逊也将积极配合地方政府，并寻找其他可以提供帮助的途径，为疫情中心地区的医疗人员提供人道主义援助。同时，我们向所有奋战在疫情一线的工作者致敬！也将持续关注疫情发展，与社会各界共同努力，为共克疫情贡献一份自己的力量！

    亚马逊捐赠的医疗防疫物资陆续抵达中国：为支持新型冠状病毒肺炎抗疫工作，亚马逊利用全球物流和运营网络，积极筹措医疗防护防疫用品。目前，从美国、欧洲等国家和地区起运的首批抗疫物资已抵达中国，后续物资也将于近期运抵。

亚马逊此次捐赠的抗疫物资包括隔离服、医用防护口罩、医用外科口罩、防护面罩，以及一次性医用帽、医用手套和鞋套等，总数逾 100 万件，相关物资将通过各地方政府送往疫区城市。

亚马逊将积极配合各地政府为疫情中心地区的医疗人员提供人道主义援助，并与社会各界携手共克疫情，共渡难关!

Amazon Donates Millions of Items to Healthcare Professionals of Affected Cities in China

Amazon leverage our worldwide logistics and operations network to donate millions of items comprising of medical-grade protective masks, isolation suits, disposable gloves, and other medical supplies to healthcare professionals of affected cities in China to help with the Novel Coronavirus outbreak relief efforts. Amazon support the Novel Coronavirus outbreak humanitarian efforts by working with China local government and donating millions of medical relief items to support the on-the-ground healthcare professionals.

耐克捐资 1000 万元支持抗击疫情

耐克集团

【2020-02-04】

微信公众号： 耐克媒体中心

公司介绍： 耐克（NIKE）是全球著名的体育运动品牌，英文原意指希腊胜利女神，中文译为耐克。公司成立于 1972 年，总部位于美国俄勒冈州波特兰市。

2020 年初，耐克集团向中国青少年发展基金会捐款 1000 万元。耐克的捐款帮助中国青少年发展基金会为前线医护人员提供安抚患者、控制新冠病毒蔓延所需的物资和设备。该笔资金重点关注最需要支持的领域，以及持续的救援工作和未来长期的恢复工作。

2 月 9 日，由苏州市各医院组建的援助湖北医疗队 260 人赴鄂支援。当天凌晨，耐克公司迅速调配医疗队员尺码的耐克运动鞋，赶在医疗队出征前进行了捐赠。

此外，当了解到一线的医务人员缺少羽绒服和运动衫时，耐克立刻行动起来，通过中国青少年发展基金会向武汉第一医院的医务人员捐赠千余件耐克羽绒服和耐克运动衫，并紧急调配其位于太仓的耐克中国物流中心的物流能力，于 2 月 21 日将捐赠物送抵医院。

Nike Donates RMB 10 Million to Help Wuhan against COVID-19

NIKE, Inc. made a 10 million RMB donation to the China Youth Development Foundation . Nike's donation to the China Youth Development Foundation helped provide frontline health and medical workers with the supplies and equipment they needed to comfort patients and address the spread of the coronavirus. Focused on areas of highest need, the funding also supports ongoing relief and longer-term recovery efforts.

On 9 February, 260 volunteer medical staff from different hospitals in Suzhou were leaving to provide medical help in Wuhan. Hearing this, Nike swiftly put together a batch of Nike shoes with the right sizes and donated them to the volunteer medical team before they set off.

When feedback from the frontline revealed that the medical staff was running short of down coats and dry tops because of intense working conditions, Nike again decided to step up. Nike collaborated with CYDF to donate and distribute more than one thousand coats and tops to Wu Han No.1 Hospital. To overcome the difficulty in delivery at the time, Nike expedited the logistics by working with its TaiCang CLC (Nike China Logistics Center) team and delivered the products to the hospital on 21 February.

BP 中国捐赠逾 300 万元人民币的物资和现金，为抗击疫情贡献一臂之力

BP 中国

【2020-02-04】

微信号： BP_BPCHINA

公司介绍： 英国石油（BP）是一家全球性的能源企业，由威廉·诺克斯·达西于 1909 年创立，总部位于英国，主要业务有油气勘探开发、炼油、天然气销售和发电、油品零售和运输以及石油化工产品生产和销售。此外，公司在可再生能源方面的业务也在快速发展。

自新冠病毒感染的肺炎疫情发生以来，BP 中国秉承安全的理念，实现无同事感染，保障业务持续运营。与此同时，BP 中国捐赠逾 300 万元的物资和现金，为抗击疫情贡献一臂之力。

- BP 中国已向中华慈善总会专项捐款 100 万元。
- BP 中国通过全球采购与物流渠道，已向武汉第九医院、潜江二医院、北京协和医院等机构捐赠价值总计 170 万元的医疗防护物资。
- BP 中国通过员工捐款以及 BP 基金会配捐，向中华慈善总会专项基金追加捐款 42 万元。
- BP 集团向世界卫生组织 COVID-19 团结应对基金专项捐款 200 万美元。

BP 中国董事长兼总裁杨筱萍表示："古语有云：'志合者，不以山海为远。'面对疫情的严峻挑战，我们 BP 与全国人民携手前行，共克难关，打赢这次疫情防控阻击战！"

一方有难，八方支援

自新型冠状病毒感染的肺炎疫情暴发以来，来自全国乃至世界各地的救援物资纷纷运抵湖北，驰援一线。作为最早参与中国经济建设以及中国能源领域最大的外商投资企业之一，BP 是唯一参与中国航空油料供应的外资能源公司，并通过两家合资企业——华南蓝天航空油料有限公司与深圳承远航空油料有限公司，为华中及华南地区共计 29 个机场提供航空燃料和相关服务，为疫情发生地区的航空物资运输注入动力与支持。

华南蓝天：勇为冲锋军，在湖北最前线为救援物资的航空运输保驾护航

华南蓝天航空油料有限公司成立于 1997 年。作为疫情暴发的中心区域，华南蓝天的团队们承担起保障湖北省内包括武汉机场的 5 座机场，以及邻近省市数个机场的航油供应重任。截至 3 月中旬，蓝天的湖北团队已为 800 多架次飞机（包括疫情防控、撤侨、专机等）保障加油，共约 5000 吨。

信息网格，确保健康

为了确保每一位员工的身体健康，华南蓝天将公司辖区内的所有员工划分成 135 个网格，并在每个网格内设立"网格管理员"，负责管理该网格内员工的疫情防控工作。与此同时，各网格管理员定期向上一层级的"网格长"汇报。不仅如此，公司还第一时间基于微信开发了员工健康信息小程序，与 OA 系统对接，实现员工健康信息数据的信息化收集与统一管理。

聚焦武汉，全力以赴

自 1 月 23 日武汉封城之后，由于客运航班暂停，华南蓝天的安全生产从保障民航航班，转为以疫情救援保障为主。虽然整体的业务量有所下降，但保障供应和防控疫情的责任更为艰巨。随着医疗救援、物资运输、医护包机、撤侨航班等飞机的增加，团队面临的最大挑战就是飞机起降的未知性。无计划的航班往往说来就来。为了更好地应对挑战，华南蓝天的湖北团队制定了全新的"武汉机场航空加油站值守及应急值班方案"，确定了由 6~8 人组成一个值守小组，小组之间以 10 天为一个轮班进行 24 小时不间断轮值作业，主要负责飞机供油、调度协调、加油设施设备的检查维修等工作。与以往不同的是，在非常时期为飞机加油，需要经过漫长的等待：等待人员陆续下机，等待机载物资全部搬运，等待机组完成不留死角的消毒。华南蓝天的团队们往往在湿冷的寒夜中，有时甚至是在雨雪天里一站就是两三个小时。尽管如此，能够保障成百上千名医护人员的乘机，以及无数救援物资的顺利运抵，是每一位华南蓝天人所坚守的昂扬斗志。

克服困难，保障供应

与湖北相邻的河南，亦有华南蓝天所服务的现场，其中信阳机场的航油恰是由湖北荆门运至的。由于省际交通受阻，运油车在驶入河南时被禁止通行。为保证机场供油稳定，华南蓝天的团队一边与当地民航局，一边与途经的镇政府和村民进行双向沟通，最终取得理解并解决了运输通行的问题。

奋勇向前，真情无畏

华南蓝天的员工当中，有同事的妻子正是呼吸科的护士。在为妻子剪去长发送往收治新冠病毒肺炎感染者的医院之后，自己主动回到机场值班。夫妻二人在这个非同寻常的春节虽然没有团聚，但共同战胜疫情的决心将彼此紧紧相连。

深圳承远：争做生力军，在后方为驰援前线与人员复工航班提供有力配合

深圳承远航空油料有限公司成立于 1991 年，是 BP 在中国的第一家航空燃油合资企业，为深圳机场提供航油供应和服务。深圳机场作为中国南方重要的交通运输枢纽之一，深圳承远公司将驰援武汉物资航班供油保障任务作为抗击疫情的重要举措，持续关注航班信息，始终与深圳机场运行指挥中心密切联系，确保供油万无一失，全力保障特殊航班需求。与此同时，自全国各地陆续复工以来，如何避免人员在返工途中的感染，是各地政府和企业所面临的一大难题。作为外来务工人员最密集的地区之一，深圳的许多企业纷纷采取包机将员工接回的方法。截至 3 月初，深圳承远共保障驰援武汉物资航班 50 余架次，加油 400 多吨；保障复工包机近 30 架次，加油 100 多吨。

通用航空：敢当后备军，发挥灵活性为难以触及地区抗疫提供高效支援

值得一提的是，在此次湖北抗击疫情的救援任务当中，一支特殊的通用航空编队发挥着重要的支持作用。通用航空是指使用民用航空器从事公共航空运输以外的民用航空活动，包括农林渔牧领域的作业，以及医疗卫生、抢险救灾等飞行活动。区别于一般的公共运输飞机，通用航空的飞机往往更加轻巧灵便，更容易飞抵无法降落大型航空器的区域。而湖北省地势大致为东、西、北三面环山，中间低平。在全省总面积中，山地与丘陵共占 80%。

自新冠肺炎疫情防控战疫打响以来，湖北通用航空在紧急运送医疗物资等方面做出了积极贡献，目前已累计飞行 312 小时，累计运输物资近 50 吨。华南蓝天湖北分公司则承担了省内通航航班近百架次、供油超 50 吨的救灾重任。2019 年 6 月，BP 航空与中国航空油料集团有限公司签署合资经营合同，双方将携手拓展在中国西南地区的通用航空油料业务。在不久的将来，BP 将更加全面地为更多中国百姓的民生提供运输能源保障。

疫情无情人有情，注入动力保飞行！BP 向奋战在一线的全体工作者致以最崇高的敬意与最深切的祝福。我们竭尽全力，与全国人民一起携手前行，共克时艰！

BP Donated RMB 3 Million worth of Medical Protective Materials and Funds to the Epic Center to Fight against the COVID-19 Pandemic

Since the outbreak of COVID-19 in mid-January, with safety remaining our core value and people's wellbeing our central concern, we have been working very hard to protect our employees and their families and to keep business continuity throughout the challenging period. BP has donated around 3 million RMB worth of medical protective materials and funds to areas hit by the disease and Chinese charities respectively, playing a small part in helping the local communities in ways we can, to get through the hardship, including:

- BP China has donated RMB 1 million to China Charity Federation;
- BP China has donated RMB 1.7-million-worth of protective equipment to Wuhan NO.9 Hospital, Qianjiang NO. 2 Hospital, Peking Union Medical College Hospital, etc.;
- BP China employees, matched by the BP Foundation, donated an additional RMB 420 thousand to China Charity Federation;
- BP is donating USD 2 million to WHO COVID-19 Solidarity Response Fund.

Xiaoping Yang, Chairman and President of BP China said that, "As ancient Chinese saying goes that, 'Nothing, not even mountains and oceans, can separate people with shared aspirations.' We are joining hands with Chinese communities to face the challenges of and win the fight against the COVID-19."

One in difficulties, all will help

As China is united as one team in this hard time, all Business Units and staff of BP China have worked closely to contribute their share to the fight against the novel coronavirus pneumonia.

Since the outbreak of COVID-19, relief supplies from all over the country and around the world keep flowing to Hubei, the frontline of the battle against the epidemic. As one of the first foreign-funded enterprises to contribute to China's economic development and one of the largest foreign-funded enterprises in China's energy sector, BP is the only company engaging in China's aviation fuel supply. Through two joint ventures, South China Blue Sky Aviation Oil Co., Ltd. and Shenzhen Chengyuan Aviation Oil Co., Ltd., BP provides aviation fuel and related services for 29 airports in Central and South China, supporting air transportation in the epidemic-hit areas.

South China Blue Sky: a "storm troop" to support the transportation of relief materials to hubei

South China Blue Sky Aviation Oil Co., Ltd. was founded in 1997. The teams of South China Blue Sky undertake the task of ensuring aviation oil supply of five airports in Hubei Province, including the provincial capital Wuhan, and several airports in the neighboring provinces and cities. By mid-March, South China Blue Sky had fueled more than 800 flights dedicated to epidemic relief, retreat of expats and chartered flights, totaling around 5000 tons of fuel in Hubei province.

Information grids established ensuring staff health

In order to ensure the health of every employee, South China Blue Sky divides all the employees into 135 grids, appointing one head for each grid to manage the epidemic prevention and control work. All the "grid heads" report to the upper level "grid chief" on a regular basis. Moreover, the company has developed the employee health information mini program based on Wechat at the possibly earliest time. By linking with the OA system, the applet realized the IT-based collection and unified management of the employee health information.

Making full efforts in supporting wuhan

Since Wuhan was put on lockdown on January 23 and passenger flights from and to Wuhan have been suspended ever since, South China Blue Sky has shifted its priority from supporting civil aviation flights to epidemic relief. Although its overall business volume has declined, its responsibility for ensuring fuel supply and controlling the epidemic is even more arduous. With the increase in the flights for medical rescue, material transportation, and evacuation and in the charter flights for medical staff, the biggest challenge facing the work team is the uncertainty about the aircraft take-off and landing schedule. Unscheduled flights often come as they do. In order to better cope with the challenges, the team of South China Blue Sky in Hubei has set-up "The Wuhan Airport Emergency Duty Plan" and assigned 6-8 people to form a shift. The teams will work in shifts around the clock in a period of 10 days, mainly responsible for aircraft oil supply, scheduling coordination, and inspection and maintenance of fuel facilities and equipment. But in the current special period, it takes an extraordinarily long time to refuel the aircraft since the staff need to wait for the passengers to get off the aircraft, for all the onboard materials to be downloaded, and for the crew to complete thorough disinfection of the aircraft. South China Blue Sky Team often stand for two to three hours at a stretch in the cold humid night, sometimes even in rainy and snowy days. Nevertheless, every South China Blue Sky employee is dedicated to ensuring the successful flight of thousands of medical staff and the smooth delivery of the huge quantities of relief materials.

Overcome difficulties to ensure supply

Henan province, adjacent to Hubei, has airports served by South China Blue Sky. Among them, Xinyang Airport's aviation fuel are transported from Jingmen, Hubei Province. Because of inter-provincial traffic control, the tanker was forbidden to enter Henan. In order to ensure the stable oil supply of the airport, the team of South China Blue Sky not only have to communicate with the local civil aviation bureau, but also keep a close contact with the township governments and villagers along the way. After thorough communications, the authorities were convinced, and transportation barrier was removed.

Supporting family members and marching ahead bravely

The wife of one of South China Blue Sky employees is a nurse with the Respiratory Department. After helping his wife cut her long hair and seeing her to the hospital which houses patients suffering the COVID-19, he returned to the site and volunteered to work. Although the couple were physically separated during unusual Spring Festival, their hearts were linked by the same determination to combat the epidemic.

Shenzhen Chengyuan: vigorously supporting epidemic relief and work resumption chartered flights

Established in 1991, Shenzhen Chengyuan Aviation Oil Co., Ltd. is BP's first aviation oil joint venture in China, supplying fuel and services for Shenzhen Airport, one of the major transportation hubs in South China. During the outbreak, Shenzhen Chengyuan ensured oil supply for the chartered flights carrying relief materials to Wuhan, making it their top working priorities. The team kept monitoring flight information closely, and always kept contact with the Shenzhen Airport operation control center, so as to ensure unfailing oil supply and meet the flights' special demand. At the same time, with many workers return to work after the Spring Festival, how to avoid the person-to-person transmission of the virus on their way to work is a big challenge faced by the government and enterprises. As one of the areas most densely populated by migrant workers, Shenzhen sees many chartered flights to pick up employees returning to work. of March, Shenzhen Chengyuan has fueled more than 50 flights carrying relief materials to Wuhan, with 400 tons of oil, and fueled nearly 30 charter flights for work-bound people, with more than 100 tons of oil.

In face of the ruthless epidemic, BP has injected power in support of disaster-relief flights! BP gives the highest respect and the best wishes to those fighting on the frontline. We will join hands to the people and make every effort to tide over this hard time!

与时间竞速，施耐德电气紧急援建火神山、雷神山医院

施耐德电气

【2020-02-04】

微信号： schneider-electriccn

公司介绍： 施耐德电气是一家全球能效管理专家，为 100 多个国家的能源及基础设施、工业、数据中心及网络、楼宇和住宅市场提供整体解决方案。成立于 1836 年，一直是法国的工业先锋之一，总部位于法国巴黎。

2020 年 2 月 3 日，武汉火神山医院开始接诊，施耐德电气（中国）有限公司紧急援建的电气设备已经用于火神山、雷神山医院。

近日来，新型冠状病毒引发的肺炎疫情牵动整个中国，施耐德电气全力以赴支援疫情防控工作。1 月 23 日，武汉市决定建立火神山医院。1 月 24 日，接到通知的施耐德电气员工自愿放弃休假，开始与施工单位及设计师沟通技术问题，并与合作伙伴一起紧急筹措电力保障所需的各种电气设备，包括配电各级开关元件、UPS 不间断电源和精密空调等。

现在，在雷神山与火神山医院，施耐德电气的环网柜、UPS 不间断电源等都开始运作，保障了用电的安全。截至 2 月 2 日，所有批次产品的调货、运输、组装、接线、调试、发货等工作都已完成，并全部到达施工现场。这些紧急支援的配电产品被安装在火神山和雷神山医院的病房、手术室和休息区。

与此同时，施耐德电气承担了为北京小汤山医院 B 区改造项目紧急调配元器件的任务，两小时内就完成了所需要的可编程控制器（PLC）及开

关电源的调配和发货，一天之内施耐德万高完成 iSCB 电涌保护器后备保护装置的生产交付，为小汤山医院快速修缮改造提供助力。

除了为医院提供用电保障外，施耐德电气已向武汉红十字会定向捐款人民币 100 万元。捐款将拨付给武汉金银潭医院、武汉儿童医院等医疗机构，用于购买抗击疫情所需的医疗用品、应急设备等紧缺物资以及开展相关的救助工作。同时公司还在法国和欧洲各地帮助提供医用紧缺物资。

让我们齐心协力，抗击并战胜疫情！

2020 年 2 月 1 日，北京小汤山：在距离武汉 1000 公里外的北京，为了防范疫情，北京市启动了小汤山医院修缮项目，以备不时之需。2 月 1 日下午 4 点，施家员工接到任务，需要为医院改造项目紧急调配 PLC 和开关电源。经过与合作伙伴的通力合作，调货和发货任务在两个小时内就圆满完成。

同样是在当天，北京小汤山医院应急感染救助项目急需施家提供 iSCB 电涌保护器后备保护装置，施耐德万高经过两个小时紧急协调，安排生产。次日一早，产品制作完毕，紧急发往项目工地。

Schneider Electric Provides Emergency Support for Huoshenshan Hospital and Leishenshan Hospital in Wuhan

When the Huoshenshan Hospital in Wuhan began to receive patients on February 3, 2020, the electric equipment by Schneider Electric China as an emergent supply played a very important role in ensuring its operation, the most urgent issue at the time. So did our supply of electric equipment to Leishenshan Hospital.

As the novel coronavirus outbreak made a massive impact throughout China, Schneider Electric spared no effort to help combat the epidemic. When Wuhan decided to build the Huoshenshan Hospital on January 23, on the following day, Schneider Electric staff immediately jumped out of their vacation and began to work on the technical details with the construction organizations and designers. They also worked with partners to make available various items of electric equipment needed for power supply, including a range of Electrical Distribution Switches, Uninterrupted Power Supplies (UPS), and precision air conditioners.

All the systems provided by Schneider Electric such as RMU (Ring Main Units) and UPS are now working to support the stable power supply at Huoshenshan Hospital and Leishenshan Hosptial. As of February 2, the dispatch, transport, assembly, connection, testing and delivery for all products had been completed, and the equipment had arrived at the construction sites. The power distribution products from Schneider Electric were installed in the wards, operating rooms and rest areas of the two hospitals.

Meanwhile, Schneider Electric also undertook the urgent task of providing electric parts and components for the remodeling of Beijing's Xiaotangshan Hospital-Area B. The company completed the dispatch and delivery of the required Programmable Logic Controllers (PLC) and switch mode power supplies in just two hours. Schneider Wingoal completed the production and delivery of the Surge Protection Device (SPD) iSCB in just one day. These efforts enabled renovating the hospital quickly.

In addition to ensuring the power supply for the hospitals, Schneider Electric also donated RMB 1 million to the Red Cross of Wuhan. The donation will be allocated to medical institutions including the Wuhan Jinyintan Hospital and Wuhan Children's Hospital, for purchasing key materials such as medical supplies and emergency equipment, and for associated relief efforts. The company has also mobilized its branch companies in France and other European countries to continue source needed medical supplies.

Let's work together to combat the epidemic and win this battle!

February 1, Beijing Xiaotangshan Hospital: In Beijing, over 1000km away from Wuhan, to prevent and combat against the epidemic, the city launched the renovation of the Xiaotangshan Hospital in case of need. Schneider Electric was tasked with providing Programmable Logic Controllers (PLCs) and switch power supplies for the program at 4 pm on February 1. Through close collaboration with partners, the dispatch and shipment were completed within just two hours.

The Beijing Xiaotangshan Hospital had an urgent need for a Surge Protection Device (SPD) iSCB from Schneider Electric on the same day, for a program designed to provide emergency help. Schneider Wingoal managed to arrange production in just two hours. The products were ready and immediately shipped to the construction site early the next morning.

高盛集团捐赠 100 万美元支持中国
应对新型冠状病毒

高盛

【2020-02-05】

微信号： gh_f6d6fa6e2a5b

公司介绍： 高盛集团是世界领先的投资银行、证券和投资管理公司，为企业、金融机构、政府、个人等众多客户提供一系列金融服务，成立于 1869 年，总部位于美国纽约市。

高盛集团宣布承诺捐赠总计 100 万美元的资金以支持中国应对新型冠状病毒肺炎疫情的工作。高盛一直在与非营利合作伙伴密切合作，以确保我们为最有需要的社群提供最有效的援助。这项捐款将用于医疗救治以及为受影响地区后续的恢复工作提供支持。

"这次新型肺炎疫情对大家的日常生活和工作都产生了影响，我们致力于在这个困难时期为大家提供支持。"高盛集团董事长兼首席执行官苏德巍（David Solomon）表示。

高盛一直密切关注新冠肺炎疫情的发展，也竭尽所能保障及支持我们员工和客户的健康安全和福祉，并鼓励员工关注及配合公司在抗击疫情所采取的一系列持续性预防及辅助措施。

Goldman Sachs Committing A Total of US$1 Million to Support China's Efforts to Tackle the Coronavirus Outbreak

Goldman Sachs announced it is committing a total of US$1 million to support China's efforts to tackle the coronavirus outbreak. The firm has been working closely with nonprofit partners to determine where our assistance can be most effective. The donation will be used to support relief and recovery efforts in affected areas.

"This global health situation is affecting many of our employees and their local communities both personally and professionally, and we are committed to providing support during this difficult period," said Chairman and Chief Executive Officer David Solomon.

Goldman Sachs is closely monitoring the situation and doing everything we can to support the wellbeing of our people and our clients. We have taken precautionary measures as developments about the outbreak continue to emerge.

并肩战"疫"！力拓助力中国抗击新型冠状病毒疫情

力拓集团

【2020-02-06】

微信号： RioTintoChina

公司介绍： 力拓集团（Rio Tinto Group），西班牙文"Rio Tinto"意思是红色的河流。1873 年成立于西班牙，集团总部在英国，是全球最具影响力的矿业公司之一，也被称为铁矿石三巨头之一。

力拓集团将向中国红十字基金会捐赠 100 万美元，以支持中国抗击新型冠状病毒疫情。捐赠款项将用于支持疫情重灾区的医院和病房建设，以及采购口罩、防护服、护目镜等急需的医疗物资。

力拓首席执行官夏杰思（J-S Jacques）表示："此次新型肺炎疫情状况令人担忧，许多我们的中国合作伙伴正奋战在抗击疫情的前线，我们心系所有受到疫情影响的中国家庭。作为中国的长期合作伙伴，力拓致力于为那些亟须帮助的人们提供全力支持。"

力拓也正在与中国合作伙伴保持密切沟通，确保提供其他切实可行的支援。

我们向奋战在抗击疫情前线的全体工作者致以最诚挚的敬意！

此时共克时艰

只待同赏春光

加油！

Rio Tinto Supports China's Fight against COVID-19 Outbreak

Rio Tinto has donated USD 1 million to the Chinese Red Cross Foundation to support China's fight against the COVID-19 outbreak. The fund will be used to support the construction of hospitals and wards in the areas most affected by the epidemic , and the procurement of urgently needed medical supplies such as negative pressure ambulances, masks, protective clothing, and goggles.

Rio Tinto chief executive officer J-S Jacques said, "It is deeply concerning to see events unfolding in relation to the coronavirus outbreak, and our thoughts are with the people and families impacted. Many of our Chinese partners are playing a vital role on the frontline of containing the outbreak and, as a company with a long-standing partnership with China, we are committed to helping those who need help right now."

In addition to the donation, Rio Tinto is working with Chinese partners to identify other practical ways Rio Tinto may be able to offer support.

We extend our most sincere tribute to all workers on the front lines of the fight against the epidemic. We are in this together – and we will get through this, together. Stay strong China!

"蒂"结同心 共"克"时艰

——蒂森克虏伯积极支持抗击新冠肺炎疫情

蒂森克虏伯中国

【2020-02-07】

微信号： thyssenKrupp_China

公司介绍： 蒂森克虏伯是一家德国多元化工业集团。创始于1811年，后由蒂森股份公司和克虏伯股份公司于1999年合并而成，总部位于德国埃森。公司的业务涉及钢铁、汽车技术、工厂技术、材料贸易和电梯技术等领域。

自新冠肺炎疫情暴发以来，蒂森克虏伯18000名员工心系疫区，密切关注疫情的发展。2020年2月7日，蒂森克虏伯宣布其在华运营公司向中华慈善总会捐赠200万元人民币，驰援湖北省尤其是武汉等重灾区抗击新冠肺炎疫情。

集团旗下的曼隆蒂森克虏伯电梯在得知武汉雷神山医院急需消毒物资后，第一时间做出反应，克服物资紧缺以及物流不畅等困难，采购了价值20万元的二氧化氯消毒液，紧急支援武汉雷神山医院疫情防控。

在疫情暴发的"风暴眼"武汉，蒂森克虏伯电梯维保技术团队迅速响应各医院的紧急需求，积极启动驻点值守工作，深入重症病人救治医疗机构开展维保工作，为武汉市金银潭医院、武汉中心医院等定点医院的疫情防控工作保驾护航。

在做好疫情防控、满足复工条件的情况下，蒂森克虏伯发动机系统（大连）有限公司应当地政府需求紧急调度安全库存，积极应对原材料紧缺等挑战，为江铃汽车负压救护车提供配套凸轮轴产品，助力完成该重点应急物资的保供任务。

"作为一家与中国拥有长达 150 多年良好合作历史的工业集团，我们根植中国市场，参与并见证着中国社会和经济的发展。在这个特殊时期，蒂森克虏伯义不容辞，勇于承担企业社会责任，实现对员工、对客户以及对社会的承诺，为疫情防控贡献一份绵薄之力。"蒂森克虏伯大中华区首席执行官高岩博士表示。

除了捐赠和保障工作的有序开展，蒂森克虏伯各运营公司也在第一时间积极响应各地政府号召，制定防疫应急方案，在确保员工安全健康的前提下，逐步恢复生产经营；各职能部门通力合作，保证员工沟通、防护物资采购分发等工作的有序进行；各业务团队也与客户和合作伙伴保持密切沟通，积极响应客户需求，尽可能将疫情对客户和合作伙伴业务的影响降至最低。

对于中国市场和合作伙伴的理解和尊重，是蒂森克虏伯在此深耕超过百年、实现高度本地化的重要基石。Engineering（工程实力）、Tomorrow（面向未来）、Together（同心同行），不仅是公司传承 200 多年的 DNA，更是对员工、对合作伙伴、对社会的千钧承诺。

Be of One Mind and Overcome Difficulties Together - thyssenkrupp Actively Supports the Fight against the Coronavirus

Since the outbreak of coronavirus, thyssenkrupp's operating companies in China and 18000 employees in China are much concerned about the people in the affected area. On February 7, thyssenkrupp announced that its groups companies in China donated two million RMB to China Charity Federation, in an effort to assist Hubei province, especially the worst hit areas like Wuhan to combat the novel coronavirus.

The group's subsidiary, Marohn thyssenkrupp Elevator, also donated chlorine dioxide disinfectant worth 200 thousand RMB to provide emergency support for the prevention and control of the epidemic in Wuhan Leishenshan Hospital, after overcoming a few difficulties such as shortage of materials and blocked transportation.

In the epicenter of Wuhan, thyssenkrupp Elevator maintenance team quickly responded to the urgent needs of hospitals, proactively provided on-site standby maintenance services in medical organizations that receive severely infected patients, and safeguarded epidemic prevention and control in a number of designated hospitals including Jinyintan Hospital and Wuhan Central Hospital.

Besides, in quick response to the request of local government, thyssenkrupp Presta Dalian Co., Ltd. urgently dispatched safety stock for component supply and supported Jiangling Motors to produce negative pressure ambulances, despite the challenges like shortage of raw material.

"As a company that has a good relationship with China for more than 150 years, thyssenkrupp is deeply rooted in China market and has been contributing and witnessing China's society and economic development. Under such tough situation, thyssenkrupp for no doubt will take corporate social responsibility, live up to its commitment to employees, customers and the society and make a contribution to prevent and control the epidemic." said Dr. Gao Yan, CEO thyssenkrupp Greater China.

In addition to the donation and emergency support, group companies of thyssenkrupp also actively responded to the requirement of local authorities, formulated emergency plans for epidemic prevention, and gradually resumed production and operation on the premise of employees' safety and health. Function departments worked together to ensure in-time communication and the supply of protective materials. Business teams also kept close communication with customers and partners, actively responded to their needs, and tried to minimize the impact on their businesses.

The understanding of and respect for local market and partners is an important cornerstone for thyssenkrupp to take roots and realize localization in China. Engineering. Tomorrow, Together, is not only the company's DNA that has been passed on for more than 200 years, but also a strong commitment to employees, partners and the society.

ABB 支持抗击疫情，积极复工复产

ABB 中国

【2020-02-10】

微信号： ABB_in_China

公司介绍： ABB 是全球技术领导企业，致力于推动行业数字化转型升级。基于超过 130 年的创新历史，ABB 以客户为中心，拥有全球领先的四大业务——电气、工业自动化、运动控制、机器人与离散自动化，以及 ABB Ability™ 数字化平台。ABB 由两家拥有 100 多年历史的国际性企业——瑞典的阿西亚公司和瑞士的布朗勃法瑞公司在 1988 年合并而成，总部位于瑞士苏黎世。

新冠肺炎疫情暴发后，ABB 一直坚守在与疫情抗争的各条战线，密切关注防控所需，在确保员工健康与安全的基础上，积极履行企业社会责任，与社会各界携手同心，共战疫情。

疫情之初，面对严峻的防控形势，ABB 第一时间向中国扶贫基金会捐赠 100 万元，设立了 ABB 医院后援基金，定向用于疫区医院、医务人员的疫情抗击及防治工作。同时，ABB 迅速启动特殊商品应急预案，全力调配全球物资，将第一批抵京的 10000 只医用级 N95 口罩借助全国抗疫救灾绿色运输通道直接送达武汉疫情一线，捐赠给了华中科技大学同济医学院附属协和医院。随后，ABB 又向北京、上海、厦门、重庆等地医院捐赠了多批 N95 口罩，为一线医护人员提供安全防护保障。

在疫情防控期间，ABB 利用在技术、产品、供应链和服务等领域的优势，与客户及合作伙伴共同努力，参与了多项重点疫情防控项目，如紧急调拨产品，火线支援武汉多家方舱医院改建、贵州版"小汤山"医院改扩建、上海金山医院扩容等项目；携手中国北斗卫星导航系统，提供高精准燃气泄漏检测系统，保障医院及周边地区燃气管网稳定运行；等等。同时，ABB 及时恢复了在线服务，提供远程支持，确保电力供应及基础设施安全运行，数字化解决方案与技术也在各个行业中大显身手，共同努力将疫情影响降至最低。

ABB 集团高级副总裁、ABB 中国总裁张志强表示："中国防控疫情的有力举措展示了中国的实力与中国人的担当，让我们对中国经济的未来更加充满信心。我们将继续植根中国，与各界携手努力，共克时艰。"

从 2020 年 2 月初开始，在各地政府的支持与各方的努力下，ABB 在全国各地的工厂、分公司、办事处已陆续复工复产，ABB 投资 10 亿元的上海机器人新工厂建设项目也于 3 月 11 日全面复工。目前，ABB 各企业、各部门一手抓防控，一手抓复工，积极协同上下游供应链，运营平稳有序。未来，ABB 将继续投资中国市场，携手客户伙伴，共同为中国经济持续稳定发展贡献力量。

ABB Supports Fight against COVID-19 and Actively Resumes Work and Production

ABB has been very concerned about the COVID-19 outbreak, paying close attention to the needs of the frontline, and standing firm alongside all parties to support the efforts in containing the virus while ensuring the health and safety of its employees.

Immediately after the outbreak, ABB announced a donation of 1 million yuan to the China Foundation for Poverty to support the needs of frontline medical staff in the affected areas. ABB also used its global supply chain and delivered a first batch of 10000 medical N95 face masks to the Union Hospital affiliated to Tongji Medical College of Huazhong University of Science and Technology which is located in Wuhan, and further donated more N95 masks to the hospitals in Beijing, Shanghai, Xiamen, Chongqing and other places, to support safety protection for the frontline medical staff.

Meanwhile, ABB team has contributed to many virus-prevention projects by working closely with the customers and partners and leveraging its advantages in technology, products, services and supply chain. The projects included the renovation of several module hospitals in Wuhan, the construction of Xiaotangshan-style hospital in Guizhou, the expansion of Shanghai Jinshan Hospital and more. In cooperation with China Beidou Satellite Navigation System, ABB provided the Mobile Gas Leak Detection System to safeguard the operation of urban gas networks. ABB also timely resumed its online services and provided remote support to ensure the impact for the customers is as minimal as possible.

"The decisive measures China has taken to combat the epidemic have fully demonstrated the country's strength and resolve to take on responsibilities, which have made us more confident in the future of the Chinese economy." said ZZ Zhang, Senior Vice President of ABB Group and Managing Director of ABB China, "Deeply rooted in China, ABB will continue to join hands with China to overcome the difficulties and win the battle together. "

With the strong support of local governments and authorities, ABB's factories, branches and offices around the country have re-started work and production since early February. On March 11, ABB has also resumed the construction of ABB's new robotics factory, a key investment of 1 billion yuan in Shanghai. ABB is driving forward the battle against the virus and production resumption simultaneously, actively coordinating the supply chain to ensure a smooth recovery of business and operation. Looking forward, ABB will continue expanding its investment in China and contribute to the long-term stable and sustainable development of China.

群策群力，为武汉加油！为中国加油！

埃克森美孚中国

【2020-02-10】

微信号： ExxonMobil-China

公司介绍： 埃克森美孚公司是全球知名的能源上市公司，成立于 1882 年，总部位于美国得克萨斯州爱文市。

继埃克森美孚中国工会于 2020 年 1 月 28 日向中华慈善总会捐赠人民币 20 万元之后，埃克森美孚宣布继续协调全球资源，再向受疫情影响的社区及中华慈善总会捐赠价值人民币 210 万元的医疗急需物资以及现金，专门用于对新型冠状病毒肺炎的防治工作。同时，埃克森美孚各分支机构也迅速积极调配资源，向属地社区捐赠物资。病毒无情人有情，在举国抗疫的时刻，时间就是生命。从 1 月 24 日设备进场，到 2 月 2 日完工，火神山医院十天内拔地而起。不为人知的是在建设过程中生产建设用钢材的湖北一钢厂备用润滑油曾经一度告急。埃克森美孚接到紧急求助信息后，为确保钢材生产设备的不停机运转，与经销商紧密合作，从审批到执行再到仓储物流配合，一路绿灯，以最快速度将 171 桶"急救"润滑油运抵钢铁企业。"我（当时）都绝望了，没想到美孚的支持力度这么大。"埃克森美孚合作经销商事后表示，"知道我们这批油是服务医院建设之后，（埃克森美孚）完全是不计成本、不辞辛劳，从前台到后台，全面支持"。"在武汉封城的艰苦条件下完成任务，没耽误生产，没有上下一心的协作真的完成不了。"埃克森美孚负责协调的同事说："当时没想别的，就觉得在这个时候能出一份力就好。"

1月27日，埃克森美孚接到紧急订单，要为正在紧急生产的负压监护型救护车提供初装机油以确保救护车按时交付疫区。润滑油团队立即牺牲假期，顶着压力与时间赛跑，紧急调配库存资源，开具证明，申请应急物资人员车辆特别通行证，寻找卡车、司机，备货，在客户、经销商和供应商的共同努力下，1月31日43桶发动机油及时运送到目的地，完成了几乎不可能完成的任务。埃克森美孚北亚润滑油业务总裁张松彬表示："全国上下的众志成城激励着我们，而整个团队'迎难而上有担当'的精神帮我们克服了所有的困难。"

我们的工作伙伴，身处不同国家、不同城市，一起加班加点，最终克服了所有的困难，将油品准时送达客户。在这特殊时期，上下一心，台前幕后每一个人的付出和努力都帮助我们战胜一个个障碍，与时间赛跑，和疫情战斗！自新冠肺炎疫情暴发以来，埃克森美孚一直密切关注疫情的发展，及时跟踪并响应中央及地方政府的指导和要求。同时，根据疫情在公司运营所在地的具体情况和当地政府要求，埃克森美孚第一时间启动了应急响应机制及业务连续性保障计划，在确保员工健康安全的情况下，保障公司业务的正常运营。埃克森美孚中国董事长万立帆表示："在密切跟踪局势发展并严格执行各级政府要求的同时，我们也希望尽我们所能利用埃克森美孚的全球资源为防治疫情贡献一份力量。"群策群力，共抗疫情。在这场没有硝烟的战"疫"中，医务人员在一线与疫情奋力抗争，而各行各业的建设者、生产者以及服务者也全力投入这场战"疫"。我们坚信在全国人民的共同努力下，抗疫必将取得最终的胜利！埃克森美孚将持续与社会各界携手同心，共克时艰！武汉加油！中国加油！

Pool the Wisdom and Efforts of All to Fight against COVID-19

After the ExxonMobil China Union donated RMB 200000 to the China Charity Federation on January 28, ExxonMobil announced that it continues to coordinate global resources and donate RMB 2100000 yuan worth of cash and medical supplies that are urgently needed for the prevention and treatment of COVID-19 to China Charity Federation and local communities. At the same time, affiliates of ExxonMobil China also quickly and actively deployed resources to donate materials to communities where they operate.

From January 24 to completion on February 2, Huoshenshan Hospital designated for treatment of confirmed cases stood up in Wuhan within ten days. This is widely complimented. However, what is little known is many stories behind the speedy construction. For example, the spare lubricants at a steel plant in Hubei, which produced construction steel for the Hospital, were once in shortage. After ExxonMobil received urgent orders, in order to ensure the non-stop operation of the steel production, it worked closely with distributors, from approval to implementation to storage and logistics, all the way with green lights. The 171 barrels of "first aid" lubricants arrived at steel plant at the fastest speed. "I was (at the time) desperate. I did not expect Mobil to support so much." ExxonMobil's partner dealers said afterwards, "Knowing that our batch of oil is serving the hospital construction, (ExxonMobil) provided full support from the front desk to the back office despite all the costs." "Completing tasks without delaying production under the difficult conditions of the Wuhan lockdown is impossible if without the cooperation from all lines." The ExxonMobil colleague for coordination said, "I didn't think of anything else at that time. All of my focus is on how to get things done during this difficult time."

On January 27, ExxonMobil received an urgent order to provide initial installation lubricants for negative pressure monitoring ambulances in emergency production to ensure that the ambulances could be delivered to the affected areas on time. The lubricant team immediately sacrificed vacations, raced against pressure and time, deployed inventory resources urgently, issued certifications, applied for permits for vehicles and drivers of emergency supplies, searched for trucks, drivers, and stocked goods. With the joint efforts of customers, dealers and suppliers, on January 31, 43 barrels of engine oil were delivered to the destination in time, completing a task almost impossible. Teoh Song-Ping, President of ExxonMobil North Asia Lubricant Business, said: "Excellent "can-do" spirit is demonstrated by the collective team, even though they are located in various cities of different countries and at different time zones. They put customers first and overcome huge obstacles in a very short time: transportation block, extensive shutdown, shortage of logistics services and so on. Finally, all these orders have been fulfilled timely and flawlessly."

Our working partners, who are located in different countries and cities, work overtime and work together to finally overcome all the difficulties and deliver the lubricants to customers on time. In this challenging time, efforts and contributions from every one help us overcome obstacles, race against time, and fight the epidemic! Since the COVID-19 outbreak, ExxonMobil has been closely monitoring the development of the epidemic, following up and responding to the guidance and requirements from the central and local governments in a timely manner. At the same time, according to the situations of our operations at different sites and local governments' requirements, ExxonMobil has initiated the emergency response mechanism and business continuity plan in the first place to ensure the normal operation of the business while ensuring the health and safety of all employees. Mr. Fernando Vallina, the Chairman of ExxonMobil (China)

Investment Co., Ltd. said, "We hope we can do our part to support China's efforts on stopping the spread of the novel coronavirus in the community by leveraging ExxonMobil's global resources while closely monitor the situation and follow the requests and instructions from Chinese governments at all levels." Work together to fight the epidemic. In this battle without gunpowder, medical staff were fighting tirelessly the virus on the front line, and construction workers, producers and service providers from all walks of life also devoted to this battle. We firmly believe that with the joint efforts of the people across the country, we will surely win the fight against COVID-19! ExxonMobil will continue to work with everyone in the communities during this difficult time! Go Wuhan! Go China!

标普全球捐赠 100 万元人民币支持抗击新型冠状病毒

标普全球

【2020-02-10】

微信号：标普全球、标普信评

公司介绍：标普全球（S&P Global）（NYSE: SPGI）是一家全球领先的金融信息提供商，在全球资本市场及商品市场中为客户提供评级服务、市场化基准及分析服务。它包含以下品牌：标普全球评级（S&P Global Ratings）、标普全球市场财智（S&P Global Market Intelligence）、标普道琼斯指数（S&P Dow Jones Indices）和标普全球普氏（S&P Global Platts）。

标普全球宣布向国际非营利组织 Give2Asia（赠予亚洲）捐赠 15 万美元（约合 100 万元），以支持中国抗击新冠肺炎疫情。Give2Asia 将与中国领先公共卫生组织合作，支持在抗击疫情一线的医护人员和医院。此次捐款将用于采购应对疫情所需的医疗物资，并为奋战在疫情最严重地区的医护人员提供支持。

同时，标普全球也鼓励员工为抗击疫情贡献力量。对于员工捐赠，标普全球将提供 1:1 等额捐赠。

作为全球领先的信息提供商，标普全球为全球和中国资本市场及大宗商品市场提供决策所需的信息和分析，并致力于为社会和社区做出应有贡献。自新冠肺炎疫情暴发以来，标普全球一直密切关注疫情发展，积极采取措施保障员工和客户的安全与健康，支持疫情防控。

标普信用评级（中国）有限公司首席执行官陈红珊表示，当我们了解到COVID-19暴发时，我们就意识到应该采取行动。我们很荣幸通过标普全球基金会捐赠约100万元（15万美元）给我们的合作伙伴Give2Asia，用以抗击疫情。标普全球在北京、上海和广州有超过250名员工，我们衷心地希望疫情早日结束。

S&P Global Awards A Grant of RMB 1 Million to Support Frontline Health Workers and Hospitals

In response to the Wuhan coronavirus outbreak, the S&P Global Foundation is awarding a grant of USD$150000 (1 million yuan) to partner agency Give2Asia that is partnering with leading Chinese public health organizations to support frontline health workers and hospitals responding to the crisis. Our donation will be used to procure the necessary equipment for the treatment and containment of the virus and support the health care workers who are traveling to the areas most affected by the outbreak.

Meanwhile, we have communicated closely with our global employees about our Foundation's contribution and encouraged them to consider making their personal contributions. Through our company's employee giving program, any direct monetary contribution our employees make to the same organization is being matched dollar-for-dollar by S&P Global.

As a world-leading information provider, S&P Global provides information and intelligence for decision making on the global and China capital market and commodity market and is committed to contributing to the society and communities. Since the break-out of the COVID-19, S&P Global has been monitoring the epidemic development, actively takes action to protect the security and health of the employees and clients from supporting the epidemic prevention and control.

Chen Hongshan, CEO of S&P Global (China) Ratings, said, "When we learned about the outbreak of the COVID-19 virus, we felt moved to take action. We were pleased to contribute approximately 1,000,000 RMB (US$150,000), via the S&P Global Foundation, to partner agency Give2Asia, to fight against the epidemic. S&P Global has more than 250 people across in Beijing, Shanghai, and Guangzhou; we hope the issue could be solved soon."

必和必拓支援中国战"疫"，与中国共克时艰

必和必拓公司

【2020-02-11】

微信号： bhp_billiton

公司介绍： 必和必拓是一家以经营石油和矿石为主的跨国公司，成立于1860年，总部位于澳大利亚墨尔本。

必和必拓集团于今日与中国红十字基金会签署协议，捐赠人民币1000万元，用以支持中国新冠肺炎治疗及防控工作。捐赠款项将主要用于为"战疫"前线的医护人员和其他医务工作者提供人道主义援助，同时为抗击疫情的其他必要行动提供支持。

必和必拓首席执行官韩慕睿先生表示："必和必拓一直心系中国和中国人民，我们将与其他在华跨国公司一起，携手社会各界，坚定地与中国客户、供应商、合作伙伴以及全体中国人民站在一起，共克时艰、抗击疫情，尽早恢复正常的生产和生活。"

必和必拓正在同中国客户和供应商紧密合作，力求稳定生产和市场供应，从而保证业务的正常运营。同时，我们也将持续与各利益相关方一起，为进一步支持疫情结束后的恢复工作而共同努力。

BHP Makes a Donation to Fight Coronavirus

BHP has donated RMB 10 million to the Chinese Red Cross Foundation to support its novel Coronavirus response efforts. The donation will be focussed towards humanitarian support for doctors, nurses and medical personnel treating Coronavirus patients, as well as other response actions necessary to fight the effects of the Coronavirus.

Chief Executive Officer, Mike Henry said, BHP is deeply committed to China and its people, and like many multinational companies with local operations, is supporting China in overcoming this challenge together. We stand with our Chinese customers, suppliers, colleagues and all citizens to fight and recover from this outbreak, Mr Henry said.

BHP will continue to engage with stakeholders throughout the response and recovery process to offer support and is working closely with its Chinese customers and suppliers to maintain stable production and supply to the market for business continuity.

共同抗疫，杜邦始终在前线

杜邦中国

【2020-02-17】

微信号： DUPONT_1802

公司简介： 杜邦是一家具有 200 多年历史的多元化科学公司，成立于 1802 年，提供以科技为基础的材料、原料和解决方案，业务涵盖四大板块：营养与生物科技、交通与工业、电子与成像、安全与建筑。总部位于美国特拉华州威明顿市。

杜邦拥有业界备受信任的个人防护装备解决方案，杜邦防护服是疫情防控最重要、紧缺的医疗物资之一。杜邦深知肩上责任重大，疫情伊始，杜邦就成立专项小组，指挥防护服工厂紧急复工，加班加点为前线医护人员以及相关人员提供防护服及其他防护设备，并从全球其他国家和地区调配货源，通过协调杜邦国内外资源与疫情争夺时间，支援医疗物资供应。与此同时，坚决不发国难财，杜邦第一时间发表声明郑重承诺相关防护产品的出厂价格绝不上调。

2020 年 1 月 31 日，杜邦宣布将通过中国红十字基金会捐赠总价值超过 255 万元的紧急物资，包括最急需的防护服逾 16000 件，用以保护医护工作者以及工作在第一线的人员，以及价值超过人民币 80 万元的益生菌产品，用以帮助调节人体免疫力。

在疫情防控阻击战中，杜邦密切配合国务院疫情联防联控机制医疗物资保障组的工作，支持本地统一管理、统一调拨，紧急协调越南、柬埔寨等地防护服支援中国。杜邦还特别建立新的业务模式，通过为中国提供 360 吨防护服面料给本地代工厂加工的合作方式，助力中国提升高等级防护服的产量，增援疫情防控物资。2月17日，工信部苗圩部长签署感谢信，代表国务院疫情联防联控机制医疗物资保障组感谢并赞扬杜邦的积极贡献。

疫情防控阻击战的最前线，始终都有杜邦的深度参与，杜邦积极与政府组织以及各个民间团体协力合作，尽全力以最快的速度将一批批防护物资运送至前线。中央赴湖北等疫情严重地区指导组也褒奖杜邦以"战时状态"，迅速反应，快速支援，有效保障了湖北省尤其是武汉市抗击疫情所需重要物资设备，为全面打赢疫情防控人民战争、总体战、阻击战做出重要贡献。

DuPont in the Frontline of Epidemic Control

DuPont provides trustable solutions in personal protective equipment (PPE), which became one of the most critical and most needed medical supplies during the epidemic control. Being aware of this great responsibility, DuPont established a Core Team to lead production resumption at converters to produce protective equipment for the frontline medical works, and to coordinate and import garments from other countries and regions. To race against the 2019-nCoV, DuPont tried all the efforts to support China's medical supply, maximizing all DuPont's possible resources at home and abroad. Meanwhile, DuPont committed not to raise the factory price of PPE products in corporate announcement.

On January 31, 2020, DuPont announced to donate medical supplies valuing RMB 2.55 million, including over 16,000 pieces of personal protective garments to protect frontline medical workers, and probiotic products worth more than RMB 800,000 to help regulate the immunity.

In the battle against COVID-19, DuPont collaborated firmly with Medical Supply Team of the State Council Joint Prevention & Control Mechanism, supporting its unified management and unified allocation, and importing protective garments from Vietnam and Cambodia urgently to aid China. To increase local production of high-quality protective garments, DuPont particularly set up a new business model of importing materials for local converters' processing. Miao Wei, the Minister of Industry and Information Technology (MIIT), singed a Thanks Letter to DuPont on behalf of Medical Supply Team of the State Council Joint Prevention & Control Mechanism, speaking highly of DuPont's great contributions.

DuPont involved deeply in the China's flight against 2019-nCoV, working closely with government authorities and non-government organizations to deliver batches of protective equipment to the forefront at top speed. Supply Supervision Team of Central Government to most Affected Regions including Hubei also spoke highly of DuPont's efforts in medical material supply for Wuhan and Hubei, and contributions to China's epidemic prevention and control with high efficiency and great passion.

卡特彼勒陈其华：中国终将打赢这场艰难的战"疫"

卡特彼勒

【2020-02-19】

微信号： caterpillarinchina

公司介绍： 卡特彼勒公司是一家工程机械和矿山设备的生产公司，于 1925 年成立，总部位于美国伊利诺伊州。

卡特彼勒全球副总裁陈其华表示："中国人民坚韧不拔的品格一直令人钦佩。我们坚信，中国终将打赢这场艰难的战'疫'。在确保卡特彼勒员工的安全和健康始终作为我们工作重心的同时，我们将继续与客户和产业链合作伙伴一起共同努力，建设一个更加美好的世界。"据悉，卡特彼勒在中国的大部分工厂已于 2020 年 2 月 10 日复工。

卡特彼勒基金会捐款 25 万美元

新冠肺炎疫情发生后，卡特彼勒基金会于 1 月 31 日向中国妇女发展基金会捐赠了 25 万美元，用于支持抗击新冠肺炎疫情的医疗工作，为前线医疗机构提供急需的医疗防护用品，并为一线医护人员和贫困患者提供支持。据悉，该笔款项将用于湖北省内武汉市、随州市、黄石市、荆门市及咸宁市定点收治新冠肺炎患者的相关医院。

卡特彼勒代理商积极投入抗击疫情行动中

2020年2月2日下午，卡特彼勒在中国的四大代理商之一利星行机械接到中国建筑第三局急需4台柴油发电机组为2月6日雷神山医院启动运营提供电力的通知。利星行机械集团立即启动应急程序，迅速整合资源，最终协调到4台成套发电机组。项目组从调货、测试、包装以及装运等各方面保障发电机组的及时出运，设备终于在24小时内抵达雷神山医院现场。

Qihua Chen of Caterpillar: China will Persevere during this Difficult Time

Qihua Chen, Caterpillar Vice President for China Operations, said: "Caterpillar has been impressed by the resilience of the people in this country, and we are confident that China will persevere during this difficult time. Be assured, the safety and well-being of our employees remains our top priority. We continue to follow government direction on remaining openings and assess daily to ensure the safety of our employees. And we will continue to work with our customers and industry partners to build a better world." It is reported that most of Caterpillar's Chinese operations reopened February 10.

Caterpillar foundation donates $250000

Since the COVID-19 outbreak began, the Caterpillar Foundation has supported the relief efforts with a $250000 donation to the China Women's Development Foundation (CWDF) to provide healthcare facilities with critical medical protective materials and support to medical staff and patients. The donation will be used in city hospitals in Hubei province which are designated for COVID-19 patient treatment, including Wuhan, Suizhou, Huangshi, Jinmen and Xian'ning.

Caterpillar dealer actively supports efforts against coronavirus

On the afternoon of February 2, Lei Shing Hong Machinery (LSHM), one of Caterpillar's four dealers in China, was contacted by the China Construction Third Engineering Bureau, which urgently needed four diesel generators for Leishenshan Hospital. The generators needed to be ready before the opening of the hospital on February 6. LSHM immediately arranged four Perkins generators for the hospital. The four generators arrived in Wuhan within 24 hours, including the testing, packaging, and transport by the LSHM team.

聚焦落实　放眼长远

——梅赛德斯－奔驰星愿基金公布首笔捐款落实细则宣布再捐 2000 万元用于持续战疫

奔驰星愿

【2020-02-25】

微信号： mbcircle

公司介绍： 梅赛德斯－奔驰是一家以豪华和高性能著称的德国汽车品牌，创立于 1871 年，总部位于德国斯图加特，是戴姆勒公司旗下的成员之一，旗下产品有各式乘用车、中大型商用车辆。

梅赛德斯－奔驰及其经销商合作伙伴于 2020 年 1 月 26 日捐赠的 1000 万元爱心资金，在经过近一个月的紧张工作之后，已经转化为大批防疫控疫物资运抵相关单位，疫情防控阶段的项目依照部署得到了全面落实。与此同时，梅赛德斯－奔驰星愿基金再次代表梅赛德斯－奔驰品牌及其经销商合作伙伴向"抗击新型冠状病毒肺炎"项目拨款 2000 万元；继火速以首笔捐款资助防控急需物资之后，第二笔捐款将支持疫情防控现期和后期的长效工作，侧重全国防疫应急工作的长效提升，为抗疫防疫阻击战再添一份力量。

新冠肺炎疫情发生后，梅赛德斯－奔驰星愿基金管委会迅速启动了重大疫情应对机制，进行抗疫捐款，第一时间驰援一线，为疫情防控贡献一份扎实的力量。在过去的一个月中，在国家卫健委、民政部的指导下和中国青少年发展基金会的协助下，梅赛德斯－奔驰星愿基金根据疫情防控的实际需求，秉持高效严谨、科学务实的原则，在三天内落实捐赠款项的拨付，并与执行机构建立进度更新机制，每 48 小时进行进度更新，全面追踪物资采购、资质核验、分配运输、医院接收等环节，确保每一笔善款都秉承透明、务实、高效的原则，得以快拨付、稳落实。

目前，首笔 1000 万元爱心资金项目全部落实且大部分已经执行完毕。其中，500 万元已拨付至湖北省包括武汉在内的 17 个市区的疫情防控指挥部统筹使用；100 万元用于支持河南、湖南、重庆、浙江、广东 5 个省（区、市）的医疗物资绝大部分已经送达新冠肺炎定点收治医院；200 万元用于采购定向支援国家医疗队的医疗物资，其中第一批已到达武汉协和医院并投入使用，第二批将针对目前实际需求加快采买和运输流程；100 万元已拨付支持疫情防控应急青年志愿服务队购置防护物资，已拨款落实至湖北、四川、河南、云南四省青少年发展基金会；100 万元率先响应由共青团中央发起的"'同舟共济 青春偕进'——希望工程关爱抗疫一线医务人员子女及因疫致困青少年特别行动"，用于关爱抗疫一线医务人员（特别是在支援防控疫情中感染疫病或牺牲的医务人员）家庭及其子女，以及资助因疫致困青少年。

戴姆勒股份公司董事会成员，负责大中华区业务的唐仕凯先生表示："过去的一个多月中，新冠肺炎疫情牵动着我们每个人的心，中国政府和人民为抗击疫情所付出的巨大努力，举世瞩目。我们看到，中国持大国担当，举前所未有之力，采取最全面、最严格、最彻底的防控措施应对疫情，阻止其进一步发展；我们看到，每一位医务工作者鞠躬尽瘁，每一个普通人守望相助，共同守卫着神州家园；我们还看到社会各界团结一心，全力以赴，竭尽己能为防疫工作筑起坚强后盾。"

根据疫情防控的最新形势和长效社会需求，梅赛德斯－奔驰星愿基金再追加捐款 2000 万元爱心资金。该笔捐款除了继续支持抗疫一线防控工作，更将重点关注疫情现期及后期长效工作，进一步助力提升国家公共卫生应急管理水平、健全公共卫生管理体系。在国家卫健委、相关主管单位和专业机构的指导下，此次主要支持的项目将包括：资助开展全国"疫情防控和公共卫生应急"专项培训；协助武汉及湖北疫情严重的地（市）和县级指定医院提升防疫水平；资助北京师范大学"抗击疫情心理健康支持项目"；资助北京市相关机构开展疫情防控科研及公共卫生项目；定向资助北京定点医院采购新冠肺炎诊断、治疗相关医疗设备；保障部分受疫情影响的进城务工人员子女学校和希望小学正常运转，资助受疫情影响的家庭经济困难学生。

唐仕凯先生强调："作为扎根中国社会的一分子，戴姆勒及梅赛德斯－奔驰值此时艰，将更加勇担社会责任，携手在华合作伙伴、全体员工以及社会各界，团结一心，共克难关。同时，我们也与各界一道积极响应政府恢复生产运营的号召，以助力汽车行业逐步回归有序发展。我们相信，以中国强大的抗疫决心和综合实力，整个中国社会及汽车工业凭借强劲的韧性和不懈的勇气，一定能打赢这场疫情防控阻击战。"

战"疫"时刻，戴姆勒及梅赛德斯－奔驰代表在华合作伙伴、全体员工及经销商向抗击疫情一线的白衣战士及所有工作人员致以崇高的敬意和衷心的感谢。在中国这个第二故乡，戴姆勒和梅赛德斯－奔驰扎根于此，与整个社会休戚与共、心手相牵；为了全面打赢疫情防控总体战、阻击战，将坚决遵照国家相关部门的统一部署，继续毫不放松抓紧抓实各项防控工作，有序恢复生产生活秩序，为切实推动行业进步和实现社会发展目标而继续贡献自己的一份力量。

梅赛德斯－奔驰星愿基金首批 1000 万元爱心资金，执行情况如下：

500 万元已拨付至湖北省青基会
- 300 万元拨付至武汉市新冠肺炎疫情防控指挥部统筹使用。
- 200 万元拨付至黄石、十堰、襄阳、宜昌等 16 市区新冠肺炎疫情防控指挥部统筹使用。

100 万元已拨付至河南、湖南、重庆、浙江、广东省市青基会，每省市 20 万元
- 河南：2 月 10 日交付防护服、口罩等医疗物资至河南省商城县人民医院、新县人民医院、光山县人民医院、信阳市第五人民医院。

- 湖南：2月17日交付免洗手消毒液、医用消毒液等物资至湖南省岳阳市第一人民医院、常德市第二人民医院、湖南医药学院第一附属医院。
- 重庆：2月17日交付医用消毒液、消毒酒精等物资至重庆市公共卫生医疗救治中心、重庆三峡中心医院、重庆医科大学附属永川医院、重庆市黔江中心医院及重庆区县疾控中心四所定点医院。
- 浙江：2月14日拨付资金至浙江大学附属第一医院，该医院统筹使用约600万元资金（含梅赛德斯－奔驰星愿基金20万元）采买了医用控温仪、呼吸湿化治疗仪、呼吸机、中央监护系统、等离子空气消毒机、红外线热像仪、正压呼吸器、口罩、防护服等医疗械物资。
- 广东：已采买医疗用品水体胶敷料，用于预防抗击疫情的医护人员的皮肤压力性损伤。物资将于2月26日发货，支持广东16家定点医院。

200万元已拨付至中国人口福利基金会

- 100万元定向支援国家医疗队6000件手术衣采买，2月19日到达武汉协和医院投入使用。
- 100万元定向支援国家医疗队其他医疗物资采买，正针对目前实际需求执行采购及后续流程。

100万元已拨付至湖北、四川、河南、云南省青基会

- 湖北50万元，四川20万元，河南20万元，云南10万元。
- 用于购置配发给基层应急青年志愿服务队的防护物资，包括口罩、医疗手套、消毒液、防护服、护目镜等，及其他必要的保障性支出。

100万元已确认投入共青团中央发起的相关特别行动

- 向抗疫一线医务人员（特别是在支援防控疫情中感染疫病或牺牲的医务人员）家庭及其子女提供关爱补助，资助因疫致困青少年。
- 中国青少年发展基金会根据实际情况落实，将关爱资金以银行转账方式划拨至个人账户。

Mercedes-Benz Star Fund Donates an Additional RMB 20 Million against COVID-19 and Shares Initial Donation Execution

Beijing — Mercedes-Benz and its dealer partner's RMB 10 million donation against COVID-19 announced on Jan. 26 has been implemented with purchased medical supplies delivered to the intended recipients. Over the past month, the Mercedes-Benz Star Fund and relevant executors have acted in a highly efficient manner and ensured a solid delivery of all donations. Today, Mercedes-Benz Star Fund, on behalf of Mercedes-Benz brand and its dealer partners, has announced it will donate an additional RMB 20 million to fight against COVID-19. The initial donation made in January is being used to provide urgently needed virus prevention and medical supplies. To reinforce the battle against COVID-19, the new donation prioritizes long-term improvements to China's national capabilities in epidemic prevention and emergency response.

When the outbreak of COVID-19 occurred, Mercedes-Benz Star Fund Management Committee immediately launched a major epidemic response mechanism to support the battle against the virus. In the past month, under the supervision of China's National Health Commission and Ministry of Civil Affairs, the Mercedes-Benz Star Fund finalized the appropriation plan for the initial donation within three days. With support from the China Youth Development Foundation, the Star Fund has acted with an efficient, disciplined, scientific-based and pragmatic approach to ensure actual demands during the outbreak will be met. Together with donation execution organizations, a tracking mechanism was set up to report the latest progress every 48 hours for areas including supply purchases, qualification verification, distribution and logistics as well as hospital acceptance. This is being done to ensure quick payment and stable delivery of the donation funds in a transparent, pragmatic and efficient manner.

So far, the initial RMB 10 million donation has been delivered as planned, most of which has been transferred into actual suppliers for frontline fight. This includes RMB 5 million allocated to the Command Center for COVID-19 Prevention and Control in 17 cities in Hubei, including Wuhan; medical supplies valued at RMB 1 million which are on the way to the designated hospitals in Henan, Hunan, Chongqing, Zhejiang, and Guangdong; supplies valued at RMB 2 million which are designated for the national medical team for supplies, the first batch has arrived at Wuhan Union Hospital and the second batch is under purchasing based on current actual needs; and RMB 1 million that has been allocated to support the CYDF's Emergency Youth Volunteer Service Team for virus prevention and control which have been allocated to the provincial Youth Development Foundation of Hubei, Sichuan, Henan and Yunnan. The remaining RMB 1 million has been used to response the Project Hope's Caring Program to the Children of Frontline Medical Workers, launched by the Central Committee of the Communist Youth League, to support the families and children of the medical workers on the frontline (especially the decreased media workers and those hit by the virus), also unprivileged youth hit by the virus.

Mr. Hubertus Troska, Member of the Board of Management of Daimler AG, Chairman and CEO of Daimler Greater China Ltd. said: "Over the past month, everyone in China has kept a close watch on COVID-19. The tremendous efforts made by the Chinese government and Chinese people to fight against the outbreak has been witness by all. China has undertaken unprecedented efforts to mobilize enormous resources nationwide and adopt the strictest, the most comprehensive and the most radical measures in containing the virus from further development. We have seen medical workers make extraordinary efforts and ordinary people help each other in the fight against the virus. We have seen the entire society act together to spare no effort to support virus prevention."

In the face of the current situation and long-term social needs, Mercedes-Benz Star Fund has announced an additional RMB 20 million donation through the Star Fund. In addition to continuously supporting the frontline in virus prevention and control, the funds will be allocated to efforts focused on long-term solutions after the virus has been contained, and eliminating negative effects caused by the outbreak. It will be used to help improve the national public health emergency management and enhance the public health management system.

Under the guidance of the National Health Commission, relevant departments and professional institutions, projects funded by this donation will include: nationwide training on "epidemic prevention and control and public health emergency" when the outbreak is contained; epidemic prevention capability improvement in designated hospitals in Wuhan and other severely affected cities and counties in Hubei; the "Mental Health Assistance Project to Fight Against the Virus" at Beijing Normal University; scientific research on epidemic prevention and control by the Beijing related institutions, purchases of medical equipment for the virus diagnosis and treatment to designated hospitals in Beijing; and maintaining normal operations at affected schools and supporting affected students, including those from schools for children of migrant workers and Hope Schools.

Troska added: "We will further intensify our social responsibilities and stand with our partners in China, our employees and all segments of society to overcome the challenges. That's why we have also actively responded to the government's call to resume work and production and have gradually resumed our main production activities to restore the orderly development of the automotive industry. I firmly believe that with China's firm commitment and its strength, and with resilience and unremitting courage, the entire society as well as the Chinese automobile industry will win the battle against the current challenge."

In the face of extreme challenges, Daimler and Mercedes-Benz, on behalf of their partners in China, as well as all employees and dealers, offer the highest respect and sincerest thanks to medical workers and all staff on the frontlines fighting COVID-19. China is our second home, and Daimler and Mercedes-Benz are always with the Chinese people in both good and challenging times. To ultimately win the war against COVID-19, we will follow the direction and action of national departments, strive to ensure strict prevention and control of the disease, orderly resume normal work and production, and make greater contributions to industrial progress and social development.

Execution status of Mercedes-Benz Star Fund's initial RMB 10 million donation:

RMB 5 million delivered to Hubei Youth Development Foundation

- RMB 3 million was delivered to the Command Center for Prevention and Control of COVID-19 in Wuhan City to be used according to overall planning.
- RMB 2 million was delivered to the Command Centers for Prevention and Control of COVID-19 in 16 cities, including Huangshi, Shiyan, Xiangyang, Yichang, to be used according to overall planning.

RMB 1 million delivered to Provincial/Municipal Youth Development Foundations of Henan, Hunan, Chongqing, Zhejiang, and Guangdong with RMB 200,000 for each province/city

- Henan: Medical supplies including protective clothing and masks were delivered to Shangcheng County People's Hospital, Xinxian People's Hospital, Guangshan County People's Hospital, and Xinyang Fifth People's Hospital in on February 10.
- Hunan: Supplies including hand disinfectant and medical disinfectant were delivered to the First People's Hospital of Yueyang City, the Second People's Hospital of Changde City, and the First Affiliated Hospital of Hunan University of Medicine on February 17.
- Chongqing: Supplies including medical disinfection solution and alcohol were delivered to Chongqing Public Health Medical Treatment Center, Chongqing Three Gorges Central Hospital, Yongchuan Hospital of Chongqing Medical University, Chongqing Qianjiang Central Hospital and four designated hospitals in Chongqing District/ County Disease Control Center on February 17.

- Zhejiang: Donation was delivered to the First Affiliated Hospital of Zhejiang University on February 14. The hospital spent about RMB 6 million (including RMB 200,000 from Mercedes-Benz Star Fund) to purchase medical temperature controllers and respiratory humidification treatment apparatus, ventilators, central monitoring systems, plasma air sterilizers, infrared cameras, positive pressure respirators, masks, protective clothing and other medical equipment and supplies.
- Guangdong: Supplies of water gel dressing used to prevent pressure injury of medial workers have been purchased, that will be sent out to 16 designated hospitals on February 26.

RMB 2 million delivered to the China Population Welfare Foundation

- RMB 1 million designated for the National Medical Team was used to purchase 6,000 surgical gowns which were sent to Wuhan Union Hospital on February 19.
- RMB 1 million designated for the National Medical Team for other supplies which is under purchasing based on current actual needs.

RMB 1 million delivered to Youth Development Foundations of Hubei, Sichuan, Henan and Yunnan Provinces

- RMB 500,000 was delivered to Hubei Province; RMB 200,000 to Sichuan Province, RMB 200,000 to Henan Province, and RMB 100,000 to Yunnan Province.
- To purchase protective supplies including masks, medical gloves, disinfectants, protective clothing, and goggle for community-level emergency youth volunteer service teams to undertake necessary rear-service work.

RMB 1 million confirmed to support special program initiated by the Central Committee of the Communist Youth League

- To support the families and children of the medical workers on the frontline (especially the decreased media workers and those hit by the virus), also unprivileged youth hit by the virus.
- CYDF will allocate the fund to recipients' personal account through bank transfer, based on actual needs.

帝斯曼中国捐款 100 万元人民币并分批捐赠超过一亿片维生素 C 产品驰援疫情防控

帝斯曼中国

【2020-02-26】

微信号： DSM_China

公司介绍： 荷兰皇家帝斯曼公司是一家以使命为导向，在全球范围内活跃于营养、健康和绿色生活的全球科学公司，致力于以缤纷科技开创美好生活。成立于 1902 年，业务涵盖为人类营养、动物营养、个人护理与香原料、医疗设备、绿色产品与应用提供创新解决方案。总部位于荷兰海尔伦市。

专注于营养、健康和绿色生活的全球科学公司帝斯曼（中国）有限公司宣布将捐赠第二批物资——100 万瓶（1 亿片）维生素 C 片以帮助抗疫医护人员提升人体免疫力，支持新型冠状病毒肺炎疫情防控工作。此前，帝斯曼中国已捐赠人民币 100 万元现金及 10 万瓶（600 万片）维生素 C 咀嚼片。通过此项捐赠，帝斯曼中国秉承对中国的承诺，运用其在健康领域的专长守护奋战于一线的医护人员。

新型冠状病毒引发的肺炎疫情自暴发以来，牵动着全国人民的心。帝斯曼中国作为企业公民，积极助力前线共抗疫情，已向中国红十字基金会捐赠人民币 100 万元，专项用于满足疫情防控及一线医务人员需求，购买紧缺医疗物资和设备以及疫情地区一线医护人员的人道救助。此外，帝斯曼中国还为奋战在一线抗击疫情的医护人员分批捐赠维生素 C 产品。第一批 10 万瓶维生素 C 咀嚼片赠予武汉协和医院各院区、荆州当地的医院，支援全国其他地区的抗疫工作者。帝斯曼中国还将捐赠 100 万瓶维生素 C 片，产品由帝斯曼江山制药（江苏）有限公司制造的原料所生产。这 100 万瓶维生素 C 片将捐赠给武汉、荆州和湖北其他疫情严重城市的医院，以及帝斯曼生产基地所在的 6 个省（区、市）多个城市和地区。维生素 C 对于支持人体免疫系统运作起着不可替代的作用。在强大的病毒面前，良好的免疫系统不仅是防止感染的一道重要防线，也是感染后控制病情发展、恢复身体健康极为关键的一环。帝斯曼中国作为营养、健康领域的全球领先企业，发挥自身优势为医护人员的工作和健康提供支持。

帝斯曼中国总裁蒋惟明博士表示："帝斯曼全体员工都心系疫情发展，视助力抗击疫情为己任。我们深知每一次病例数字跳动的背后都是鲜活的个人和家庭，在疫情发生后第一时间响应并高效支援防疫工作。随着防疫进入攻坚时刻，帝斯曼中国将竭尽所能，凭借专业、及时的服务以及全球生产和供应链网络为疫情防控做出贡献，与中国一起共渡难关。"

长期以来，帝斯曼中国在应对全球诸多严峻挑战中扮演着积极角色。疫情当前，帝斯曼中国责无旁贷，将继续关注其进展并采取后续相关行动，全力支持这场战"疫"。

DSM China Donates to Support Efforts Amidst COVID-19 Outbreak

DSM China, part of Royal DSM, a global science-based company in Nutrition, Health & Sustainable Living, today announced that it will donate a second batch of goods, 100 million Vitamin C pills, to help boost citizen's immune systems amid the COVID-19 outbreak. Prior to this, DSM has donated 1 million RMB in cash and 6 million Vitamin C chewable tablets. With these donations, DSM affirms its commitment to China and its people, applying its expertise to protect the medical staff in the frontlines.

In the wake of the COVID-19 outbreak, sentiments of support have stirred within the country. DSM has pledged to actively support the frontline fight against the spread of the virus with a donation of 1 million RMB to the Chinese Red Cross Foundation. The funds are to be used to purchase medical supplies and equipment in short supply according to the requirement of COVID-19 prevention and control and supplement the needs of frontline medical personnel.

In addition, DSM donates two batches of Vitamin C products for medical personnel working tirelessly to contain the virus. The first batch of 6 million Vitamin C chewable tablets is donated to Wuhan Union Hospital of China and its branches and hospitals in Jingzhou, Hubei Province and other provinces. DSM will also donate a second batch of 100 million Vitamin C pills, the raw material of which is manufactured by DSM Jiangshan Pharmaceutical (Jiangsu) Co., Ltd. These 100 million Vitamin C pills will be donated to hospitals in Wuhan, Jingzhou and other cities where DSM production sites and offices are located in.

Vitamin C plays an irreplaceable role in supporting the operation of the immune system. A strong immune system is not only an important defense line to prevent infection, but also the key to controlling disease development and restoring health after infection. DSM uses its strengths as a leading global company in nutrition and health to provide support for the work and health of medical staff.

Dr. Jiang Weiming, DSM China President says, "This is a hard time for the people of China and our thoughts are with those that have been affected. DSM is closely monitoring the outbreak, so we can respond and play our part. As prevention and control works enter a crucial stage, we are eager and committed to providing our full support and make contributions through our expertise and global production networks. DSM will stand with China in these difficult times."

同心协力，抗击疫情

陶氏公司

【2020-02-29】

微信号： DowChemicalChina

公司简介： 陶氏化学是一家研制及生产系列化工产品的化学公司，成立于 1897 年，总部位于美国密歇根州米特兰。

2020 年 1 月 29 日，为帮助抗击新型冠状病毒引发的肺炎疫情，陶氏化学宣布向深圳壹基金公益基金会捐赠人民币 100 万元，用于为湖北省武汉市及周边地区提供急需的医疗物资及服务支持。

随着疫情的发展，陶氏又于 2 月 19 日、2 月 28 日、3 月 13 日分别向湖北省咸宁市捐赠 56 吨消毒产品，向武汉和孝感市 1 家医院和 8 个志愿者服务组织捐赠 1000 瓶免洗抑菌洗手凝露，向上海华山医院武汉医疗队捐赠 1000 件高等级防护服。

"中国不仅是我们的全球第二大市场，也是 3200 多名员工的祖国，本次疫情牵动了每一个陶氏员工的心。通过捐赠，我们希望能够为在前线奋战的医务和社区工作者提供支持和保护"，陶氏化学大中华区总裁林育麟说。

"陶氏在中国开展业务已有近百年历史，我们同中国的合作伙伴和同事结下了深厚的情谊。陶氏化学中国团队的韧性让我感动，我非常钦佩中国人民的毅力和决心。我们非常急切地期待看到商务活动、社会和个人生活恢复正常，这场尚未结束的危机告诉我们一个道理：人类的命运是不可分割的——影响到我们伙伴和朋友的事，也会影响到我们自己。武汉加油！"陶氏公司 CEO 吉姆·菲特林说。

In the Fight Together

On Jan 29th, Dow Greater China announced to donate RMB1 million via the Shenzhen One Foundation to support the Corona Virus control efforts in Wuhan and nearby cities in Hubei province. The donation was used to buy medical supplies and fund community voluntary services.

Later on, respectively on Feb 19th, Feb 28th, and Mar 13th, Dow provided additional aid of 56 tons of disinfectants, 1000 bottles of hand sanitizers and 1000 medical coveralls respectively to Xianning City, 1 hospital and 8 volunteers groups as well as the Wuhan Medical Team of Shanghai Huashan Hospital to protect the "China is Dow's 2nd largest market world-wide and home to more than 3200 Dow people. Our thoughts go to everyone affected by the outbreak. I am glad that Dow is able to do something to help protect the medical workers and volunteers in the frontline ," said Yoke Loon Lim, president of Dow Greater China.

"Dow has been doing business in China for nearly 100 years. In that time, we've developed a strong commitment to our partners, friends, and colleagues throughout the region. I've been impressed by the resilience of Dow's Chinese colleagues, just as I've been impressed with China's perseverance and determination to manage this crisis. We are eager to see business, social, and family life return to normal. Even while this crisis continues to unfold, it has reminded us of one truth about the world we live in today: We are interconnected in ways both large and small. What impacts our partners and friends, impacts all of us. Wuhan, Jia You!" said Jim Fitterling, CEO of Dow Inc.

众志成城，共克时艰！捷豹路虎多措并举，驰援中国抗"疫"

捷豹路虎中国

【2020-03-06】

微信号： gh_6a01b986b37f

公司介绍： 捷豹路虎（英文简称 JLR）是一家拥有两个顶级奢华品牌的英国汽车制造商。从赛道传奇到人生旅迹，从探险利器到挑战奇迹，捷豹路虎中国与你一起尽享英伦风范，前瞻未来出行。

近日，1000 件从英国发出的杜邦 Tyvek 600 Plus 专业医用防护服运抵上海，将通过浦东新区商委捐赠给上海市东方医院、第七人民医院、浦东医院等 6 家设有发热门诊的医疗机构，用于支援上海市抗击新冠肺炎工作，完善抗"疫"一线医护人员的防护措施。这是捷豹路虎中国自疫情发生以来采取的又一援助举措。

在疫情防控的战线上，捷豹路虎持续通过各项实际行动，助力中国抗击新冠肺炎。此次疫情暴发后，捷豹路虎中国第一时间联合奇瑞捷豹路虎，向湖北省慈善总会捐赠 500 万元，用于疫情严重地区的防控物资采购、医护工作者及志愿者的身心健康保障。此外，捷豹路虎更是着眼于未来，向中国宋庆龄基金会捐赠 300 万元，用于开展后续重大流行疾病中小学校园预防工作，目前已在积极落实中。

与此同时，为了确保复工的有序进行，捷豹路虎中国还紧急从英国调配 10 万余只口罩及消毒防护用品，分发给全国 240 多家经销商店一线员工以及位于上海、北京、广州及成都办公室的员工，并支援常熟生产基地，切实保障经销商及公司员工的身体健康，从而有力维持企业正常运转，支持社会和国民经济正常发展。

为了助力中国抗"疫"，捷豹路虎董事会成员、位于英国布罗米奇堡（Castle Bromwich）和哈利伍德（Halewood）工厂的员工此前也纷纷发起声援行动，以"我们与你同在，中国加油！"字样的横幅，表达了对中国人民的深切关怀和全力支持。

捷豹路虎全球董事、捷豹路虎中国总裁潘庆先生指出："此次疫情对于全球所有国家而言，都是一个严峻的挑战。捷豹路虎从英国总部到中国的每一位员工都密切关注着疫情发展，并通过自身努力为抗'疫'贡献力量。在疫情防控取得显著成效的紧要关头，让我们继续携手，众志成城，早日打赢这场没有硝烟的战'疫'！"

捷豹路虎中国将持续关注疫情动态，在积极组织复工生产的同时，继续做好防疫医疗物资组织、医护人员保障以及后续校园预防等相关工作，为抗击新冠肺炎疫情贡献力量。

Jaguar Land Rover Takes Consecutive Actions to Support the Fight against COVID-19 in China

Recently, Jaguar Land Rover China working with its supplier Beeswift purchased 1000 pieces of Dupont Tyvek 600 Plus medical protective clothing from the UK and has shipped them to Shanghai. With the help of Pudong New District Commission of Commerce, these protective clothing will be donated to 6 hospitals with fever outpatient, including Shanghai East hospital, Shanghai Seventh People's hospital and Shanghai Pudong Hospital, to provide strong protection for the frontline medical staff. This is one of the aid actions by JLR China since the outbreak of the disease.

Jaguar Land Rover (JLR) has taken consecutive actions to support the prevention and control against COVID-19 in China. After the outbreak, JLR China and Chery JLR jointly donated 5 million yuan to Hubei Charity Federation for procurement of urgently needed medical and living materials for severely affected regions in Hubei Province as well as for the support of frontline medical personnel. In addition, JLR China also donated 3 million yuan to China Soong Ching Ling Foundation for the future prevention of epidemic diseases at primary and middle schools, which is under implementation now.

To ensure the safety of dealer's staff and its own employees' returning to work, JLR China procured 100000 facemasks from the UK, which has been distributed to its 240 dealers' frontline employees across the country and the employees in JLRC offices of Shanghai, Beijing, Guangzhou, Chengdu, as well as to support the production base in Changshu. In this way, the brand seeks to guarantee the health of every employee, so as to maintain the operation of business and contribute to national stability and development.

JLR board members and plant staff at Castle Bromwich and Halewood in Britain also expressed their deep care and concern for the Chinese people by showcasing a banner that reads "Our thoughts are with you, our Chinese friends!"

Mr. Qing Pan, a board member of JLR and executive director of JLR China, said, "The epidemic is a serious challenge for any country. Every JLR employee from the UK to China is closely following the development of the epidemic and contributing to combat it through their own efforts. Though some remarkable achievements have been made, we still need to join hands and work together to claim the ultimate victory."

JLR China will pay close attention to the epidemic. While organizing the resumption of production, it will continue to support the control of COVID-19 and the future prevention of epidemic diseases, contributing to the battle against the disease.

辉瑞中国心系抗疫一线

辉瑞公司

【2020-03-16】

微信号： 辉瑞制药

公司介绍： 辉瑞公司是一家以研发为基础的生物制药公司，创建于1849年，总部位于美国纽约市。公司产品包括降胆固醇药、口服抗真菌药、抗生素等。

在防治新冠肺炎疫情的关键时刻，辉瑞公司竭尽所能支持、协助中国政府及卫生医疗伙伴抗击疫情。持续关注新冠肺炎疫情的进展并尽所能为患者和医护人员提供帮助，到目前为止累计捐赠了总价值超过900万元的救治药品和防护物资。

疫情初期，随着确诊病人数字的不断增加，对相关药品的需求量大增。而在专家给出的治疗方案中，辉瑞的几个主要抗生素都在其中。对此，辉瑞中国立刻组织召开紧急跨部门会议，并迅速决定通过武汉红十字会向武汉市相关医疗机构捐赠价值220万元的抗感染产品，用于感染病人的抢救和治疗。

本次捐赠过程中，辉瑞各部门全力合作，连夜工作，无缝对接，经过20多个小时与时间赛跑，迅速完成捐赠所需内外部流程，在大年三十当天上午将第一批抗感染药物送达武汉红十字会，用辉瑞速度体现了责任和关爱。

随着疫情的进展，医用防护物资日益短缺。辉瑞基金会向相关国际公益组织捐赠50万美元，用于支持其在全球范围内募集和运输急需防护物资，包括医用口罩、医用手套、防护服等医用防护用品。这些物资已通过相关机构捐赠至武汉当地的多家。

新冠肺炎疫情的蔓延初步得到遏制，然而来自辉瑞的支援却丝毫没有止步。在此之后，辉瑞又陆续向陕西、辽宁、湖北等地的多家医院以及杭州红十字会多次捐赠医用防护物资。截至 2020 年 2 月 25 日，累计捐赠药品和物资价值已超过 900 万元。

辉瑞生物制药集团中国区总经理 Andreas Penk 先生表示："辉瑞一直把履行企业社会责任作为在华的重要使命之一。这次捐赠再次体现了'一方有难、八方相助'的精神，是全体辉瑞员工应尽的义务。"

辉瑞普强大中华区总裁苗天祥先生表示："我们将密切关注疫情的进展，并尽我们所能为患者和医务人员提供帮助，为挽救患者的生命尽一份力。"

作为目前领先的在华外资制药公司，辉瑞一直致力于提高中国人民健康水平，并积极参与人道主义救助和支持。在包括非典流行、汶川地震、玉树地震、雅安地震、昭通地震、昆山爆炸事故、江苏响水化工厂爆炸事故等历次重特大社会事件和自然灾害中，辉瑞公司都在第一时间积极伸出援助之手，与各相关机构合作，提供包括药品捐赠、财务支持、人员培训等在内的紧急救助和专业支持，并由此多次获得有关部门和公益组织的嘉奖。

Pfizer China Supported Anti-Coronavirus Battle in China

At the critical moment of prevention and treatment of COVID-19, Pfizer China offered support and assistance to the Chinese government and health care providers (HCPs) in fighting against the epidemic. The company continues to pay attention to the progress of the COVID-19, helps patients and HCPs as much as possible. So far, Pfizer has donated emergency drugs and protective materials with a total value of over 9 million yuan.

With the increasing number of diagnosed cases early in the epidemic, the demand for relevant drugs is increasing rapidly. In the treatment plan proposed by experts, several of the major antibiotics are manufactured by Pfizer. Thereupon, Pfizer China immediately held an emergency cross-department meeting, quickly decided to donate 2.2-million-yuan worth of anti-infective products to the hospitals in Wuhan through the Red Cross Society of China Wuhan Branch, for the rescue and treatment of infected patients.

In the donation process, various Pfizer departments worked day and night, and seamlessly. After more than 20 hours of running against time, the internal and external processes needed for donation were completed quickly. The first batch of anti-infective drugs were delivered to the Wuhan Red Cross Society in the morning of the New Year's Eve, reflecting responsibility and care with Pfizer's speed.

With the development of the epidemic situation, medical protective materials are in short supply. The Pfizer Foundation granted USD500,000 to international NGOs to support the delivery of urgently needed medical protective supplies, which including medical masks, gloves, protective suits , etc. These materials have been delivered to several hospitals in Wuhan.

The spread of COVID-19 was initially curbed, but the support from Pfizer did not stop. After that, Pfizer successively donated medical protective materials to several hospitals in Shaanxi, Liaoning, Hubei and other places as well as the Hangzhou Red Cross Society. Up to February 25, 2020, the cumulative value of donated drugs and materials from Pfizer had exceeded 9 million yuan.

Mr. Andreas Penk, Pfizer biopharmaceutical group China President, said: "Pfizer has always regarded fulfilling corporate social responsibility as one of its important missions in China. This donation once again demonstrated the spirit of 'helps come from all sides', which is the obligation of all Pfizer employees. "

"We will pay close attention to the progress of the epidemic situation, do our best to help patients and medical staff, and to help save patients 'lives," said Mr. Miao Tianxiang, President of Pfizer Upjohn Greater China.

As a leading multinational pharmaceutical company in China, Pfizer has been committed to improving the health and well being of the Chinese people and actively participating in humanitarian assistance and support. In the past major social events and natural disasters, including the SARS, Wenchuan earthquake, Yushu earthquake, Ya'an earthquake, Zhaotong earthquake, Kunshan explosion accident, Jiangsu Xiangshui chemical plant explosion accident, Pfizer actively gave its assistance at the first time, collaborated with all relevant organizations to provide emergency aid and professional support including drug donation, financial support, personnel training, etc., and thus won positive feedbacks from relevant authorities and public service organizations for many times.

马士基集团捐赠价值超 200 万元医用物资并助力救援物资运输，共抗疫情

马士基集团

【2020-03-17】

微信号： Maersk Group

公司介绍： A.P. 穆勒 – 马士基成立于 1904 年，总部位于丹麦哥本哈根，是一家综合的集装箱航运物流企业，已服务于中国的对外贸易 95 年，旗下马士基是全球最大的集装箱航运公司。

通过多方努力和支持，A.P.穆勒 – 马士基通过湖北省慈善总会等机构，向黄冈市、襄阳市和孝感市定点医院捐赠的物资已于近日陆续运抵湖北，用以支持新冠病毒的防控工作。捐赠物资总价值超过 200 万元（约 30 万美元），包含医用防护服 4000 套、医用外科口罩 10 万只以及救护车 3 辆。

在疫情暴发后，马士基集团偕同旗下品牌积极采取措施为中国提供物流支持。旗下品牌丹马士加入紧急物资运输行列，响应菜鸟"免费向武汉运输救援物资绿色通道"倡议，与多个物流企业一起，免费从海内外为武汉地区运输社会捐赠的救援物资。除此之外，丹马士携全球网络提供国际物流方案，通过空运服务，将海外救援物资从美国、英国、德国、土耳其、捷克、以色列、印度尼西亚、日本、新加坡、马来西亚等国家送达前线。截至 2020 年 3 月 12 日，丹马士协助海外物资进口物流服务，已运送了 83 吨救援物资，其中包括超过 130 万只口罩及 3000 件防护服。

马士基还通过提供免费空运和陆侧物流等方式协助客户及相关机构进行驰援物资运输，其中包括马士基通过免费空运服务承运亚马逊捐赠的抗

疫物资；马士基车队协助多个基金会进行物资运输，将 330 台制氧机等物资从江苏丹阳运送至武汉市黄陂区的中华慈善总会蒙牛应急物资中心。

此外，马士基为中国大陆客户额外提供了 2020 年 1 月 24 日至 2020 年 2 月 9 日特殊的进口免箱期，帮助客户减轻负担。

马士基旗下全资子公司宜欧物流也积极参与驰援疫情救助，为支援疫区的进口国际医疗物资提供免费的进口通关及配套的仓储配送服务措施，以协助加快急需防控物资的运输。

马士基集团将继续密切关注疫情发展，全力配合政府和相关机构共抗疫情，并将继续深耕中国市场，和客户以及合作伙伴一起，寻找商机，加深合作！

A.P. Moller – Maersk Donates Medical Materials with Value over RMB 2 Million and Assists in the Transportation of Relief Supplies to Fight against the Epidemic

After weeks of efforts, A.P. Moller – Maersk's donated materials towards Hubei province, have been successfully delivered to the corresponding hospitals in Huanggang, Xiangyang and Xiaogan through Hubei Charity Federations and the related organizations. These relief supplies with a total value of more than RMB 2 million (around USD 300,000) include 100,000 medical surgical masks, 4,000 sets of medical protective clothing and living supplies, and three ambulances."

After the outbreak of the coronavirus, A.P. Moller-Maersk, together with its brands, actively take initiatives to provide logistics support to China. A.P. Moller-Maersk, together with its brand Damco Freight Forwarding, actively respond to advocacy from Cainiao, Alibaba's logistics affiliate to provide free transportation for emergency supplies to Wuhan. Damco collaborates with multiple logistics companies to transport relief materials both home and abroad to the epidemic center. Through its air freight service, Damco successfully delivered the medical materials to the epidemic center in China, from US, UK, Germany, Turkey, Czech Republic, Israel, Indonesia, Japan, Singapore, Malaysia and other countries. As of March 12, it has delivered 83 tons of relief materials including more than 1.3 million masks and 3,000 protective clothes.

Maersk is also providing free air transportation and land-side logistics to support a number of our clients (such as Amazon) and organizations with facilitating the delivery of medical supplies for the affected areas; Maersk trucking team assists different foundations in the transportation of materials, e.g. 330 oxygen generators were transported from Danyang, Jiangsu, to Mengniu Emergency Materials Center of China Charity Federation located in Huangpi District, Wuhan.

In addition, between January 24th, 2020 and February 9th, 2020, Maersk skips the Import Detention & Demurrage (DnD) calculation for customers in Mainland China, helping customers to mitigate the impact of the coronavirus.

OceanEast, a Maersk's fully owned warehousing and distribution company, also joins the efforts. From February 1st, OceanEast provides free import customs clearance and relevant warehousing and distribution services for imported international medical materials, assisting customers to fasten the speed of transporting the urgently needed goods.

A.P. Moller-Maersk will continue to follow the situation closely and cooperate with the government as well as the relevant organizations in this regard. A.P. Moller-Maersk is as committed to China as ever and we are looking forward to re-engaging with our customers as well as partners.

阿斯利康捐赠雾化祛痰药物增援疫情防控

阿斯利康中国

【2020-03-18】

微信号： 阿斯利康中国

公司介绍： 阿斯利康是一家全球性生物制药企业，由前瑞典阿斯特拉公司和前英国捷利康公司于 1999 年合并而成，总部位于英国剑桥。公司专注于研发、生产及销售处方类药品，重点关注肿瘤、心血管、肾脏及代谢、呼吸等主要疾病领域。

今日，阿斯利康宣布向中国初级卫生保健基金会捐赠价值超过 600 万元的雾化祛痰药物，用于新冠肺炎患者的对症治疗及疾病防控。本次捐赠覆盖包括湖北、武汉在内的全国多个省市，其中逾半药品将驰援县域医院，惠及广大基层患者。

随着疫情的发展和对新冠肺炎研究的持续深入，祛痰药物在诊疗中得到更多重视。中国初级卫生保健基金会在劝募函中也提到，现有部分新冠肺炎诊治医院及县域医院仍然缺少祛痰相关药物。

疫情防控就是责任，在了解到医院及患者需求后，阿斯利康第一时间决定向中国初级卫生保健基金会捐赠雾化祛痰药物（吸入用乙酰半胱氨酸溶液），并加大向基层医院的捐赠力度，以缓解各级医院药物压力，助力新冠肺炎防控。

捐赠药品完成打包装箱，准备运输，经过争分夺秒的筹备，首批药品已运抵江苏省丹阳市云阳人民医院及安徽省宣城市泾县医院，支持当地疫情防控。

疫情不灭，行动不止：自新冠肺炎疫情发生以来，阿斯利康第一时间响应，积极参与到抗击疫情的战役之中并已开展了 7 次总计超过 1000 万元的捐赠，持续不断地为疫情防控提供支援。

- 1 月 24 日除夕，阿斯利康向红十字会捐款 100 万元，成为最早向新冠肺炎防控提供援助的跨国制药公司之一。
- 1 月 28 日，首批捐赠的 15000 只口罩发放给了武汉的 15 家医院，为一线医护人员提供防护。
- 2 月 2 日，阿斯利康捐赠价值 550 万元的药品已经送达武汉的雷神山医院和火神山医院，为受灾最严重地区的医务人员和患者及时提供了帮助。
- 2 月 10 日，阿斯利康捐赠了超过 90000 副医用手套，提供给湖北、上海、无锡、广州、杭州、成都、安徽、河北、湖南、云南、陕西和山西省，缓解前线医护人员的燃眉之急，为医护人员提供防护。
- 阿斯利康全国各地员工捐款总计超过 260 万元，用于采购爱心物资并已及时送达疫情一线。
- 2 月 24 日，和珐博进（中国）共同向中国初级卫生保健基金会捐赠价值近 100 万元用于治疗肾性贫血的创新药品
- 3 月 18 日，向中国初级卫生保健基金会捐赠价值超过 600 万元的雾化祛痰药物，用于新冠肺炎患者的对症治疗及疾病防控。

阿斯利康全球执行副总裁、国际业务及中国总裁王磊表示："阿斯利康持续关注疫情发展，根据实际需求，为疫情防控提供力所能及的支援。我们相信这场战疫终将胜利，更相信中国经济的极强韧性。我们始终看好中国强大的经济潜能，将继续在行动上支持中国经济的发展并与之共同成长。"

AstraZeneca's Added Donation of Atomization Expectorant Medicines to Fight COVID-19

Today, AstraZeneca announced that it has donated atomization expectorant medicines worthy of over RMB 6 million to the China Primary Health Care Foundation for treatment of COVID-19 patients and disease prevention and control. This donation covers a number of provinces and cities including Wuhan, Hubei. More than half of the medicines will benefit primary patients in the county areas.

With the development of the epidemic and the deepening of research on COVID-19, expectorant drugs have played an increasingly important role in treatment. China Primary Health Care Foundation also mentioned in the solicitation letter that some COVID-19 treatment hospitals and county hospitals still lack expectorant drugs.

It's our responsibility to help fight the COVID-19 epidemic. After learning about the needs of the hospital and patients, AstraZeneca immediately decided to donate an atomizing expectorant (acetylcysteine solution for inhalation) to the China Primary Health Care Foundation, in an effort to alleviate pressure of drugs in hospitals at all levels, particularly grassroots hospitals.

After packing & transporting medicines against the time, the first batch of medicines have been delivered to Yunyang People's Hospital in Danyang City, Jiangsu Province and Yixian Hospital in Xuancheng City, Anhui Province to support local epidemic prevention and control.

Since the outbreak of the COVID-19, AstraZeneca has made swift response and actively participated in the battle against the epidemic. Up till March 18, it has launched 7 donations totaling more than RBM 10 million continuously supporting the combat against COVID-19:

- On the New Year's Eve of January 24, we were among the first multinational pharmaceutical companies to donate RMB 1 million to the Red Cross, supporting the local prevention and control of pneumonia;
- On January 28, the first batch of 15,000 medical masks donated were handed over to 15 hospitals in Wuhan, providing protection for the frontline medical staff;
- On February 2, the medicines we donated, which are worthy of RMB 5.5 million, has reached the Huoshenshan Hospital and Leishenshan Hospital in Wuhan, hoping to assist medical staff and patients in the most affected areas;
- On February 10, AstraZeneca donated over 90,000 pairs of medical gloves to Hubei, Shanghai, Wuxi, Guangzhou, Hangzhou, and Chengdu to support the protection of local frontline medical staff, as well as regions relatively short of medical resources including Anhui, Hebei, Hunan, Yunnan, Shaanxi and Shanxi Province;
- AstraZeneca's employees voluntarily donated RMB 2.6 million;
- On February 24, the medicines donated by AstraZeneca and FibroGen China, which are worthy of about RMB 1 million, arrived at Wuhan to meet the treatment needs of local patients with chronic renal diseases and suffering from anemia;
- On March 18, AstraZeneca donated atomization expectorant medicines worthy of over RMB 6 million to China Primary Health Care Foundation. The donation covered various areas including Wuhan, Hubei province, with half of the medicine to benefit primary patients in county areas.

Wang Lei, executive vice-president, international and China president of AstraZeneca, said: "AstraZeneca follows closely the development of the epidemic, and provides its continuous assistance according to actual needs. We believe that this war against epidemic will eventually triumph. With belief in the strong and resilient Chinese economy, we are always optimistic about China's strong economic potential and will continue to support China's economic development as we grow together with it."

思爱普追加千万抗"疫"捐赠，数字化助力湖北中小企业复产复工，再现活力

SAP 天天事

【2020-03-18】

微信号： sapdaily

公司介绍： 思爱普公司成立于 1972 年，是德国市值最高的企业，欧洲最大的科技公司，目前为全球最大的企业应用软件提供商。总部位于德国沃尔多夫。

思爱普今天宣布，将捐赠总值超过 1500 万元的软件产品和配套服务，帮助武汉及湖北地区中小企业，建立数字化体系，实现灾后重建。此外，还将追加超过 300 万元现金捐赠。截至目前，思爱普（SAP）为抗击疫情累计捐助总额已超过 2000 万元，充分展现出 SAP"在中国、为中国"的企业社会责任担当。

思爱普全球高级副总裁、中国总经理李强先生说："植根中国 25 年来，SAP 始终致力于携手合作伙伴，用数字化能力和全球最佳实践，为中国客户的成功保驾护航。危机当下，我们更要发挥核心业务优势，为客户的利益筑起坚固防线，为抗击疫情、助力复工复产、护航实体经济再添一份力量。"

新冠肺炎疫情暴发至今，给中小企业造成极大经营困扰，甚至是生存危机。为助其渡过难关，恢复生产，SAP 借助 2019 年与武汉市硚口区合作成立的"SAP 武汉赋能中心"为平台，为武汉及湖北地区的中小企业提供软件和服务，打造数字化能力，实现端到端运营。此举有助于缓解中小企业现金流紧张、数字化转型资金不足的问题。也将惠及整个武汉市的区

域经济，实现快速复苏繁荣的目标。

此前，思爱普已在疫情暴发第一时间向湖北慈善总会捐款 300 万元，支持武汉疫情中心的五家医院。此次追加的逾 300 万元现金，将定点捐给武汉火神山、雷神山医院，以及湖北随州、孝感、黄冈等地医院，购买防护和消杀用品，继续用于疫情防控。

思爱普联席首席执行官柯睿安（Christian Klein）也向中国员工、客户及合作伙伴发来真挚问候，对中国在疫情期间展现的建设速度和应对能力表示赞赏。他说："相信疫情之后，中国以及 SAP 中国的员工、客户和合作伙伴都将变得更为强大。我们对中国的中长期经济前景充满信心，并将继续致力于支持中国市场。"

随着疫情在全球的蔓延，供应链的中断给企业带来极大压力。为了维护供应链的可靠性和透明度，确保关键物资能到达最急需它们的地方，思爱普董事会日前决定，将联结着 400 多万家企业的全球领先 B2B 业务匹配平台——SAP Ariba Discovery 的访问权限，向所有企业免费开放 90 天，免费发布，免费响应，帮助采购方与供应商建立联系，寻找商机，改善困境。

SAP Donates Millions More in Pandemic Support – Using Digital Means to Empower Hubei SMEs Regain Vitality

SAP announced today that it will donate software products and supporting services valued at more than RMB 15 million to help small and medium enterprises in Wuhan and Hubei to establish a digital system and realize post-disaster reconstruction. In addition, SAP is providing an additional RMB 3 million cash donations on top of an already-donated RMB 3 million. The total SAP donation now exceeds RMB 20 million, fully demonstrating SAP's corporate social responsibility in China.

Sam Li, SAP Global Senior Vice President and General Manager of China, said: "Having taken root in China 25 years ago, SAP has always been committed to working with partners to safeguard the success of Chinese customers. In time of crisis, we will leverage our core business to build a solid line of defense for customers, and make further contributions to help China get back to work and aid in economic recovery."

The outbreak of the COVID-19 which has become a global pandemic. The situation has caused deep business challenges to SMEs. To help them survive the difficult period and resume production, SAP is leveraging the "SAP Wuhan Empowerment Center" established in cooperation with Wuhan's Qiaokou District in 2019. They will use the center as a platform to provide software and services for SMEs in Wuhan and Hubei to build digital capabilities and achieve end-to-end operations. This will help alleviate the problem of tight cash flows for SMEs and insufficient funds for digital transformation. This move will also benefit the regional economy of Wuhan and help achieve the goal of rapid recovery and prosperity.

Previously, SAP had donated 3 million to the Hubei Charity Federation to support five hospitals of the Wuhan Epidemic Center. The additional cash of more than 3 million will be donated to "Huoshenshan" and "Leishenshan" hospitals in Wuhan, as well as hospitals in Suizhou, Xiaogan, Huanggang and other places in Hubei, to purchase protection and disinfection supplies for virus prevention and control.

Christian Klein, the co-CEO of SAP, also personally sent sincere greetings to Chinese employees, customers and partners, and expressed his appreciation for the speed and response capacity of China during the epidemic. He said: "I believe that after the epidemic, employees, customers and partners in China and SAP China will become stronger. We are confident in China's medium and long-term economic prospects and will continue to support the Chinese market."

The COVID-19 outbreak has disrupted supply chains and is putting great pressure on Chinese companies. In order to maintain the reliability and transparency of their supply chains and ensure that critical materials can reach where they are most needed, the SAP Board of Directors has decided to open SAP Ariba Discovery, the world's leading B2B business matching platform that connects more than 4 million businesses worldwide. Access, open to all enterprises for 90 days free of charge, will help buyers to quickly establish contacts with suppliers, find business opportunities, and improve their business situations.

诺基亚与中国携手共克时艰

诺基亚

【2020-03-18】

微信号： Nokia_in_China

公司介绍： 诺基亚是一家主要从事移动通信设备生产和相关服务、智能解决方案的公司，由弗雷德里克·艾德斯坦于 1865 年创立，总部位于芬兰埃斯波。

2020 年 3 月 18 日，诺基亚宣布设立新冠病毒全球捐赠基金，助力抗疫一线，向各国最需要帮助的地方提供援助。

早在 2 月 7 日，诺基亚贝尔（诺基亚在华合资子公司）就向中国扶贫基金会捐赠 300 万元，设立诺基亚贝尔紧急救援基金，用于协调开展在武汉紧急救援及后期恢复重建工作。

诺基亚贝尔紧急救援基金向卫健委定点防疫防治医院捐赠共 8 辆负压监护型救护车，协助防治救援主战场开展工作，避免医务人员交叉感染，防止疫情进一步扩散。诺基亚贝尔紧急救援基金所购买的 8 辆负压监护型救护车分别交付于湖北省第三人民医院（湖北省中山医院）、武汉大学人民医院（湖北省人民医院）、黄冈市红安县人民医院、荆州市广东医科大学附属医院、宜昌市中心人民医院、十堰市西苑医院。

自疫情发生，诺基亚就和中国客户及合作伙伴一起，坚守在战"疫"第一线。1 月 25 日，全力助力武汉电信，仅用了一天半时间率先开通武汉火神山医院第一个 5G 基站；1 月 29 日，携手辽宁联通仅用一天时间就为辽宁省人民医院新型冠状病毒感染肺炎隔离楼部署了无线网络，成功实现远程查房、远程监控、远程探视、远程对话等功能；1 月 30 日，按照宁夏移动统一部署，仅3天时间就完成以银川市原望远胸科医院为新型冠状病毒肺炎隔离临时急救医院所需的无线网络部署的全部任务；2月12日，再次为辽宁省人民医院扩增的隔离楼搭建无线网络，支持新病房的远程智能监控系统运作；2月19日，仅用48小时，就支持安徽联通成功实现宿州"小汤山医院"部署5G覆盖，"高速运转"完成了工程建设的极速战、总体战、攻坚战；截至目前，诺基亚积极支持中国三大运营商及铁塔公司，共投入近5000人、设备超33000件，设立7×24保障值守岗位，按既定的应急响应机制，确保了全国如北京、广东、浙江、福建、贵州、河南等地由诺基亚建设的通信网络安全平稳运行。

除此之外，诺基亚积极提供新技术新方案助力各地抗击疫情。1月27日，仅用一天时间，就帮助四川移动完成了新冠肺炎疫情大数据监控分析平台的上线，可用于识别疫情人员是否最近一月内返程人员，针对疑似患者所到高频地址之处进行全面预防消毒及排查处理、针对确诊病例高频驻留的居民区、楼宇进行消毒及监控布防处理，针对已确诊且病情严重的患者所驻留累计次数较多的居民区、楼宇进行隔离十天观察处理，获得四川省省长尹力的高度认可；迅速推出高精度、远距离、大范围的红外体温检测方案（通过AI自动识别与处理，可在人流密集的公共场所实现无接触式测温、大规模人群实时体温测量、自动抓取发热人群等，且能做到精准识别，确保不遗漏目标），目前，红外体温检测方案已在上海、湖南、四川等多地部署。

正如诺基亚集团总裁、首席执行官苏立在2月3日致中国政府及客户的信中所说："诺基亚在过去四十年服务中国的历程中，与我们的核心价值客户共同创造过如2008年奥运会、2010年世博会通信保障的辉煌，也一起携手共渡过如2003年的SARS、2008年的汶川地震等艰难时期。这次我们依然会满怀信心与中国共度时艰，再次打赢这场疫情对抗战。中国，加油！"

Nokia Joining Forces with China to Go Through the Difficult Times

On March 18th, Nokia announced the establishment of Global Coronavirus Endowment Fund to help fight the epidemic and provide assistance to countries in need.

As early as February 7, Nokia Shanghai Bell (Nokia 's joint venture subsidiary in China) donated 3 million RMB to the China Foundation for Poverty Alleviation, and established the Nokia Shanghai Bell Emergency Relief Fund, to coordinate emergency rescue and the end of epidemic recovery and reconstruction efforts in Wuhan.

Nokia Shanghai Bell Emergency Relief Fund donated a total of 8 negative pressure ambulances and other medical supplies under the guidance of National Health Commission and other government agencies to support epidemic control for hospitals in Hubei, to prevent cross-infection of healthcare workers, and to prevent the further spread of the virus. The eight ambulances were delivered to the Third People's Hospital of Hubei Province (Zhongshan Hospital of Hubei Province), People's Hospital of Wuhan University (People's Hospital of Hubei Province), Huanggang People's Hospital of Hongan County, Affiliated Hospital of Jingzhou Guangdong Medical University, Central People's Hospital of Yichang City and Xiyuan Hospital of Shiyan City.

Since the happening of the epidemic, Nokia along with our Chinese customers and partners, have been standing on the front lines of epidemic control. On January 25th, we assisted Wuhan Telecom to open the first 5G base station for Wuhan "Huoshenshan" hospital in only one and a half days . On January

29th, we joined forces with Liaoning Unicom to setup wireless connection for the Liaoning Provincial People's Hospital Coronavirus isolation ward in just 1 day. We successfully implemented technologies to enable functions such as remote patient checkup, remote monitoring, remote patient visits, and remote communications. On January 30, we completed the wireless connection network construction for Yinchuan Coronavirus temporary isolation and ICU hospital in just 3 days, under the overall direction of Ningxia Mobile.

On February 12, we supported Liaoning Unicom again to assist expanded wireless network coverage and remote monitoring capabilities, to support the expansion of the isolation ward of Liaoning Provincial People's Hospital. On February 12, we opened 5G network coverage for Suzhou "Xiaotangshan" Hospital, and overcame difficulties for "high-speed operation" and the requirements for expedited and comprehensive network construction. As of now, Nokia has actively supported China's three major operators and China Tower companies, while investing a total of 5000 personnel and 33,000 sets of equipment to set up 7 * 24 guaranteed network security monitoring stations, while fully adhering to the emergency response mandates to ensure continued stable network operations for all key service areas in China, such as in Beijing, Guangdong, Zhejiang, Fujian, Guizhou and Henan.

In addition, Nokia has actively provided new technologies and solutions to help fight the Coronavirus epidemic. On January 27, it only took one day to help Sichuan Mobile to complete the launch of the new big data monitoring and analysis platform for Coronavirus prevention. This system can be used to identify whether the infected person was someone with a travel history within the last month, and also target locations with high-frequency for suspected patients, so healthcare workers can carry out comprehensive preventive disinfection and inspection and treatment of residential areas and buildings where confirmed cases reside frequently, and isolate residential areas and buildings for 10 day monitoring where there are an accumulation of patients or identified severe cases of illness. Nokia's Big Data solution was highly recognized by the Governor Yin Li of Sichuan Province.

In addition, Nokia quickly launched the high-precision, long-distance, large-scale infrared body temperature detection solution (through AI automatic identification and processing, and can achieve non-contact temperature measurement in crowded public places, large-scale crowd real-time temperature measurement, automatic capture of fever individuals with accuracy while ensuring no targets are missed), Nokia's infrared body temperature detection solutions have now been deployed in Shanghai, Hunan, Sichuan and other places.

As Nokia CEO Rajeev Suri stated in a letter to the Chinese government and customers on February 3, "Nokia has been in service to China over the past 40 years and has experienced together many good and also difficult times together with our customers and communities in China, such as the SARS outbreak in 2003, Wenchuan earthquake and the Olympic Games in the same year in 2008, as well as World Expo in 2010. This time we remain confident that by working together, we will overcome the challenges jointly once again! China, Be Strong!"

一切都会好起来！

可口可乐公司

【2020-03-19】

微信号： coke1886

公司介绍： 可口可乐是世界上最大的全品类饮料公司，成立于 1886 年，总部位于美国佐治亚州亚特兰大市。

新冠肺炎疫情发生以来，可口可乐中国系统紧急调动全球资源为受影响的地区提供重要的救援帮助，支持中国抗击疫情。截至 2020 年 3 月 1 日，可口可乐中国系统累计捐款 450 万元，可口可乐基金会累计捐赠 50 万美元现金和 50 万美元的医用物资。此外，可口可乐中国系统通过"净水 24 小时"行动，共捐助饮用水及饮料超过 126 万瓶。

在全国范围内，可口可乐中国系统的"净水 24 小时"还在持续行动，为当地一线人员和社区急送饮用水和其他饮料产品。"净水 24 小时"是 2013 年可口可乐中国和壹基金发起的应急饮用水救援机制，充分利用经营业务多年积累的本地化生产和分销渠道优势，力争在 24 小时内将饮用水送达救灾一线。

以下为可口可乐中国发布的部分信息：

- 1 月 27 日"可口可乐中国"微信官方账号：一定会好起来！
- 2 月 10 日"可口可乐中国"微信官方账号：可口可乐中国在行动！
- 2 月 11 日"可口可乐中国"微信官方账号：150 万只口罩已从旧金山发货
- 2 月 14 日"可口可乐中国"微信官方账号：今天的礼物到了
- 2 月 16 日"可口可乐中国"微信官方账号：给雷神山送可乐

I Will Be There for You!

Till March 1st, The Coca-Cola China System has contributed 4.5 million RMB to assist the efforts fighting the virus and provided some 1.26 million bottles of beverage by activating Clean Water 14, a disaster relief mechanism aiming to bring clean drinking water to disaster victims within 24 hours. The Coca-Cola Foundation has donated half a million US dollars and another half a million worth of medical protective supplies.

Clean Water 24 is still delivering bottled water and other beverages to medical professionals and other people at the frontline. Clean Water 24 was launched by Coca-Cola China in partnership with One Foundation to deliver drinking water to disaster-stricken area, leveraging the Coca-Cola distribution network reaching the very grassroot communities in the country.

UPS 向中国运送超过 400 万只口罩及防护装备，助力中国抗击疫情

UPS

【2020-03-20】

微信号： gh_e4cOb31a45e3

公司介绍： UPS 快递（United Parcel Service）是 1907 年成立于美国华盛顿州西雅图的一家全球性公司，主要业务是快递承运商与包裹递送公司，同时也是专业的运输、物流、资本与电子商务服务的领导性的提供者。

2020 年第一季度，UPS 与 UPS 基金会、医疗产品捐赠方和救援合作伙伴 MAP International、MedShare 等为助力武汉新型冠状病毒感染的肺炎疫情防控，提供免费空运和地面运输支持，向中国的医疗工作者捐赠了逾 400 万只防护口罩、11000 套防护服和 280000 双防护手套。

UPS 基金会主席兼 UPS 首席多元化和融合推广官爱德华多·马丁内斯（Eduardo Martinez）说："世界需要强有力的公私合作伙伴关系来共同遏制该致命病毒的传播扩散。UPS 基金会正扩大其人道主义救援网络，提供供应链专业知识和航空运送服务以支持我们的合作伙伴。"

"UPS 基金会是流行病供应链网络（以下简称'PSCN'）和流行病防备全球卫生安全小组私营部门圆桌会议（以下简称'PSRT'）的成员。我们已建立了全球救援机构网络，向处于危机中的社区提供援助支持，包括此次向中国的医护人员提供医疗援助。"

UPS 基金会同时宣布扩大对新冠肺炎疫情的应对措施，包括新的拨款分配，使用超过 600 万美元用于联合国机构、人道主义救援伙伴、以社区

为基础的非营利组织和国际非政府组织。

救援支持包括与十余个组织合作提供货物运输、供应链咨询和现金捐助，以加快向医疗工作者分发个人防护装备，并为受影响的个人和社区提供其他人道援助。

爱德华多·马丁内斯表示："UPS 基金会与 UPS 的丰富经验可以帮助社区通过建设与规划来抵御未来灾难且具备灾后复原能力。这种专长使我们能够在这个前所未有的需要时刻向我们的合作伙伴提供至关重要的支持。"

"我们在世界各地建立的公私伙伴关系有时长达数年甚至数十年。并且，我们能够共同努力，互相激励，并将我们专业的后勤知识用于有意义的行动，迅速支持生命救援。"

UPS Airlifted More than 4 Million Masks and Protective Gear to China to Help Combat the Spread of the Coronavirus

Over the first quarter of 2020, working with medical product donors and relief partners including MAP International and MedShare, UPS and The UPS Foundation, provided free air transportation of more than 4 million respirator masks and 11000 protective coveralls and 280000 nitrile gloves to China to help combat the spread of the coronavirus.

UPS airlifted more than 4 million masks and protective gear to China President of the UPS Foundation and UPS Chief Diversity and Inclusion Officer. Eduardo Martinez: "The world needs strong public-private partnerships to help contain the spread of this deadly virus and The UPS Foundation is expanding its humanitarian relief network to support our partners in providing supply chain expertise and air transport."

The UPS Foundation is a member of the Pandemic Supply Chain Network (PSCN) and the Private Sector Round Table (PSRT) for the Global Health Security Group on Pandemic Preparedness. We have developed a global network of relief agencies to help bring aid to communities in crisis, in this case, to bring medical aid to healthcare workers in China.

The UPS Foundation has also expanded its response to the coronavirus, including new grant allocations, surpassing $6 million to United Nations agencies, humanitarian relief partners and community-based non-profit and international non-government organizations.

The relief support includes collaboration with more than a dozen organizations and the provision of in-kind transportation, supply chain consultation, and cash contributions to expedite the distribution of personal protective equipment for healthcare workers and other life-sustaining activities for impacted individuals and communities.

"The UPS Foundation and UPS have extensive experience in helping communities prepare for, respond to, and recover from sudden onset and prolonged crises. That expertise enables us to provide critical support to our partners during this unprecedented time of need," said Eduardo Martinez, president of The UPS Foundation and UPS chief diversity and inclusion officer.

"The public-private partnerships we have developed around the world span years – even decades in some cases. We're able to work together, inspire each other, and rapidly deploy our support and logistics expertise toward meaningful actions to drive life-sustaining results," he continued.

渣打捐款 260 万元支持中国抗击新冠肺炎疫情

渣打中国

【2020-03-23】

微信号： StandardcharteredCN

公司介绍： 渣打是一家领先的国际银行集团，业务网络遍及全球 59 个最有活力的市场，为 144 个市场的客户提供服务。渣打网络与"一带一路"沿线市场的重合度超过 75%。渣打成立于 1853 年，总部位于英国伦敦。

渣打银行（中国）有限公司（"渣打中国"）于 2020 年 1 月 28 日向上海市慈善基金会捐款人民币 100 万元，支持由上海市慈善基金会发起的"抗击新型冠状病毒肺炎疫情专项行动"，为武汉的 7 所医院购买了 50 台抗击疫情急需的心电检测仪。

2 月 19 日，渣打集团在全球范围内发起员工捐款，共募集善款人民币 81 万元。渣打集团同时配比捐赠 10 万美元（约合人民币 69 万元）。该笔捐赠用于为湖北提供一线医护人员防护装备及针对社区的疫后心理援助。

渣打环球商业服务有限公司也在 2 月向天津开发区慈善协会捐款人民币 13 万元，用于支持当地抗疫一线。

为抗击新冠肺炎疫情，渣打共计捐赠 263 万元。

自新冠肺炎疫情发生以来，渣打中国遵照政府及监管部门指导，做好针对性的业务运营计划和应急预案，采取多项措施，始终注重保护员工和客户的健康和安全，注重为客户持续提供高质量金融服务。

1 月 28 日，一家中国企业需要紧急在海外采购抗击新冠肺炎所需物资。渣打中国的业务团队充分发挥其网络优势和业务专长，密切协调渣打新加坡和韩国的多个团队，群策群力，顺利突破 T+1 的交易时效，成功帮助客户在当天顺利完成交易。

此外，对向防疫专用账户捐款和汇划防疫专用款项的企业和个人，渣打中国一律免收手续费。

Standard Chartered Donated RMB 2.6 Million Supporting the Fight against COVID-19 in China

Standard Chartered China donated RMB 1 million to Shanghai Charity Foundation on 28th January to support its "Special Initiative to support disaster relief of COVID-19". The fund was used to purchase 50 electrocardiogram monitors to 7 Wuhan hospitals, meeting their urgent needs while fighting against COVID-19.

After the Spring Festival holiday, Standard Chartered launched a global staff fundraising, and raised the total RMB 830000 from employees. Standard Chartered Group also matched US$ 100000 (approx. RMB 690000) to the fundraising. By collaborating with Shanghai United Foundation and Shanghai Fosun Foundation, some of the fund was used to support the first-line medical staff in Hubei with protective equipment, and the rest was used to provide post epidemic psychological assistance to Hubei local communities.

Standard Chartered Global Business Service Center also donated RMB 130000 in February to TEDA Charity Association to support the prevention of Coronavirus outbreak.

Standard Chartered donated total RMB 2.63 million yuan to fight the COVID-19 in China.

Since COVID-19's outbreak, Standard Chartered Bank developed targeted business operation plan and emergency plan with guidance from the government and regulator. The Bank took multiple measures to constantly protect the health and safety of employees and clients, while providing high-quality financial service to our clients.

On 28 January, a Chinese company made an urgent request to purchase resources overseas for fighting against COVID-19. Standard Chartered Bank successfully assisted the client to complete the transaction on the same day, a breakthrough for usual "T+1" trading period, by fully leveraging the Bank's global network and financial capabilities, and coordinating the resources and multiple teams in Singapore and South Korea.

In addition, Standard Chartered Bank waivered the management fee for donation to specialised COVID-19 prevention account and specialised payment transfer for COVID-19 prevention.

阿尔斯通战"疫"任务之口罩供给：
一个也不能少

阿尔斯通

【2020-04-02】

微信号： 阿尔斯通招聘

公司介绍： 阿尔斯通是一家致力于打造引领更加绿色、智能的交通出行解决方案，开发并推广适用于未来可持续发展交通模式集成系统的供应商。成立于1928 年，业务板块包括应用于高速及超高速列车、地铁、有轨电车、电动公交车等领域的系统、设备和服务，覆盖系统集成、定制服务、基础设施、信号和数字化解决方案等。总部位于法国巴黎。

自新冠肺炎疫情暴发以来，越来越多的民众开始佩戴口罩，以保护自己不受感染，这导致包括中国在内的世界各国陆续发生口罩供不应求的情况。全球范围内，即使是在抗疫一线的医务人员，也面临着口罩等医疗防护物资匮乏的困境。

在这一前所未有的非常时期，阿尔斯通全球展现出"同舟共济，团结一致"的精神，在同心协力的跨国合作下，经受住时间的考验，成功应对各地由 N95 口罩短缺带来的影响。

当时正值中国农历新年，阿尔斯通团队已然夜以继日地投入口罩采购工作当中：寻找合格的供应商和货源（甚至调用了阿尔斯通其他国家工厂的口罩储备），协调供应链和物流；分批从全球六大洲逾 20 个国家采购到 9.5 万只口罩，有力保障了中国企业员工和亲属的健康和安全。从询价、下单到运输，仅仅 10 天时间，首批口罩于 2020 年 2 月 12 日顺利抵达各工作场所。在严格执行防疫措施前提下，阿尔斯通中国各工厂于 2 月 10 日开始有序复工。

与此同时，阿尔斯通中国大力支持其合作伙伴，共同对抗疫情：先后支援北京、成都、南京、上海和西安地铁及铁路职工 1.2 万只口罩。此外，阿尔斯通基金会向湖北省慈善总会捐款总值 1.5 万欧元（约 12 万元人民币）用于疫情防控。

两个月过去了，中国疫情形势得以缓解，这一世界主要口罩供应商已恢复生产。而全球其他国家正面临着一场硬战：从边境管控、供应链中断，到口罩供给严重不足。然而，阿尔斯通其他国家的员工可能并不知道，阿尔斯通中国已在争分夺秒地联络本地厂商、供货商和货运代理，为全球各地的阿尔斯通企业提供约 150 万只口罩。这些口罩除供给各国深受疫情影响的员工及其家属之外，将优先提供给医务人员、坚守岗位的铁路职工和制造业的工人们。

阿尔斯通亚太区总裁方玲表示："此次阿尔斯通全球团队倾力互助，团结一致，共同抗疫，充分体现了'同一个阿尔斯通'的互助互爱精神。感谢世界各地同事们的努力，携手共济，在极短时间内为中国和海外员工以及合作伙伴筹集到充足的口罩等物资和疫情防控基金。阿尔斯通每一位员工的健康，是我们战胜此次疫情以及今后任何病毒的核心'武器'——这取决于我们对所有同事和当地社区的关怀。我们将不遗余力地保障每位员工的健康，确保安全的工作环境，集结全球力量，肩并肩打赢这场世界性的疫情防控阻击战。"

Alstom's Coronavirus Mask Mission – Ensuring No One is Left Behind

As the coronavirus explodes, more people have begun wearing face masks to protect themselves, leading to not only a China-wide, but also a global shortage of the product. Across the world, even frontline medical staff are clamouring for face masks and other personal protective equipment.

During such unprecedented times, a different kind of "health"– the health of Alstom's global community bonds – has thankfully stood the test of time, as our teams collectively respond to the shortage of N95-type masks worldwide.

During the extended Chinese New Year holidays, Alstom teams in over 20 countries across six continents stepped up to secure over 95,000 masks for colleagues in China offices and industrial sites. These efforts ranged from sourcing manufacturers and suppliers, coordinating the supply chain and logistics to even tapping onto the sites' spare supply. With Alstom's operations in China resuming on 10 February in line with heightened precautionary measures, the first batch of masks successfully reached the sites on 12 February. All this took only 10 days after the onset of activation amid the outbreak!

During this period, Alstom also made a commitment to support our partners in China. Thus, around 12000 masks were dispatched to frontline rail workers in Beijing, Chengdu, Nanjing, Shanghai and Xi'an. At the same time, Alstom Foundation donated €15000 (approximately RMB120000) to Hubei Charity Federation in order to help to stop the epidemy.

Two months on, even as China, the world's main supplier, comes back onstream, companies around the globe are battling a host of obstacles, from control borders disrupting supply chain to a supply squeeze on masks. Little did we know, Alstom team in China would now be mobilising local mask manufacturers, traders and forwarders, to supply some 1.5 million masks to our other major sites worldwide. These masks would not only go to Alstom employees and families, but also in priority to medical services, frontline transport workers and manufacturing suppliers in coronavirus-hit countries where possible.

Ling Fang, Senior Vice President for Alstom in Asia Pacific, says: "The immense support coming from Alstom teams all over the world shows our One Alstom team spirit. Thanks to timely joint efforts of our colleagues worldwide, masks and funds were available to our employees and stakeholders from and beyond China within a very short span of time. The health of our Alstom community is an essential weapon in the fight against this and any future viruses – how much we care for our fellow colleagues and local communities. We will spare no effort in keeping our environment safe for all employees and our communities, and standing together in the global fight against this public health crisis."

雅培中国捐赠总额超 4100 万元现金和医疗物资助力抗击疫情

雅培中国

【2020-04-17】

微信号： abbott_china

公司介绍： 雅培是全球医疗健康行业领导者，业务涵盖诊断、医疗器械、营养品、药品等各个医疗健康领域的前沿科技。成立于 1888 年，总部位于美国芝加哥。

全球领先的医疗健康公司雅培自 2020 年 1 月 28 日起连续发起数轮捐赠，包括现金、医疗物资，以及医学、婴幼儿营养品，和全国人民和医务人员共同抗击新型冠状病毒，为奋战在一线的医护人员及其子女、儿童病患提供全面的科学营养支持，也为需要营养支持的宝宝家庭提供营养援助，帮助全国妈妈复工，迄今捐赠总额累计已超过 4100 万元。

雅培中国的捐赠如下

- 雅培婴幼儿及医学营养品，包括雅培医学营养品全安素和特殊膳食用营养基粉，以全面营养支持的专业解决方案，为夜以继日奋战在治疗一线的医务人员提供科学配比的全面均衡营养，为病患康复铸就强有力的营养后盾；倍得力电解质冲剂（Pedialyte），为处于高强度工作有脱水风险的一线医护人员快捷补充糖盐水，帮助其迅速恢复体力；儿童营养品小安素，为全国主要重点医院的医务人员子女，以及有风险感染疫情的儿童病患提供营养支持；以及雅培菁挚和铂优恩美力婴幼儿配方奶粉，为有宝宝喂养困难的家庭提供营养支持，帮助全国妈妈复工。

- 雅培全自动生化分析仪（ARCHITECT c8000 System），这是一款世界领先的全能身体指征检测设备，可用于对患者血液疾病指标和多项健康指标的检测，从而了解其身体情况、危重症及恢复情况，属于疾控中心必需的检验设备。

- 雅培 i-STAT 手持式血液分析仪，被广泛应用于灾难急救、急诊、重症监护室和手术室等临床第一线。可满足隔离患者的即时床旁检测，更迅速地帮助医生救治危重病人，为病患争取黄金救治时间。

- CentriMag™ 循环支持系统 ① 将用于武汉市华中科技大学同济医学院附属协和医院对于危重症患者的救治。该系统能满足广泛的临床需求和应用，为患者提供更为全面、更为优化的心肺循环支持。配合外接氧合器时，CentriMag™ 循环支持系统能够实现 ECMO 的相关功能。同时，其还能够作为心室辅助装置为急性心衰竭病患提供左心室、右心室、双心室辅助。此外，该系统还能为预后未明的病患提供过渡期心脏辅助。

- 现金捐款，根据医院一线医护人员的需求，用于采购急需的防护服、口罩、消毒液等医疗防护用品，帮助医护人员更加安全地救治病患。

通过捐赠，雅培中国希望能以实际行动为疫情防控贡献自己的力量，为奋战在一线的医护工作者提供支持。雅培中国将持续关注疫情的防控情况，携手各方，众志成城，守护健康中国！

---

① 雅培 CentriMag™ 循环支持系统尚未在中国大陆上市。

Abbott Donates RMB 41 Million Worth of Medical Supplies and Funding to Support Relief Efforts for the Coronavirus Outbreak in China

Since Jan 28th, Abbott, a global healthcare company, has made rounds of consecutive donation including funding grants, medical supplies, medical and pediatric nutrition products to contain the coronavirus outbreak in China. The donation has been used to offer science-based nutritional support to both children at infection risk and to medics who are fighting on the front line against the virus. It also aims to assist Chinese mothers who return to work and need help to take care of infant's healthy growth. To date Abbott's donation has exceeded 41 million yuan.

Abbott's donation includes:

- Abbott's science-based nutrition products, including medical nutrition products Ensure Complete and base powder, to provide nutritional support to patients and medical professionals who are working day and night to contain the coronavirus; Pedialyte, an advanced rehydration drink that can help medics efficiently balance vital minerals and nutrients under intensive work to recover strength; Pediasure, a full nutritional formula product to children of medics in major hospitals and children patients at infection risk; Eleva and Similac Infant Formula for working mothers who need help of nutritional support to their infants. Abbott's ARCHITECT c8000 clinical chemistry system. The diagnostic system is essential for hospitals while they manage patients who are kept in quarantine.

ARCHITECT c8000 features efficient tests that can evaluate multiple health indicators. It can help doctors understand whether patients are critically ill and the progress of their recovery.

- Abbott's i-STAT system. The handheld blood analyzer system enables doctors to obtain fast test results for multiple health indicators for patients in quarantine, saving more time for the treatment of patients. The system can be widely applied in emergency rooms, intensive care units and surgery rooms.

- Abbott's CentriMag™ Acute Circulatory support system [1] for the Union Hospital of Tongji Medical School affiliated from Huazhong University of Science and Technology in Wuhan. The CentriMag™ Circulatory support system can meet a wide range of clinical needs and applications, providing patients with more comprehensive and optimized cardiopulmonary circulatory support. With an external oxygenator, CentriMag™ could provide ECMO functionality. Meanwhile, it can also be used as a ventricular assist device to provide left ventricular, right ventricular and double ventricular assist for patients with acute heart failure. In addition, the system can provide transitional cardiac assistance for patients with unknown prognosis.

- Funding grants used to purchase medical necessities including protective suits, masks and disinfectant.

Abbott will continue to pay close attention to developments related to the coronavirus outbreak and will continue to help support the healthcare system to safeguard people's health in China.

---

[1] CentriMag™ Acute Circulatory support system is not available in China

部分跨国公司捐赠中国"抗疫"一览 *

公司名称	捐赠时间	捐 赠 金 额
赛诺菲 Sanofi	2020-01-24	捐资 100 万元，捐助价值 50 万检测物质
葛兰素史克 GSK	2020-01-24	捐资 200 万元
星巴克 Starbucks	2020-01-25	捐资 300 万元
蔻驰 Coach	2020-01-25	捐资 100 万元
嘉吉 Cargill	2020-01-26	捐资 250 万元、捐助价值 100 万元的防护物质
宝马 BMW	2020-01-26	捐资 500 万元
金光 APP	2020-01-26	捐资 1 亿元
艾默生 Emerson	2020-01-26	捐资 70 万元
路易达孚 LDC	2020-01-27	捐资 100 万元、捐助价值 40 万元物质
欧莱雅 L'OREAL	2020-01-27	捐资 500 万元
百事 Pepsi	2020-01-28	捐资 800 万元
高通 Qualcomm	2020-01-29	捐资 700 万元
通用电气 GE	2020-01-29	捐助价值 2000 万元医用物资及现金，其中包括 1000 万元专项资金，用于购买疫区急需的物资及满足疫区部分紧急现金需求
拜尔 Bayer	2020-01-29	捐赠总值超过 1000 万元的急需医疗物资及资金

---

* 说明：此表内容主要根据公司官网、主流媒体报道整理而成，并按照时间先后排序。

公司名称	捐赠时间	捐 赠 金 额
诺华 Novartis	2020-01-29	捐资 200 万元
国际商业机器 IBM	2020-01-30	捐资 200 万元
英特尔 Intel	2020-01-30	捐资 100 万美元
特斯拉 Tesla	2020-01-30	捐资 500 万元
摩根大通 JPMorgan Chase	2020-01-30	捐资 100 万美元
霍尼韦尔 Honeywell	2020-01-31	捐助价值 200 万美元的物资，包括空净和水净产品、ICU 空气管理系统、医院管理扫描、打印设备、口罩等
杜邦 DuPont	2020-01-31	捐助价值 255 万元的紧急物资，包括逾 16000 件防护服和益生菌产品
飞利浦 Philips	2020-01-31	捐助 1500 万元价值的设备，包括医院急需的设备和空气净化器等
卡特彼勒 Caterpillar	2020-01-31	捐资 25 万美元
凯雷 Carlyle	2020-01-31	捐资 300 万元
三星 Samsung	2020-01-31	捐资 3000 万元
丰田 Toyota	2020-01-31	捐资 1000 万元
安博 Prologis	2020-02-02	捐助 50 万只普通医疗口罩、2 万只 N95 医疗口罩、3 万只 N95 普通口罩、750 套医疗防护衣
安联 Allianz	2020-02-02	捐资 400 万元
大众汽车集团（中国） Volkswagen group	2020-02-03	捐资 1.2 亿元（携旗下大众、奥迪、保时捷、宾利和斯柯达与合资企业共同捐助）
亚马逊 Amazon	2020-02-03	捐助超过 100 万件包括医用防护口罩、医疗防护服、医用手套等医疗防护防疫用品
康明斯 Cummins	2020-02-03	捐资 300 万元

公司名称	捐赠时间	捐 赠 金 额
默沙东 Merck	2020-02-03	捐资 100 万元
瑞银 UBS	2020-02-03	捐资 100 万美元
耐克 Nike	2020-02-04	捐资 1000 万元
施耐德 Schneider-Electric	2020-02-04	捐资 100 万元，同时支持火神山、雷神山和小汤山等地建设，提供电气产品和设备
高盛 Goldman Sachs	2020-02-05	捐资 100 万美元
巴斯夫 BASF	2020-02-05	捐资 100 万元
汇丰 HSBC	2020-02-05	捐资 700 万元
力拓 Rio Tinto	2020-02-06	捐资 100 万美元
诺基亚 Nokia	2020-02-07	捐资 300 万元、捐助 8 辆负压监护型救护车、支持武汉火神山医院第一个 5G 基站开通
蒂森克虏伯 ThyssenKrupp	2020-02-07	捐资 200 万元和价值 20 万元抗疫物资
德银 Deutsche Bank	2020-02-07	捐资 100 万元
ABB	2020-02-10	捐资 100 万元、捐助 16000 只口罩
标普全球 S&P Global	2020-02-10	捐资 100 万元
摩根士丹利 Morgan Stanley	2020-02-10	捐资 100 万美元
埃克森美孚 ExxonMobil	2020-02-10	捐助价值 230 万元的现金和医疗物资
壳牌 Shell	截至 2020-02-10	捐资 200 万元、捐赠 30 吨医用酒精
必和必拓 BHP Billiton	2020-02-11	捐资 1000 万元

公司名称	捐赠时间	捐 赠 金 额
微软 Microsoft	截至 2020-02-12	捐赠总额超过 4578 万元
太古集团 Swire	截至 2020-02-13	捐资 2200 万元
花旗 CitiBank	2020-02-13	捐资 25 万美元（约合人民币 70 万元）
东芝 Toshiba	2020-02-14	捐资 100 万元
强生 Johnson & Johnson	截至 2020-02-15	捐资 100 万元、捐助价值 2600 万人民币的紧缺 医疗防护物质
宝洁 P&G	截至 2020-02-24	捐资 100 万元、捐助价值 1400 万元的物资
梅赛德斯 - 奔驰 Mercedes-Benz	截至 2020-02-25	捐资 3000 万元
道达尔 Total	2020-02-28	捐资 200 万元
博世 Bosch	2020-02-28	捐助价值 800 万元的物资
可口可乐 Coca-Cola	截至 2020-03-01	捐资 450 万元、捐资 50 万美元、捐助价值 50 万 美元医用物资、捐助饮用水及饮料超过 126 万瓶
雀巢 Nestles	截至 2020-03-04	捐赠总额超过 6000 万元
罗氏 Roche	截至 2020-03-04	捐赠总额 2400 万元，包括现金、药品和物资
捷豹路虎 Jaguar/Land Rover	2020-03-06	捐资 800 万元、捐助 1000 件防护服
雅诗兰黛 Estee Lauder	截至 2020-03-08	捐资 500 万元、捐助价值 1000 万元的护肤用品
普利司通 Bridgestone	2020-03-10	捐资 300 万元
沃尔沃 Volvo	截至 2020-03-15	捐资 145 万元、捐助价值 1000 万元的紧急医疗 物资与设备、捐赠 100 万元专项疫苗研发资金
马士基 A．P Moller Maersk	2020-03-17	捐助价值 200 万元的医用物资

公司名称	捐赠时间	捐赠金额
思爱普 SAP	2020-03-18	捐资 615 万元、捐助价值 1500 万元的软件产品和配套服务。捐赠总额 2100 万元
阿斯利康 AstraZeneca	截至 2020-03-18	捐赠总额超过 1700 万元的现金、药品和防疫物资，包括 360 万元、15000 只口罩和 90000 副医用手套、价值 550 万元的药品、价值近 100 万元治疗肾性贫血的创新药品、价值超过 600 万的雾化祛痰药物
帝斯曼 DSM	截至 2020-03-18	捐资 200 万元，捐助 110 万瓶维生素 C 产品
陶氏 Dow	截至 2020-03-19	捐资 100 万元、捐助 60 吨消毒液、1000 瓶免洗洗手液、1000 件防护服
联合包裹速递服务 UPS	2020-03-20	捐助 450 万只口罩、11000 套防护服
渣打 Standard Chartered	截至 2020-03-23	捐资 260 万元
戴尔科技 Dell Technologies	截至 2020-03-25	捐赠总额 900 万元，包括 200 万元现金、264 台台式电脑和笔记本电脑、价值超过 600 万人民币解决方案和和设备
正大集团 CP Group	截至 2020-03-24	捐资 3276 万元、捐助价值 3054 万元的物资
达能 Danone	截至 2020-03-30	捐赠总额近 2300 万元现金和物资，包括价值 1509 万元的脉动维生素饮料、218 万医学营养品、2 万个医用口罩、505 万元现金用于购买 3 辆负压救护车和 1 台人工肺
辉瑞 Pfizer	截至 2020-03-30	捐助价值 1100 万元的抢救药品和防护用品
英国石油 BP	截至 2020-03-30	捐赠总额逾 300 万元，包括防护服、口罩、面屏等医疗防疫物资
雅培 Abbott	截至 2020-04-17	捐赠总额 4100 万元和医疗物资

图书在版编目 (CIP) 数据

责任与担当：抗击新冠肺炎疫情中的跨国公司. 中英双语版 / 中国国际跨国公司促进会主编. -- 北京：社会科学文献出版社, 2020.10

ISBN 978-7-5201-7149-6

Ⅰ.①责… Ⅱ.①中… Ⅲ.①跨国公司-日冕形病毒-病毒病-肺炎-疫情管理-中国②跨国公司-企业管理-中国 Ⅳ.①R563.1②F279.247

中国版本图书馆CIP数据核字（2020）第183558号

责任与担当（中英双语版）
　　——抗击新冠肺炎疫情中的跨国公司

主　　　编 / 中国国际跨国公司促进会
执行主编 / 李新玉

出 版 人 / 谢寿光
组稿编辑 / 邓泳红
责任编辑 / 宋　静

出　　　版 / 社会科学文献出版社·皮书出版分社（010）59367127
　　　　　　地址：北京市北三环中路甲29号院华龙大厦　邮编：100029
　　　　　　网址：www.ssap.com.cn
发　　　行 / 市场营销中心（010）59367081　59367083
印　　　装 / 三河市龙林印务有限公司

规　　　格 / 开　本：787mm×1092mm　1/16
　　　　　　印　张：31.75　字　数：481千字
版　　　次 / 2020年10月第1版　2020年10月第1次印刷
书　　　号 / ISBN 978-7-5201-7149-6
定　　　价 / 198.00元

本书如有印装质量问题，请与读者服务中心（010-59367028）联系